Challenging Issues in the Management of Chronic Hepatitis B Virus

Editor

MITCHELL L. SHIFFMAN

CLINICS IN LIVER DISEASE

www.liver.theclinics.com

Consulting Editor
NORMAN GITLIN

November 2021 • Volume 25 • Number 4

ELSEVIER

1600 John F. Kennedy Boulevard • Suite 1800 • Philadelphia, Pennsylvania, 19103-2899

http://www.theclinics.com

CLINICS IN LIVER DISEASE Volume 25, Number 4
November 2021 ISSN 1089-3261, ISBN-13: 978-0-323-81068-5

Editor: Kerry Holland
Developmental Editor: Ann Gielou M. Posedio

Clinics in Liver Disease (ISSN 1089-3261) is published quarterly by Elsevier Inc., 360 Park Avenue South, New York, NY 10010-1710. Months of issue are February, May, August, and November. Business and Editorial Offices: 1600 John F. Kennedy Blvd., Ste. 1800, Philadelphia, PA 19103-2899. Customer Service Office: 3251 Riverport Lane, Maryland Heights, MO 63043. Periodicals postage paid at New York, NY and additional mailing offices. Subscription prices are $319.00 per year (U.S. individuals), $100.00 per year (U.S. student/resident), $752.00 per year (U.S. institutions), $409.00 per year (international individuals), $200.00 per year (international student/resident), $790.00 per year (international instituitions), $371.00 per year (Canadian individuals), $100.00 per year (Canadian student/resident), and $790.00 per year (Canadian institutions). Foreign air speed delivery is included in all *Clinics* subscription prices. All prices are subject to change without notice. **POSTMASTER:** Send address changes to *Clinics in Liver Disease*, Elsevier Health Sciences Division, Subscription Customer Service, 3251 Riverport Lane, Maryland Heights, MO 63043. **Customer Service: Telephone: 1-800-654-2452 (U.S. and Canada); 314-447-8871 (outside U.S. and Canada). Fax: 314-447-8029. E-mail: journalscustomer service-usa@elsevier.com (for print support); journalsonlinesupport-usa@elsevier.com (for online support).**

Reprints. For copies of 100 or more of articles in this publication, please contact the Commercial Reprints Department, Elsevier Inc., 360 Park Avenue South, New York, NY 10010-1710. Tel.: 212-633-3874; Fax: 212-633-3820; E-mail: reprints@elsevier.com.

Clinics in Liver Disease is covered in *MEDLINE/PubMed (Index Medicus)*, Science Citation Index Expanded, Journal Citation Reports/Science Edition, and Current Contents/Clinical Medicine.

Contributors

CONSULTING EDITOR

NORMAN GITLIN, MD, FRCP (LONDON), FRCPE (EDINBURGH), FAASLD, FACP, FACG
Head of Hepatology, Southern California Liver Centers, San Clemente, California, USA

EDITOR

MITCHELL L. SHIFFMAN, MD, FACP, FACG, FAASLD
Director, Liver Institute of Richmond, Liver Institute of Hampton Roads, Bon Secours Mercy Health, Richmond and Newport News, Virginia, USA; Professor of Medicine, Eastern Virginia Medical School, Norfolk, Virginia, USA

AUTHORS

JOSEPH AHN, MD, MS, MBA
Professor of Medicine, Division of Gastroenterology and Hepatology, Oregon Health & Science University, Portland, Oregon, USA

NELSON E. AIREWELE, MD
Liver Institute of Virginia, Bon Secours Mercy Health, Richmond; Liver Institute of Virginia, Bon Secours Mercy Health, Newport News, Virginia, USA

TARIK ASSELAH, MD, PhD
Université de Paris, Centre de Recherche sur l'inflammation, Inserm U1149, CNRS ERL8252, Paris; Department of Hepatology, AP-HP, Hôpital Beaujon, Clichy, France

MARIA BUTI, MD
Professor of Medicine, Liver Unit, Internal Medicine Department, Hospital Universitari Vall d'Hebron, Vall d'Hebron Barcelona Hospital Campus, Barcelona; Centro de Investigación Biomédica en Red de Enfermedades Hepáticas y Digestivas (CIBERehd), Instituto de Salud Carlos III, Madrid, Spain

PHUNCHAI CHARATCHAROENWITTHAYA, MD, Msc
Gastroenterology Division, Department of Internal Medicine, Faculty of Medicine, Siriraj Hospital, Mahidol University, Bangkok, Thailand

SIMONE E. DEKKER, MD, PhD
Internal Medicine Resident, Department of Medicine, Oregon Health & Science University, Portland, Oregon, USA

RAFAEL ESTEBAN, MD
Professor of Medicine, Liver Unit, Internal Medicine Department, Hospital Universitari Vall d'Hebron, Vall d'Hebron Barcelona Hospital Campus, Barcelona; Centro de Investigación Biomédica en Red de Enfermedades Hepáticas y Digestivas (CIBERehd), Instituto de Salud Carlos III, Madrid, Spain

JORDAN J. FELD, MPH, MD
Professor of Medicine, University of Toronto, Toronto Centre for Liver Disease, University Health Network, Toronto, Ontario, Canada

ELLEN W. GREEN, MD, PhD
Internal Medicine Resident, Department of Medicine, Oregon Health & Science University, Portland, Oregon, USA

GRISHMA HIRODE, MSc
Toronto Centre for Liver Disease, University Health Network, Toronto, Ontario, Canada

DANIEL Q. HUANG , MBBS, MRCP
Division of Gastroenterology and Hepatology, Department of Medicine, National University Hospital, University Medicine Cluster, National University Health System; Department of Medicine, Yong Loo Lin School of Medicine, National University of Singapore, Singapore

HARRY L.A. JANSSEN, PhD, MD
Professor of Medicine, University of Toronto, Toronto Centre for Liver Disease, University Health Network, Toronto, Ontario, Canada

APICHAT KAEWDECH, MD
Gastroenterology and Hepatology Unit, Department of Internal Medicine, Faculty of Medicine, Prince of Songkla University, Songkhla, Thailand.

JEFFREY KAHN, MD
Associate Professor of Clinical Medicine, Division of Gastrointestinal and Liver Diseases, Keck School of Medicine at University of Southern California, Los Angeles, California, USA

WILLIAM KEMP, MBBS, PhD, FRACP
Associate Professor, Consultant Hepatologist, The Alfred Hospital, Melbourne; Monash University, Melbourne, Victoria, Australia

GUAN SEN KEW, MBBS, MRCP
Division of Gastroenterology and Hepatology, Department of Medicine, National University Hospital, University Medicine Cluster, National University Health System, Singapore

SARO KHEMICHIAN, MD
Assistant Professor of Clinical Medicine, Division of Gastrointestinal and Liver Diseases, Keck School of Medicine at University of Southern California, Los Angeles, California, USA

PIETRO LAMPERTICO, MD, PhD
Division of Gastroenterology and Hepatology, Foundation IRCCS Ca' Granda Ospedale Maggiore Policlinico, Department of Pathophysiology and Transplantation, CRC "A. M. and A. Migliavacca" Center for Liver Disease, University of Milan, Milan, Italy

ASHLEY M. LANE, MD
Assistant Professor of Medicine, Division of Gastroenterology and Hepatology, Department of Medicine, University of Colorado Anschutz Medical Campus; Department of Medicine, Division of Gastroenterology and Hepatology, Rocky Mountain Regional VA Medical Center; Department of Gastroenterology and Hepatology, Rocky Mountain Regional VAMC, Aurora, Colorado, USA

SENG GEE LIM, MBBS, MD
Division of Gastroenterology and Hepatology, Department of Medicine, National
University Hospital, University Medicine Cluster, National University Health System;
Department of Medicine, Yong Loo Lin School of Medicine, National University of
Singapore, Singapore

ALESSANDRO LOGLIO, MD
Division of Gastroenterology and Hepatology, Foundation IRCCS Ca' Granda Ospedale
Maggiore Policlinico, Milan, Italy

DIMITRI LOUREIRO, PhD
Université de Paris, Centre de Recherche sur l'inflammation, Inserm U1149, CNRS
ERL8252, Paris; Department of Hepatology, AP-HP, Hôpital Beaujon, Clichy, France

AMMAR MAJEED, MD, PhD, FRACP
Associate Professor, Consultant Hepatologist, The Alfred Hospital, Melbourne; Monash
University, Melbourne, Victoria, Australia.

STEPHEN C. PAPPAS, MD, JD, FAASLD, FCLM
Department of Medicine, Baylor College of Medicine, Ben Taub General Hospital,
Houston, Texas, USA

TEERHA PIRATVISUTH, MD
Gastroenterology and Hepatology Unit, Department of Internal Medicine, Faculty of
Medicine; NKC Institute of Gastroenterology and Hepatology, Songklanagarind Hospital,
Prince of Songkla University, Songkhla, Thailand

MAR RIVEIRO-BARCIELA, MD, PhD
Liver Unit, Internal Medicine Department, Hospital Universitari Vall d'Hebron, Vall
d'Hebron Barcelona Hospital Campus, Barcelona; Centro de Investigación Biomédica en
Red de Enfermedades Hepáticas y Digestivas (CIBERehd), Instituto de Salud Carlos III,
Madrid, Spain

STUART K. ROBERTS, MBBS, MD, MPH, FRACP, FAASLD, AGAF
Professor, Head of Hepatology, The Alfred Hospital, Melbourne; Monash University,
Melbourne, Victoria, Australia.

LISA SANDMANN, MD
Department of Gastroenterology, Hepatology and Endocrinology, Hannover Medical
School, Hannover, Germany

ARIF SAROWAR, BSc
Toronto Centre for Liver Disease, University Health Network, Toronto, Ontario, Canada

MITCHELL L. SHIFFMAN, MD, FACP, FACG, FAASLD
Director, Liver Institute of Richmond, Liver Institute of Hampton Roads, Bon Secours
Mercy Health, Richmond and Newport News, Virginia, USA; Professor of Medicine,
Eastern Virginia Medical School, Norfolk, Virginia, USA

NORAH A. TERRAULT, MD, MPH
Professor of Medicine, Division of Gastrointestinal and Liver Diseases, Keck School of
Medicine at University of Southern California, Los Angeles, California, USA

ISSAM TOUT, PhD
Université de Paris, Centre de Recherche sur l'inflammation, Inserm U1149, CNRS
ERL8252, Paris; Department of Hepatology, AP-HP, Hôpital Beaujon, Clichy, France

MAURO VIGANÒ, MD, PhD
Hepatology Division, San Giuseppe Hospital Multimedica Spa, Milan, Italy

HEINER WEDEMEYER, MD
Professor, Department of Gastroenterology, Hepatology and Endocrinology, Hannover Medical School, Hannover; German Center for Infection Research (DZIF), Partner Site Hannover/Braunschweig, Germany

PHILIPPE J. ZAMOR, MD
Associate Professor of Medicine, Division of Hepatology, Carolinas Medical Center-Atrium Healthcare, Charlotte, North Carolina, USA

Contents

prevent the development of liver cirrhosis and decompensated cirrhosis, and to decrease the risk of hepatocellular carcinoma.

Pegylated interferon-alpha therapy is one of the first-line chronic hepatitis B treatment. Finite treatment duration, absence of drug resistance, delayed response, and higher hepatitis B surface antigen loss than nucleos(t)ides analog therapy are the advantages of pegylated interferon-alpha treatment. Common side effects and subcutaneous injections requirement limit its use. Identifying patients likely to respond to pegylated interferon-alpha and optimizing treatment is reasonable. Motivating patients to complete the 48-week treatment is necessary. Treatment is stopped or switched to other treatment strategies in patients with stopping rule criteria. Combination therapy with nucleos(t)ides analog may improve response, but remains controversial.

Controversial areas in chronic hepatitis B (CHB) are those where there is uncertainty, or differences of opinion in management, or where evidence may be insufficient. Areas of controversy include whether patients with high viral load but normal liver function tests should be treated to prevent hepatocellular carcinoma (HCC) or liver disease progression to cirrhosis. Another area is whether quantitative hepatitis B surface antigen (qHBsAg) can be used to better characterize phases of CHB and prognosticate. Finally, the utility of qHBsAg in the management of patients on antiviral therapy such as interferon and nucleoside analogues could improve management practices.

Hepatitis B is the leading cause of hepatocellular cancer (HCC) worldwide. Untreated, annual HCC incidence rates in chronic hepatitis B subjects are 0.4% in noncirrhotics and 2% to 3% in cirrhotics. Surveillance with ultrasound with/without α-fetoprotein at 6-month intervals is recommended in at-risk persons including children. Antiviral therapy in chronic hepatitis B with entecavir or tenofovir significantly lowers the risk of HCC across all stages of liver disease, and lowers the risk of HCC recurrence following curative therapy. There are insufficient data to recommend use of tenofovir over entecavir in the prevention of de novo or recurrent HCC postcurative therapy.

Despite effective vaccines and approved therapeutic agents, hepatitis B virus (HBV) remains a prevalent global health problem. Current guidelines rely on a combination of serologic, virological, and biochemical markers to identify the phase in the natural history of chronic HBV infection. Discordant serologic results can occur, which may lead to misclassification. Commonly encountered results that differ from the typical profiles seen in chronic HBV infection are described. For each scenario, the frequency of occurrence, possible explanations, and recommendations for clinical management are discussed. Recognition of discordant serologic findings is crucial for optimal clinical decision.

Many patients with hepatitis C virus (HCV) have also been exposed to hepatitis B virus (HBV). The 2 viruses interact and in most cases HCV suppresses HBV. When HCV is treated with direct antiviral agents, this suppressive effect is removed, HBV replication may increase, and a flare in liver enzymes with liver injury may occur. All patients with chronic HCV should therefore be checked for serologic evidence of HBV. Patients with hepatitis B surface antigen are at the highest risk for reactivation, and these patients should receive prophylactic treatment of HBV during and for 6 months after HCV treatment.

Chronic hepatitis D virus (HDV) infection is the most severe form of viral hepatitis with high rates of end-stage liver disease and hepatocellular carcinoma. Therefore, effective antiviral treatment strategies are needed desperately. Until recently, antiviral treatment was limited to pegylated interferon-alpha. With the conditional approval of the entry inhibitor bulevirtide by the European Medicines Agency, new treatment options are now available. In addition, multiple other antiviral compounds are currently tested in clinical phase II and III trials and represent promising agents for the treatment of chronic HDV infection.

The significant morbidity and mortality of people with end-stage renal, liver, heart, and lung diseases in need of transplantation provides rationale for use of organs from donors who are hepatitis B positive. The recipient's hepatitis B status plays a key role in defining the prophylactic strategy. The availability of safe and effective therapies (hepatitis B antivirals and hepatitis B immune globulin) has contributed to the safety of using hepatitis B–positive donors. The outcomes in both liver and nonliver solid organ transplant recipients given hepatitis B–positive organs have been excellent if appropriate prophylactic therapies provided.

Owing to standard precautions and initiatives for universal hepatitis B virus (HBV) vaccination in the general population and health care workers, risk of transmission of HBV infection from the patient to a health care worker (and vice versa) is very low. The need for mandatory HBV screening and vaccination in health care workers is less clear than in the past. Health care workers with chronic HBV infection neither require restrictions on professional practice nor disclosure of infection status to a patient. Further study is required to develop effective revaccination strategies to manage health care workers who are vaccine nonresponders.

Despite the significant improvement of long-term outcomes in CHB patients long-term treated with NA, none of these drugs can directly target and efficiently clear the cccDNA, which persists in the nuclei of the infected hepatocytes. New anti-HBV strategies that target directly or indirectly HBsAg to achieve "functional cure", ie. Loss of serum HBsAg coupled with serum undetectable HBV DNA, are based on the short-term administration of combination therapies with complementary and synergistics mechanisms of action, targeting in one or multiple critical steps of viral life.

CLINICS IN LIVER DISEASE

THE CLINICS ARE AVAILABLE ONLINE!
Access your subscription at:
www.theclinics.com

Preface

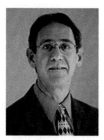

Mitchell L. Shiffman, MD, FACP, FACG, FAASLD
Editor

Chronic hepatitis B virus (HBV) is the most common cause of chronic viral liver disease throughout the world. Despite there being an effective vaccine for over 50 years, chronic HBV remains a primary cause of hepatocellular carcinoma (HCC), a common cause of cirrhosis, and leads to an estimated 880,000 deaths annually. Given the worldwide magnitude, health implications, and constant advances made in our understanding and treatment of HBV, this virus has been a recurring topic of *Clinics in Liver Disease*. This issue, "Challenging Issues in the Management of Chronic Hepatitis B Virus," addresses the most relevant issues that physicians struggle with when evaluating and treating patients with HBV infection.

One of the most striking aspects of HBV today is the marked change that continues to occur in the demographics of this disease. This is primarily due to immigration of persons from areas of the world where HBV is common to countries where HBV has traditionally been less common. The impact of migration on the worldwide prevalence of HBV is important for clinicians to consider when they provide routine medical care.

HBV exists in several different states, some of which cause chronic liver injury and require treatment. Many serologic and virologic tests are utilized to assess HBV activity and viral resolution. Mutations in the HBV virus genome may lead to confusing serologic patterns. As a result, many physicians remain uncertain of how to interpret HBV serologies and manage those patients with discordant HBV serologic patterns.

Although the recommendations for managing and treating acute and chronic HBV are contained within practice guidelines produced by various hepatology and gastroenterology societies, many patients with HBV do not fit neatly into various categories, and the practitioner is sometimes left undecided on whether to treat for prolonged periods of time. Both interferon and oral antiviral agents are available for treatment of chronic HBV. Although the vast majority of physicians and patients prefer oral therapy, interferon can be very effective and remains a viable option for some patients. Measuring HBV DNA and HB surface antigen titer may be very useful in selecting patients for treatment and assessing response to these treatments.

Chronic HBV is one of the most important risk factors for developing HCC. Patients with chronic HBV should be screened for HCC. HBV needs to be effectively managed

Clin Liver Dis 25 (2021) xiii–xiv
https://doi.org/10.1016/j.cld.2021.08.001
1089-3261/21/© 2021 Published by Elsevier Inc.
liver.theclinics.com

in patients who develop HCC. New treatments for HCC, particularly the checkpoint inhibitors, may impact HBV.

Patients with chronic HBV can be coinfected with hepatitis C virus (HCV) or hepatitis D virus (HDV). All patients with chronic HCV should be evaluated for HBV and treated or administered prophylactic therapy to prevent HBV flare if appropriate. Immigration is also changing the demographics of HBV-HDV coinfection. Managing HBV-HDV coinfection has been a challenge in the past, but a new treatment for HDV has been shown to be effective and should soon be available.

Given the effectiveness of oral antiviral therapy and the increased waiting time for patients in need of organ transplants, many liver transplant centers are now actively transplanting organs with previous exposure to HBV into patients without HBV. Whether transplant recipients who receive such organs or patients with chronic HBV who undergo liver transplantation require life-long antiviral therapy remains controversial.

Health care workers and first responders are now routinely vaccinated against HBV. However, some may not respond to the vaccine or have undetectable anti-HB surface. The medical and legal ramifications of a health care worker with chronic HBV require careful consideration.

We would very much like to have a treatment that cures HBV, like we now have for HCV. Unfortunately, HBV is a much more complicated virus and has proven itself to be a formidable enemy. However, novel therapies with different mechanisms of action and targets are being developed and tested as potential treatments that may one day cure HBV.

I would like to thank the authors, who represent 8 countries and 4 continents, for their excellent contributions to this issue of *Clinics in Liver Disease*. It is my hope that our readers will find this issue informative, clinically relevant, and helpful in the assessment and management of their patients with HBV infection.

Mitchell L. Shiffman, MD, FACP, FACG, FAASLD
Liver Institute of Richmond
Liver Institute of Hampton Roads
Bon Secours Mercy Health
Richmond and Newport News, Virginia, USA

Eastern Virginia Medical School
Norfolk, Virginia, USA

E-mail address:
Mitchell_Shiffman@bshsi.org

The Changing Demographics of Hepatitis B Virus Infection

Issam Tout, PhD[a,b], Dimitri Loureiro, PhD[a,b], Tarik Asselah, MD, PhD[a,b],*

KEYWORDS

- Hepatitis B • Migrants • Hepatitis D • Vaccination • Demographics • Prevention

KEY POINTS

- Immigration from high- to low-endemic countries increases hepatitis B virus (HBV) prevalence and the incidence of hepatocellular carcinoma.
- Most immigrants from high-endemic countries have very poor knowledge and awareness of HBV infection.
- Universal vaccination reduces HBV prevalence and HBV-attributable cancer incidence cases among children, adolescents, and young adults.
- Hepatitis delta virus infects up to 30 million people worldwide with a high risk of progression to cirrhosis.
- Reinforcement of the global vaccine coverage, improvement of access to long-term therapy with nucleos(t)ide analogues, improvement of screening and linkage to care, and development of innovative treatments are essential to eradicate HBV.

INTRODUCTION

The burden of hepatitis B virus (HBV) infection constitutes a public health threat in many areas of the world with a previous estimated global prevalence as high as 350 to 400 million and an annual mortality rate of up to 1.34 million individuals.[1,2] Chronic HBV infection is a major contributor to the development of cirrhosis, hepatocellular carcinoma, and liver-related death, with a more recent estimation of 257 million infected people worldwide despite the long-term existence of a highly effective vaccine[3] and efficient treatments.[4] The total number of hepatitis B surface antigen (HBsAg)-positive chronic hepatitis B (CHB) patients in 2005 was estimated at 240 million with a global prevalence of 3.7%, broken down into 127 million men with a prevalence of 3.9% and 113 million women with a prevalence of 3.5%. HBsAg endemicity is categorized

[a] Université de Paris, Centre de Recherche sur l'inflammation, Inserm U1149, CNRS ERL8252, 16 rue Henri Huchard, F-75018 Paris, France; [b] Department of Hepatology, AP-HP, Hôpital Beaujon, 100 boulevard du Général Leclerc, F-92110 Clichy, France
* Corresponding author. Department of Hepatology, AP-HP, Hospital Beaujon, 100 boulevard du General Leclerc, F-92110 Clichy, France
E-mail address: tarik.asselah@aphp.fr

Clin Liver Dis 25 (2021) 673–687
https://doi.org/10.1016/j.cld.2021.06.001
1089-3261/21/© 2021 Elsevier Inc. All rights reserved.

liver.theclinics.com

as low (<2%), low-intermediate (2–4.9%), high-intermediate (5–7.9%), and high (≥8%).[5] Long-term treatment with nucleos(t)ide analogues (NA) is the current first-line therapy for patients with CHB recommended by most of the current guidelines.[6–8] NA can prevent disease progression and liver failure and decrease the risk of HCC. However, they have to be administrated long-life, with low rates of on-therapy functional cure (HBsAg loss).[9] Stopping NAs can even be considered for certain categories of patients with CHB.[10] The prevalence of HBV infection in the general population was estimated to 3.61% worldwide and highly depends on the region. A highest endemicity is to be seen in countries of the African region (8.83%) and Western Pacific region (5.26%) and up to 22.3% in the Pacific region while being lower in prevalence (<2%) in North America and Western Europe.[11] In Europe, the average HBV prevalence was estimated at 1.5%, with 15 million people infected.[3]

A major variable that has only recently been considered in seroprevalence rates is the impact of migration from countries with high prevalence rates to those with low rates of HBV infection.[12] In the presence of frequent international air travel and the globalization of the world economy, mass migration has been on the upswing in the last half of the twentieth century. According to the EASL 2017 guidelines, all first-degree relatives and sexual partners of subjects with CHB should be advised to be tested for HBV serologic markers (HBsAg, anti-HBs, anti-HBc) and to be vaccinated if they are negative for these markers.[6]

In developed countries, the prevalence is higher among those who immigrated from high- or intermediate-prevalence countries (HBsAg prevalence ≥2%), and therefore, screening for HBV is recommended in all persons born in those countries under American Association for the Study of Liver Diseases (AASLD) 2018.[7] In addition, US-born persons not vaccinated as infants whose parents were born in regions with high HBV endemicity (≥8%) should also be screened.[7]

In this review, the authors evaluate the impact of recent immigration from Asian countries, Middle East, Africa and Central America to Europe, North America/USA, and Australia, on the prevalence of HBV. Moreover, the authors discuss the impact of vaccination on the incidence and prevalence of HBV over the past 50 years in various countries.

IMPACT OF RECENT IMMIGRATION FROM ASIA, MIDDLE EAST, AFRICA AND CENTRAL AMERICA TO EUROPE, NORTH AMERICA/USA, AND AUSTRALIA

At the international level, there is no universally accepted definition of the term "migrant," as it differs from country to country. Migrants may remain in the home country or host country ("settlers"), move on to another country ("transit migrants"), or move back and forth between countries ("circular migrants" such as seasonal workers) (World Health Organization [WHO]).[13] The UN Recommendations on Statistics of International Migration define a long-term migrant as a "person who moves to a country other than that of his or her usual residence for a period of at least a year."[14] These mobile, migrant populations are composed of several groups, including immigrants, seasonal workers, refugees, asylum seekers, international students, and others. According to the UN, the total number of international migrants in 2019 was 271.6 million.[15] The percentage of migrants among the population has increased from 2.8% in 2000 to 3.5% in 2019.[15] These numbers remain underestimated for not including undocumented migrants or trafficked persons.

Europe

Population movements and worldwide migration are currently changing the HBV prevalence and incidence in several low endemic countries in Europe (eg, Italy, Germany), owing to the higher HBsAg prevalence rates in migrants and refugees from outside Europe compared with the indigenous population.[16] According to the UN, the total number of migrants to Europe in 2019 was 82.3 million.[15] Chu and colleagues[12] aimed to determine the impact of the migration on HBV infection by comparing the available data on prevalence and transmission routes of HBV in the migration population and the general population in 6 Northern and North-Western European countries (the Netherlands, Germany, Finland, Denmark, Sweden, and the United Kingdom). Evident differences were found between the migration and the general population in HBV prevalence as immigrants from high/intermediate hepatitis B endemic countries constitute a substantial proportion of HBsAg(+) and chronic cases in all 6 countries. The percentage range of HBsAg+ in 3 largest migrant groups in these countries were 4% to 4.6% compared with 0.01% to 0.7% in general population.[12]

Pooled estimates of chronic HBV prevalence data from the European Center for Disease Prevention and Control surveys indicate that 53% of HBV carriers were born outside the European Union (EU).[17] For instance, a meta-analysis on HBV prevalence among immigrants to the EU found that high prevalence rates among migrants, particularly those from East Asia, sub-Saharan Africa, are similar to the countries of origin.[18]

A recent study investigated 170 HBsAg-positive immigrants living in Italy for 1 to 7 years to ascertain whether they may have become infected in the host country.[19] HBV genotype was identified in 109 of the 113 HBV-DNA-positive immigrants and HBV-genotype-E predominated (68.9%). Only 5.5% of the subjects showed an HBV genotype absent or extremely rare in their native country. Thus, it was suggested that immigrants may acquire HBV infection in Italy, and therefore, HBV vaccination programs should be extended to all immigrants living in Italy.[19]

In Spain, a multicenter study (June 2014 to May 2015) in which outpatients with CHB were seen and followed-up in 4 Hepatology units followed-up a total of 951 patients.[20] Of them 46.6% were immigrants (58.7% of them born in Africa) and were significantly younger compared with nonimmigrants, whereas indicators of metabolic comorbidities (eg, alcohol, obesity) were significantly higher in nonimmigrants. They found that chronic hepatitis B e-antigen (HBeAg)-positive infection was significantly higher in immigrants (3.9% vs 0.6%, $P = .001$), and chronic HBeAg-negative hepatitis was higher nonimmigrants (31.7% vs 21.4%, $P<.001$). Furthermore, the proportion of those with indication of effectively receiving therapy at the time of data collection was higher in nonimmigrants (83.2% vs 57.8%, $P<.001$).[20] The fact that some immigrants do not get adequately treated is due to several factors including local adaptation that precludes access to treatment. Another issue is the refusal to provide health care to immigrants in certain EU countries. A study on sub-Saharan African migrants living in the Paris area showed that the reported refusal of care was nearly twice as high in the CHB group (10%) compared with the reference group (6%, $P<.001$).[21]

In the Netherlands, 77% of chronic HBV infections are estimated to originate from outside the EU, predominantly from high and intermediate prevalence regions.[22] A study on first-generation migrants (FGM) of the Turkish community in Arnhem (Netherlands) found that 3% of Turkish FGM older than 24 years had active hepatitis B.[23] The investigators recommended that active hepatitis screening of FGM from Turkey should be part of the national health policy, as it will benefit the individual and public health in the Netherlands.[23]

Another study in Germany has shown a 15 to 25 times higher HBsAg prevalence of 3% to 5% of Turkish immigrants in comparison to the general population.[24] Moreover, the prevalence of refugees with previous exposure to hepatitis viruses was higher than that in the general German population, but lower than in other migrant populations in Germany. The vaccination status against hepatitis B was poor.[25]

In Sweden, immigration increased the incidence of HCC and raised the question whether immigrants from regions with a high incidence of HCC ought to be subjected to mandatory HBV and HCV diagnosis and consequent liver ultrasounds for diagnosis of occult HCC.[26]

On the ongoing Syrian Civil war, more than 10% of the displaced Syrian refugees (1,3 million) went to Europe (57% in Serbia and Germany compared with 31% in Sweden, Hungary, Austria, Netherlands, and Bulgaria and 12% in the remaining 37 European Countries).[27] According to the Office of Migration and Refugees in Germany, nearly one million Syrian refugees applied for asylum in 2015 alone. According to German researchers, nearly 2.3% of Syrian migrants coming into Germany have tested positive for HBV, a rate nearly 3 times higher than the rest of the country. Fewer than 20% of the refugees assessed have been immunized for HBV, and it is speculated that 63% of the Syrian population has not been vaccinated against HBV.[28]

North America/United States of America

Since the 1960s, the immigration patterns have changed. Regions supplying immigrants to Australia, Canada, and the United States, which were historically western and central European population movements, have predominantly shifted to Latin American, African, and Asian origins.[29] According to the UN, the total number of migrants to Northern America in 2019 was 58.6 million, which represents 16% of their total population.[15] Data from 1999 to 2016 reported an overall CHB prevalence of 0.35%, with a lower prevalence (0.15%) among US-born persons than foreign-born (FB) persons (1.28%), particularly among non-Hispanic Asians (3.85%).[30] About 59% of FB with CHB in the United States in 2018 emigrated from Asia, 19% from the Americas, and 15% from Africa.[31,32] According to a recent meta-analysis, the total prevalence of CHB in the United States may be as high as 2.4 million, including FB and US-born persons.[31] A study used cross-sectional data from 5982 individuals screened at community events held from 2009 to 2015 in FB immigrants living in the Baltimore Washington metropolitan area to assess HBV prevalence.[22] Most participants were born in Asia (77.8%). The prevalence of HBV infection was 6.1% in Asia-born immigrants (highest for those from Cambodia [11.9%] compared with Vietnam [8.2%], China [8.1%], Laos [6.1%], and Korea [4.6%]) compared with 3.7% and in Africa-born immigrants (highest for those from Liberia [6.7%] and Sierra Leone [6.7%], followed by Cameroon [4.4%] and Nigeria [4.2%]).[22]

A cross-sectional survey among 71 first-generation African Americans in New York City was conducted to better understand the HBV burden in this vulnerable population and to identify risk factors for the implementation of more effective prevention and treatment programs.[33] This survey found 87.50% of participants migrated from sub-Saharan Africa and 79.10% had lived in the United States for 10 or fewer years. Almost half of the participants never underwent HBV screening (44.29%) or HBV vaccination (49.23%). It was found that 60.87% of participants never received any HBV screening or vaccination recommendation from doctors. In addition, first-generation African immigrants had very limited knowledge of HBV transmission.[33]

Other issues such as health insurance coverage, worries about paying rent, and language of interview all differentially affect HBV testing and linkages to care among FB persons.[34] Culturally sensitive health promotion campaigns should be provided more, which may improve HBV-related outcomes. Among 773 investigated HBV-infected individuals, FB decedents were twice as likely as US-born decedents to have a liver-related cause of death, whereas behavioral risk factors were more often reported by US-born individuals.[35] Both populations need to receive routine HBV screening, vaccination if indicated, and medical care to limit the severity of HBV infection outcomes.[35]

Social factors were explored with community health experts working in African Immigrants (AI) communities throughout the United States It was found that religious preferences and cultural norms affect health care access, awareness of HBV, and were considered as barriers to HBV screening and care.[36]

In another study, a predictive model was created, including 3019 individuals considered at high risk for HBV in underserved communities, particularly Asian American, Pacific Islander, and African immigrant populations.[37–39] The investigators found an association between insurance status and HBV infection and that Pacific Islander and African immigrant populations had higher odds of infection compared with those from the Americas[37];this highlights the need to expand testing in high-risk populations for HBV.

Among women with HBV infection who gave birth in New York City during 1998 to 2015, the incidence of births declined significantly among US-born women but not among non–US-born women, highlighting the need for successful vaccination programs worldwide.[28]

In hepatitis B testing and linkage-to-care programs serving non–US-born persons during the period October 2014 to September 2017, prevalence of current HBV infection was high in this population and among household and sexual contacts of HBV-infected persons.[29]

Australia

In 2016, an estimated 230,000 Australians (about 0.9% of the population) were living with CHB.[40] The main populations affected by CHB in Australia include those born in endemic areas overseas (particularly the Asia-Pacific region).[41] The prevalence of CHB in Australia has increased over the past decade, predominantly related to the increases in migration from endemic areas such as the Asia -Pacific region and sub-Saharan Africa, as well as parts of southern and eastern Europe, and the Middle East.[42]

A study on HBV prevalence was conducted on women aged 15 to 44 years between 2000 and 2016.[43] Prevalence estimates were the highest among women born in Sierra Leone (11.13%, 95% confidence interval [CI]: 8.29%–13.96%), Taiwan (8.08%, 95% CI: 6.74%–9.43%), Cambodia (7.47%, 95% CI: 6.50%–8.45%), and Vietnam (7.36%, 95% CI: 6.97%–7.75%); more moderate estimates among women from North Korea (2.76%, 95% CI: 1.99%–3.53%), and Samoa (2.64%, 95% CI: 1.99%–3.29%). In comparison, prevalence was only 0.18% (95% CI: 0.17%–0.19%) in Australian-born women. Reductions in HBV prevalence were significant during this period among all women except those born in Vietnam (P = .08), South Korea (P = .41), and Sudan (P = .06).[43] Among immigrants of Chinese background, engagement with HBV screening and health care for CHB is relatively low. Jin and colleagues[44] explored sociodemographic factors that might influence this knowledge in a survey including 390 participants of this community. They found that knowledge about HBV prevention, transmission, and treatment is very limited and depended on sociodemographic variables (knowing someone living with HBV and stigma associated with HBV),[44] and this helps in the development of targeted health promotion to increase HBV knowledge in Australia.

Percentages of FB persons living with CHB in 2016 are presented in **Fig. 1**.

Hepatitis Delta Virus Infection and Migration

Hepatitis D virus (HDV) infection in patients with CHB causes the most severe form of chronic viral hepatitis and continues to represent a major health problem. The latest data show that the global prevalence is much higher than previously considered.[45]

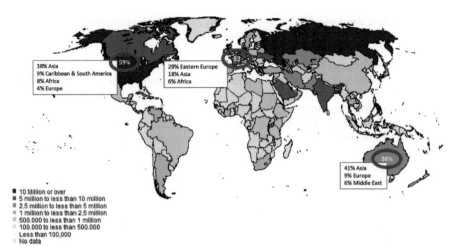

Fig. 1. Map of numbers of international migrants and percentages of foreign-born (FB) living with CHB in 2016. (*From* International Migrant Stock 2019, Geospatial Information Section, UNITED NATIONS.)

Chen and colleagues[46] recently estimated that more than 60 million individuals worldwide have been exposed to HDV. The prevalence of HDV in HBV carriers reached 10.6%, which is twice as high as previous estimations. These cases often consist of an aging cohort of domestic patients with advanced liver fibrosis who represent the end stage of the natural history of HDV and of a younger generation of immigrants from endemic countries who account for most of the new infections.[47]

Europe

In HBsAg-positive immigrants, the prevalence of HDV infection depends on the country of origin. In fact, the epidemiologic impact of HDV infection is high when immigrants from areas endemic to HDV infection (eg, Equatorial Guinea) settle in areas of low endemicity (eg, Germany or England, with a prevalence of 4%), whereas the impact is lesser or nonexistent if the migratory flows are directed toward countries with intermediate endemicity (eg, Italy and Greece, with a prevalence of around 10%).[48] A nationwide retrospective study on 1112 HDV-infected patients was conducted in France to identify prognostic factors in patients with HDV infection.[49] They found that European HDV-1 and African HDV-5 patients were more at risk of developing cirrhosis. African patients displayed better response to interferon therapy than non-African patients (46.4% vs 29.1%, $P<.001$), and HDV viral load at baseline was significantly lower in responders than in nonresponders.[49]

Northern America/Australia

In the United States, HDV surveillance data are limited and anti-HDV testing is rarely conducted, thereby limiting the validity of prevalence estimates.[50,51] In a midwestern US population of 1007 HBV-infected individuals, 3.3% were positive for anti-HDV and only 12% were tested for anti-HDV.[50] A recent analysis of the 2011–2016 National Health and Nutrition Examination Survey reported an HDV prevalence of 42% among HBsAg-positive carriers.[52] Asian and FB adults had the highest prevalence of both HBsAg and anti-HDV. In a study performed in Northern California, Gish and colleagues[52] reported an HDV prevalence of 8% in HBsAg-positive patients. Only 42% of the 1191 HBV-infected individuals were tested for HDV. Interestingly, 67% of the patients with HDV infection were diagnosed with cirrhosis compared with only 22% of the HBV monoinfected cohort.[52]

In a recent study of 4407 individuals tested for HDV between 1997 and 2016 in Queensland, Australia, 179 recorded HDV positive (prevalence of 4.1%). HDV seropositivity was associated with overseas birth, particularly in Africa.[53]

AASLD recommends risk-based screening for HDV. The "at-risk" groups include persons who inject illicit drugs, persons with HIV, those at risk for sexually transmitted diseases, and persons who emigrated from countries of high endemicity.[54] Da and colleagues[55] determined independent risk factors for HDV including intravenous drug users, HBV DNA less than 2000 IU/mL, alanine aminotransferase greater than 40 U/L, and HDV endemic country of origin. EASL recommends HDV screening for all patients with HBV infection.[6]

These data have prompted various national and regional guidelines for screening of migrants at high risk for HBV and HCV, especially in host nations that attract the largest numbers of immigrants globally. The European,[6] American,[7] and Canadian[56] guidelines for HBV screening will be summarized later (**Table 1**).

THE IMPACT OF VACCINATION ON THE INCIDENCE AND PREVALENCE OF HEPATITIS B VIRUS INFECTION

Vaccines against HBV infection are highly effective. A plasma-derived vaccine, first used in a national infant immunization program in 1984,[57] was gradually replaced by recombinant vaccines administered by a dose at birth followed by 2 to 3 doses at monthly intervals.[58]

Asia

China contributes with more than half the global burden of liver cancer, but a decline has been observed in incidence rates of CHB and HCC. It is predicted that the incidence of liver cancer attributable to HBV infection in China's population could decrease by half by 2050 if primary prevention interventions, such as vaccination, are well implemented.[59] A universal vaccination program launched by Taiwan's government in 1984 effectively decreased the rate of hepatitis B carriage and the development of HCC in the younger generation.[60] The 30-year experience of this program has been an impressive success in reducing the number of patients with HBV infection and is an invaluable reference for the rest of the world.[61]

There is a projected increase of HBV infection in China of 60 million people still living with HBV in 2030 and 10 million HBV-related deaths, including 5.7 million HBV-related cancer deaths between 2015 and 2030. Nayagam and colleagues[62] showed via a dynamic simulation model of HBV that these cases can be decreased by 2.1 million by highly active case finding and optimal antiviral treatment regimens. In India, a care model for preventive and disease-specific health care for a marginalized population in Arunachal Pradesh was developed.[63] The investigators showed it was able to effectively link that population to screening, preventive vaccination, and follow-up therapeutic care to define the migratory nature of the population and disease. This model of care can be applied to other similar settings globally.[63]

Africa

In Zimbabwe, full vaccine coverage with 3 doses and the inclusion of the birth dose is vital in reducing vertical and horizontal transmission in early life.[64] However, the birth dose is not routinely administered in Zimbabwe due to limited funds, unavailability of cold chain facilities, and difficulty in reaching infants within 24 hours of birth.[65] In a

Table 1
Recommendations on hepatitis B virus screening by the European (EASL), American (AASLD), and Canadian (CASL) guidelines

EASL	AASLD	CASL
• Initial evaluation of a subject with CHB should include a complete history, a physical examination, assessment of liver disease activity and severity, and markers of HBV infection. • All first-degree relatives and sexual partners of subjects with CHB should be advised to be tested for HBV serologic markers (HBsAg, anti-HBs, anti-HBc). • Screening for HBsAg in the first trimester of pregnancy is strongly recommended. • All candidates for chemotherapy and immunosuppressive therapy should be tested for HBV markers prior to immunosuppression.	• Patients at risk[a] for CHB who should be screened for HBV infection (HBsAg and anti-HBs). • Screening is recommended in all persons born in countries with a HBsAg seroprevalence of ≥2%, US-born persons not vaccinated as infants whose parents were born in regions with high HBV endemicity (≥8%), pregnant women, persons needing immunosuppressive therapy, and the at-risk[a] groups.	• All candidate immigrants to Canada should undergo screening for HBV during their medical evaluation. • High-risk[b] groups should be screened for CHB infection with HBsAg, anti-HBs, and anti-HBc, and their response to the vaccine should be assessed.

[a] Persons born in regions of high or intermediate HBV endemicity (HBsAg prevalence of 2%): Africa (all countries) North, Southeast, East Asia (all countries), Australia and South Pacific (all countries except Australia and New Zealand), Middle East (all countries except Cyprus and Israel), Eastern Europe (all countries except Hungary), Western Europe (Malta, Spain, and indigenous populations of Greenland), North America (Alaskan natives and indigenous populations of Northern Canada), Mexico and Central America (Guatemala and Honduras), South America (Ecuador, Guyana, Suriname, Venezuela, and Amazonian areas), Caribbean (Antigua-Barbuda, Dominica, Grenada, Haiti, Jamaica, Saint Kitts and Nevis, Saint Lucia, and Turks and Caicos Islands); US-born persons not vaccinated as an infant whose parents were born in regions with high HBV endemicity (8%); persons who have ever injected drugs; men who have sex with men; persons needing immunosuppressive therapy, including chemotherapy, immunosuppression related to organ transplantation, and immunosuppression for rheumatological or gastroenterologic disorders; individuals with elevated ALT or AST of unknown cause; donors of blood, plasma, organs, tissues, or semen; persons with end-stage renal disease, including predialysis, hemodialysis, peritoneal dialysis, and home dialysis patients; All pregnant women; infants born to HBsAg-positive mothers; persons with chronic liver disease, for example, HCV; persons with HIV; household, needle-sharing, and sexual contacts of HBsAg-positive persons; persons who are not in a long-term, mutually monogamous relationship (eg, >1 sex partner during the previous 6 mo); persons seeking evaluation or treatment for a sexually transmitted disease; health care and public safety workers at risk for occupational exposure to blood or blood-contaminated body fluids; residents and staff of facilities for developmentally disabled persons; travelers to countries with intermediate or high prevalence of HBV infection; persons who are the source of blood or body fluid exposures that might require postexposure prophylaxis; inmates of correctional facilities; unvaccinated persons with diabetes who are aged 19 through 59 y (discretion of clinician for unvaccinated adults with diabetes who are aged ≥ 60 y).

[b] Born in region where HBV is more common (Central, East, or South Asia; Australasia; Eastern Europe; South America; Sub-Saharan Africa; North Africa; or Middle East); household contacts with HBV carriers (including unvaccinated persons whose parents were from HBV-endemic countries), especially children of HBV-positive mothers; sexual contacts with multiple sexual partners; illicit injection or intranasal drug use or shared drug paraphernalia (past or present); inmates; patients with chronic renal failure who need dialysis; signs of liver disease (ie, abnormal liver enzyme tests) or other infectious diseases (ie, hepatitis C, human immunodeficiency virus; hepatomegaly, splenomegaly, thrombocytopenia, and jaundice are late findings); all pregnant women; patients needing immune modulation therapy or those who will develop immunosuppression such as cancer chemotherapy.

prospective cohort study in Burkina Faso, of 5200 pregnant women consulting for the antenatal visit, 47 out of 60 (78.3%; 65.8–87.9) children born alive were immunized for HBV within 24 hours of life, showing large gaps in HBV "mother to child transmission" (MTCT).[66] Universal access to the vaccine birth dose should be allocated in these regions. A recent study showed reduction in HBV-attributable cancer incident cases among children (from 2080 to 1430), adolescents, and young adults (from 10,890–909) mainly because of the universal HBV vaccination.[67]

Northern America

In the United States, a multicenter retrospective study (2015–2018) evaluating care among all women with HBV during pregnancy was conducted on 372 women.[68] For 33% of patients, the pregnancy encounter was the first time for HBV diagnosis, highlighting the importance of pregnancy as an opportunity for HBV linkage to care. All infants received hepatitis B immune globulin (HBIG) and the first HBV vaccine dose, 106 (81%) received the second, and 94 (74%) received the third dose but fewer at the recommended time intervals reflecting limited awareness of HBV guidelines. Overall, rates of adherence to care guidelines for HBV for mothers during pregnancy and their infants are suboptimal but seem to be improving over time.[68] Colocation of HBV care in the obstetrics department shows promise in improving adherence to maternal care measures. Earlier use (within 1 hour after birth) of HBIG and hepatitis B vaccine can provide better protection efficacy against MTCT of HBV.[69] The disparity between the number of people who are chronically infected and those who receive treatment can partially be explained by the large number of infected persons who are unscreened and thus remain undiagnosed, the lack of access, including insurance, education, and referral to appropriate medical care.[70]

Europe

A nurse-led intervention in England improved case referral rates by an additional 14% (from 86% [88/102 cases] to 99.7% [648/650 cases]).[71] The proportion of contacts tested increased from 34% to 72% to 94% with 18 new cases of HBV diagnosed. Among close contacts tested, vaccination rates of at least 3 doses increased from 77% (43/56) to 93% (452/491).

On the other hand, use of antiviral agents such as lamivudine, telbivudine, and tenofovir in several studies have been shown to reduce rates of MTCT in highly viremic mothers with CHB. A recent multicenter study showed that TAF, for highly viremic mothers, effectively prevented MTCT of hepatitis B. There were no safety concerns for either mothers or infants with 24 to 28 weeks of follow-up.[72] A study commissioned by the WHO, determined that maternal HBV DNA of greater than or equal to 5.30 $\log^{10}$ IU/mL seems to be the optimal threshold for MTCT of HBV infection despite infant immunoprophylaxis.[73] HBeAg was accurate to identify women with HBV DNA levels higher than this threshold and has high sensitivity to predict cases of immunoprophylaxis failure. Therefore, in areas where HBV DNA assays are unavailable, HBeAg can be used as an alternative to assess eligibility for antiviral prophylaxis.[73]

PERSPECTIVES

With only 9 years to go until the 2030 deadline of the WHO on eliminating viral hepatitis is reached, and although much progress has been made toward elimination, there are still some important gaps in terms of policy and progress, especially in resource-limited settings. First, we must consider the high number of people

---

Box 1
Strategies to control hepatitis B.

- Reinforce global vaccine coverage.
- Reinforce HBV screening, especially among migrants.
- Improve global access to long-term therapy with NA.
- Improve disease management.
- Broaden treatment indications to treat all viremic CHB patients..
- Increase public awareness of the burden of HBV infection..
- Advance in preclinical and clinical development of innovative treatments to achieve HBV cure.
- Develop novel biomarkers for risk stratification among HBV-infected fibrotic patients.

---

chronically infected with viral hepatitis (257 million individuals) and its catastrophic burden of disease worldwide (1.34 million annual deaths), despite an efficient vaccine. Secondly, the necessary systems and infrastructure to implement universal vaccination and to diagnose and link all infected persons to care are still missing or inadequate in many regions, including high-income countries. Furthermore, the Covid-19 pandemic and its associated economic downturn is diverting the attention and resources of all governments, health departments, and health care professionals as well as making it difficult for any commitment of new funding toward viral hepatitis elimination. In addition, many country-level barriers exist from procurement to deployment to absurd restrictions on who can prescribe or be prescribed.[74]

The overall goals of most strategies is to reduce the transmission of HBV, decrease morbidity and mortality caused by CHB, and minimize the personal and social impact of persons living with hepatitis B. Numerous steps should be firmly taken: reinforcement of the global vaccine coverage, including the vaccination of all newborn babies, preventing MTCT especially in highly endemic regions; reinforcement of HBV screening especially among HBV endemic migrants; improvement of the global access to long-term therapy with NAs; and improvement of disease management. In addition, we must broaden treatment indications to treat all viremic patients, including "immune tolerant" with extremely high viral loads.

The funding for hepatitis programs should be increased worldwide by increasing public awareness of the burden of HBV infection. New policies are required to push advancement in preclinical and clinical development of innovative treatments, especially immunotherapies and try to achieve functional cure. Finally monitoring HBV-infected fibrotic patients with novel biomarkers for risk stratification is also clinically important. Strategies with practical steps that must take place to control hepatitis B are resumed in (**Box 1**).

All the aforementioned surely requires substantial financial and political commitment and global prioritization.

CLINICS CARE POINTS

- Global vaccine coverage and efficient HBV screening should be reinforced especially among migrants.

- Global access to long-term anti-HBV therapies with NAs should be improved.
- Broadening treatment indications to treat all viremic CHB patients including immune tolerants is crucial.
- Improving public awareness of the burden of HBV infection as well as a better disease management is important.

DISCLOSURE

T. Asselah has acted as a speaker and/or advisor board and/or investigator for Abbvie, Eiger Biopharmaceutical, Janssen, Gilead, Myr Pharmaceutical, Roche, and Merck. I. Tout and D. Loureiro have nothing to disclose.

REFERENCES

1. Trépo C, Chan HLY, Lok A. Hepatitis B virus infection. Lancet 2014;384(9959): 2053–63.
2. Lavanchy D. Hepatitis B virus epidemiology, disease burden, treatment, and current and emerging prevention and control measures. J Viral Hepat 2004;11(2): 97–107.
3. Global hepatitis report. 2017. Available at: https://www.who.int/publications-detail-redirect/global-hepatitis-report-2017. Accessed April 30, 2021.
4. Asselah T, Loureiro D, Boyer N, et al. Targets and future direct-acting antiviral approaches to achieve hepatitis B virus cure. Lancet Gastroenterol Hepatol 2019; 4(11):883–92.
5. Ott JJ, Stevens GA, Groeger J, et al. Global epidemiology of hepatitis B virus infection: new estimates of age-specific HBsAg seroprevalence and endemicity. Vaccine 2012;30(12):2212–9.
6. European Association for the Study of the Liver. Electronic address: easloffice@easloffice.eu, European Association for the Study of the Liver. EASL 2017 Clinical Practice Guidelines on the management of hepatitis B virus infection. J Hepatol 2017;67(2):370–98.
7. Terrault NA, Lok ASF, McMahon BJ, et al. Update on prevention, diagnosis, and treatment of chronic hepatitis B: AASLD 2018 hepatitis B guidance. Hepatol Baltim Md 2018;67(4):1560–99.
8. Sarin SK, Kumar M, Lau GK, et al. Asian-Pacific clinical practice guidelines on the management of hepatitis B: a 2015 update. Hepatol Int 2016;10(1):1–98.
9. Tout I, Loureiro D, Mansouri A, et al. Hepatitis B surface antigen seroclearance: immune mechanisms, clinical impact, importance for drug development. J Hepatol 2020. https://doi.org/10.1016/j.jhep.2020.04.013.
10. Tout I, Lampertico P, Berg T, et al. Perspectives on stopping nucleos(t)ide analogues therapy in patients with chronic hepatitis B. Antivir Res 2021;185: 104992.
11. Schweitzer A, Horn J, Mikolajczyk RT, et al. Estimations of worldwide prevalence of chronic hepatitis B virus infection: a systematic review of data published between 1965 and 2013. Lancet 2015;386(10003):1546–55.
12. Chu JJ, Wörmann T, Popp J, et al. Changing epidemiology of hepatitis B and migration–a comparison of six Northern and North-Western European countries. Eur J Public Health 2013;23(4):642–7.
13. WHO | definitions. WHO. Available at: http://www.who.int/migrants/about/definitions/en/. Accessed May 10, 2021.

14. Recommendations on Statistics of international migration. Available at: https://unstats.un.org/unsd/publication/seriesm/seriesm_58rev1e.pdf. Accessed May 10, 2021.

15. United Nations. International migration 2019 wall chart 2019. United Nations, Department of Economic and Social Affairs, Population Division; 2019. Available at: www.unmigration.org.

16. Hampel A, Solbach P, Cornberg M, et al. [Current seroprevalence, vaccination and predictive value of liver enzymes for hepatitis B among refugees in Germany]. Bundesgesundheitsblatt Gesundheitsforschung Gesundheitsschutz 2016;59(5):578–83.

17. Rantala M, van de Laar MJ. Surveillance and epidemiology of hepatitis B and C in Europe – a review. Eurosurveillance 2008;13(21):18880.

18. Rossi C, Shrier I, Marshall L, et al. Seroprevalence of chronic hepatitis B virus infection and prior immunity in immigrants and refugees: a systematic review and meta-analysis. PLoS One 2012;7(9):e44611.

19. Sagnelli C, Ciccozzi M, Alessio L, et al. HBV molecular epidemiology and clinical condition of immigrants living in Italy. Infection 2018;46(4):523–31.

20. Miquel M, Pardo A, Forné M, et al. Current trends in access to treatment for hepatitis B in immigrants vs non-immigrants. Gastroenterol Rep 2020;8(5):362–6.

21. Vignier N, Dray Spira R, Pannetier J, et al. Refusal to provide healthcare to sub-Saharan migrants in France: a comparison according to their HIV and HBV status. Eur J Public Health 2018;28(5):904–10.

22. Marschall T, Kretzschmar M, Mangen M-JJ, et al. High impact of migration on the prevalence of chronic hepatitis B in The Netherlands. Eur J Gastroenterol Hepatol 2008;20(12):1214–25.

23. Richter C, Beest GT, Sancak I, et al. Hepatitis B prevalence in the Turkish population of Arnhem: implications for national screening policy? Epidemiol Infect 2012;140(4):724–30.

24. Burgazli KM, Mericliler M, Sen C, et al. The prevalence of hepatitis B virus (HBV) among Turkish immigrants in Germany. Eur Rev Med Pharmacol Sci 2014;18(6):869–74.

25. Jablonka A, Solbach P, Wöbse M, et al. Seroprevalence of antibodies and antigens against hepatitis A-E viruses in refugees and asylum seekers in Germany in 2015. Eur J Gastroenterol Hepatol 2017;29(8):939–45.

26. Taflin H, Hafström L, Holmberg E, et al. The impact of increased immigration to Sweden on the incidence and treatment of patients with HCC and underlying liver disease. Scand J Gastroenterol 2019;54(6):746–52.

27. Refugees UNHC for. UNHCR global appeal 2015 update - Europe summary. UNHCR. Available at: https://www.unhcr.org/publications/fundraising/5461e5f80/unhcr-global-appeal-2015-update-europe-summary.html. Accessed May 5, 2021.

28. Rubido JCA. The international liver congress, April 13-17th, 2016, Barcelona, Spain. Biotecnol Apl 2016;33(2):2501–5.

29. Gushulak BD, MacPherson DW. Globalization of infectious diseases: the impact of migration. Clin Infect Dis 2004;38(12):1742–8.

30. NHANES - about the national health and nutrition examination survey. Available at: https://www.cdc.gov/nchs/nhanes/about_nhanes.htm. Accessed May 10, 2021.

31. Wong RJ, Brosgart CL, Welch S, et al. An updated assessment of chronic hepatitis B prevalence among foreign-born persons living in the United States. Hepatology 2021. https://doi.org/10.1002/hep.31782.

32. Juon H-S, Ha E, Kim F, et al. Prevalence of viral hepatitis in foreign-born populations in the Baltimore-Washington metropolitan area, 2009-2015. J Community Health 2019;44(2):203-7.

33. Ogunwobi OO, Dibba O, Zhu L, et al. Hepatitis B virus screening and vaccination in first-generation African immigrants: a Pilot study. J Community Health 2019; 44(6):1037-43.

34. Greene KM, Duffus WA, Xing J, et al. Social determinants of health associated with HBV testing and access to care among foreign-born persons residing in the United States: 2009 - 2012. J Health Disparities Res Pract 2017;10(2):1-20.

35. Higgins DC, Kuncio DE, Johnson CC, et al. Influence of birth origin and risk factor profile on hepatitis B mortality: Philadelphia, PA 2003-2013. Ann Epidemiol 2018; 28(3):169-74.

36. Freeland C, Bodor S, Perera U, et al. Barriers to hepatitis B screening and prevention for African immigrant populations in the United States: a Qualitative study. Viruses 2020;12(3):305.

37. Freeland C, Vader D, Cohen C, et al. A predictive model for hepatitis B infection among high-risk adults using a community-based sample in greater Philadelphia. J Viral Hepat 2020;27(12):1319-25.

38. Arciuolo RJ, Lazaroff JE, Rosen JB, et al. Trends in hepatitis B surveillance among pregnant women in New York city, 1998-2015. Public Health Rep 2020;135(5): 676-84.

39. Harris AM, Link-Gelles R, Kim K, et al. Community-based services to improve testing and linkage to care among non-U.S.-Born persons with chronic hepatitis B virus infection - three U.S. Programs, october 2014-september 2017. MMWR Morb Mortal Wkly Rep 2018;67(19):541-6.

40. Annual surveillance Report on HIV, viral hepatitis and STIs in Australia 2017. Kirby Institute; 2017. Available at: https://kirby.unsw.edu.au/report/annual-surveillance-report-hiv-viral-hepatitis-and-stis-australia-2017. Accessed May 10, 2021.

41. Viral hepatitis mapping project national report 2018-2019 ASHM. Available at: https://ashm.org.au/resources/hcv-resources-list/viral-hepatitis-mapping-project-national-report-2018-2019/. Accessed May 10, 2021.

42. Prevalence and epidemiology of hepatitis B. B Positive. Available at: https://www.hepatitisb.org.au/prevalence-and-epidemiology-of-hepatitis-b/. Accessed May 10, 2021.

43. He W-Q, Duong MC, Gidding H, et al. Trends in chronic hepatitis B prevalence in Australian women by country of birth, 2000 to 2016. J Viral Hepat 2020;27(1): 74-80.

44. Jin D, Brener L, Treloar C. Knowledge and beliefs about hepatitis B virus infection and associated factors among Chinese migrants in Australia: the result of a quantitative study. Health Soc Care Community 2020. https://doi.org/10.1111/hsc. 13239.

45. Stockdale AJ, Kreuels B, Henrion MYR, et al. The global prevalence of hepatitis D virus infection: systematic review and meta-analysis. J Hepatol 2020;73(3): 523-32.

46. Chen H-Y, Shen D-T, Ji D-Z, et al. Prevalence and burden of hepatitis D virus infection in the global population: a systematic review and meta-analysis. Gut 2019;68(3):512-21.

47. Rizzetto M, Hamid S, Negro F. The changing context of hepatitis D. J Hepatol 2021;74(5):1200-11.

48. Coppola N, Alessio L, Onorato L, et al. HDV infection in immigrant populations. J Med Virol 2019;91(12):2049-58.

49. Roulot D, Brichler S, Layese R, et al. Origin, HDV genotype and persistent viremia determine outcome and treatment response in patients with chronic hepatitis delta. J Hepatol 2020;73(5):1046–62.

50. Safaie P, Razeghi S, Rouster SD, et al. Hepatitis D diagnostics: utilization and testing in the United States. Virus Res 2018;250:114–7.

51. Patel EU, Thio CL, Boon D, et al. Prevalence of hepatitis B and hepatitis D virus infections in the United States, 2011-2016. Clin Infect Dis 2019;69(4):709–12.

52. Gish RG, Yi DH, Kane S, et al. Coinfection with hepatitis B and D: epidemiology, prevalence and disease in patients in Northern California. J Gastroenterol Hepatol 2013;28(9):1521–5.

53. Coghill S, McNamara J, Woods M, et al. Epidemiology and clinical outcomes of hepatitis delta (D) virus infection in Queensland, Australia. Int J Infect Dis 2018; 74:123–7.

54. Terrault NA, Ghany MG. Enhanced screening for hepatitis D in the USA: overcoming the delta Blues. Dig Dis Sci 2020. https://doi.org/10.1007/s10620-020-06584-w.

55. Da BL, Rahman F, Lai WC, et al. Risk factors for delta hepatitis in a North American cohort: who should Be screened? Am J Gastroenterol 2021;116(1):206–9.

56. Coffin CS, Fung SK, Alvarez F, et al. Management of hepatitis B virus infection: 2018 guidelines from the Canadian association for the study of the liver and association of medical microbiology and infectious disease Canada. Can Liver J 2018. https://doi.org/10.3138/canlivj.2018-0008.

57. Chen DS, Hsu NH, Sung JL, et al. A mass vaccination program in Taiwan against hepatitis B virus infection in infants of hepatitis B surface antigen-carrier mothers. JAMA 1987;257(19):2597–603.

58. WHO recommendations for routine immunization - summary tables. Available at: https://www.who.int/teams/regulation-prequalification/eul/immunization-vaccines-and-biologicals. Accessed May 3, 2021.

59. Shi J-F, Cao M, Wang Y, et al. Is it possible to halve the incidence of liver cancer in China by 2050? Int J Cancer 2021;148(5):1051–65.

60. Liu C-J, Chen P-J. Elimination of hepatitis B in highly endemic settings: lessons learned in Taiwan and challenges Ahead. Viruses 2020;12(8):815.

61. Chiang C-J, Yang Y-W, You S-L, et al. Thirty-year outcomes of the national hepatitis B immunization program in Taiwan. JAMA 2013;310(9):974–6.

62. Nayagam S, Chan P, Zhao K, et al. Investment case for a comprehensive package of interventions against hepatitis B in China: applied modeling to help national strategy planning. Clin Infect Dis 2021;72(5):743–52.

63. Abutaleb A, Khatun M, Clement J, et al. A model of care optimized for marginalized remote population unravels migration pattern in India. Hepatology 2021; 73(4):1261–74.

64. Accrombessi M, Adetola CV, Bacharou S, et al. Assessment of the anti-HBs antibody response in Beninese infants following 4 doses of HBV vaccine, including administration at birth, compared to the standard 3 doses regime; a cross-sectional survey. Vaccine 2020;38(7):1787–93.

65. Dzingirai B, Katsidzira L, Matyanga CMJ, et al. Progress on the elimination of viral hepatitis in Zimbabwe: a review of the policies, strategies and challenges. J Viral Hepat 2021. https://doi.org/10.1111/jvh.13510.

66. Guingané AN, Bougouma A, Sombié R, et al. Identifying gaps across the cascade of care for the prevention of HBV mother-to-child transmission in Burkina Faso: findings from the real world. Liver Int 2020;40(10):2367–76.

67. Li C, He W-Q. The impact of universal hepatitis B vaccine on the trend of liver cancer from the Global Burden of Disease Study 2017. Liver Int 2021. https://doi.org/10.1111/liv.14821.

68. Kushner T, Kaplowitz E, Mei R, et al. Adherence to pregnancy hepatitis B care guidelines in women and infants in the United States and evaluation of two interventions to improve care: a multicentre hospital-based study. J Viral Hepat 2021; 28(4):582–91.

69. Huang H, Xu C, Liu L, et al. Increased protection of earlier use of immunoprophylaxis in preventing perinatal transmission of hepatitis B virus. Clin Infect Dis 2020. https://doi.org/10.1093/cid/ciaa898.

70. Cohen C, Holmberg SD, McMahon BJ, et al. Is chronic hepatitis B being undertreated in the United States? J Viral Hepat 2011;18(6):377–83.

71. Beebeejaun K, Amin-Chowdhury Z, Letley L, et al. Impact of a nurse-led enhanced monitoring, management and contact tracing intervention for chronic hepatitis B in England, 2015-2017. J Viral Hepat 2021;28(1):72–9.

72. Ding Y, Cao L, Zhu L, et al. Efficacy and safety of tenofovir alafenamide fumarate for preventing mother-to-child transmission of hepatitis B virus: a national cohort study. Aliment Pharmacol Ther 2020;52(8):1377–86.

73. Boucheron P, Lu Y, Yoshida K, et al. Accuracy of HBeAg to identify pregnant women at risk of transmitting hepatitis B virus to their neonates: a systematic review and meta-analysis. Lancet Infect Dis 2021;21(1):85–96.

74. Cox AL, El-Sayed MH, Kao J-H, et al. Progress towards elimination goals for viral hepatitis. Nat Rev Gastroenterol Hepatol 2020;17(9):533–42.

Interpretation of HBV Serologies

Philippe J. Zamor, MD[a],*, Ashley M. Lane, MD[b,c,d]

KEYWORDS

- HBV DNA • HBsAg • HBeAg-Negative • HBeAg-Positive • Acute HBV
- Chronic HBV • Anti-HBc

KEY POINTS

- HBV infection is associated with pathognomonic changes in viral proteins (antigens) and host antibody responses, which define the natural history and phases of infection.
- HBV genotypes are distributed differently throughout the world and have specific individual characteristics that can predict the progression of hepatic fibrosis and ultimately to hepatocellular carcinoma.
- There is a complicated relationship that has been characterized by the various HBV serologies and HBV DNA that has been reviewed in this article. Generally, the higher the hepatitis B viral load the risk of hepatocellular carcinoma increases, especially in patients with HBeAg-negative infection.

HISTORY OF SEROLOGIC TESTING. THE AUSTRALIA ANTIGEN

The discovery of a new previously uncharacterized protein (Au) in the serum of an Australian aboriginal person provided the answer for the yet to be addressed question regarding the etiology of viral hepatitis, now known to be hepatitis B virus (HBV). Scientific curiosity led researchers who were not directly involved with viral hepatitis research identified what we know as the HBV surface antigen (HBsAg). In 1885, Lürmann recognized the infectious nature of hepatitis during an "icterus epidemic," which occurred after a smallpox vaccination (produced from human lymph) campaign.[1] Several outbreaks of hepatitis were described in recipients of yellow fever vaccine, the largest during World War II among U.S. Army personnel with close to 50,000 clinical cases.[2] It was reported that at one Army base, 5000 soldiers were vaccinated on a single day, with over 1000 having developed jaundice.[3]

[a] Division of Hepatology, Carolinas Medical Center-Atrium Healthcare, 1025 Morehead Medical Drive, Charlotte, NC 28204, USA; [b] Division of Gastroenterology and Hepatology, Department of Medicine, University of Colorado Anschutz Medical Campus, Aurora, CO, USA; [c] Department of Medicine, Division of Gastroenterology and Hepatology, Rocky Mountain Regional VA Medical Center, Aurora, CO, USA; [d] Department of Gastroenterology and Hepatology, Rocky Mountain Regional VAMC, 1700 N. Wheeling Street, Aurora, D3-111E, CO 80045, USA
* Corresponding author.
E-mail address: Philippe.Zamor@atriumhealth.org

Clin Liver Dis 25 (2021) 689–709
https://doi.org/10.1016/j.cld.2021.06.012
1089-3261/21/© 2021 Elsevier Inc. All rights reserved.

The terms "hepatitis A" and "hepatitis B" were introduced in 1947. Baruch Blumberg was a geneticist with a research interest in identifying genetic markers for susceptibility to certain diseases. Blumberg's colleague, Harvey Alter discovered the new antigen in several samples of the huge serum collection, quite often in Australian aborigines, for whom the Australia Antigen was named. At that time, Alter was investigating sources of transfusion complications. His initial scientific curiosity was piqued by his interest in the concept of polymorphism, whereby "the persistence ...two forms of a species in the same habitat in such proportions that the rarest of them cannot be maintained by recurrent mutation." In pursuit of his scientific curiosity, he collaborated with Oxford researcher Tony Allison, who specialized in sickle-cell trait studies, and traveled to Nigeria in 1957 to collect large numbers of blood samples from several distinct human groups. Shortly after, he transitioned to the National Institutes of Health conducted field studies in Alaska to collect blood samples from diverse populations of humans and animal species. He and Allison published their findings describing experiments of using starch gel electrophoresis to identify differences in the concentration and mobility of haptoglobins and other serum proteins.[4–6]

While examining the Au antigen under electron microscopy, Dane noted that Au antigen appeared not only on the surface of the small pleomorphic particles, but also on larger, virus-like objects 42 nm in size with a clearly visible inner core.[7] Soon thereafter, researchers released the core particles from the "Dane particles" with a mild detergent and demonstrated by immune electron microscopy that HBV patients had formed antibodies (anti-HBc) against this core antigen (HBcAg).[8] This strongly indicated that the Dane particle was the actual virus causing hepatitis B. Au was certainly the surface antigen of the virus envelope and was named HBsAg thereafter. In 1973, Robinson was able to detect an endogenous DNA polymerase activity within HBV and soon thereafter identified the viral DNA itself.[9,10]

REVIEW SEROLOGIC TESTS USED TO DETECT HBV

HBV infection is associated with pathognomonic changes in the serum of affected individuals. Viral proteins (antigens) and host antibody responses define the natural history and phases of infection and guide therapeutic management.

Hepatitis B Surface Antigen and Antibody

The presence of a hepatitis B surface antigen (HBsAg) is the serologic hallmark of HBV infection and establishes the diagnosis.[11,12] HBsAg proteins form the envelope for infectious HBV particles, and are also found in the form of noninfectious spheres or filaments (subviral particles). HBsAg is a surrogate marker of infected cells, and is detected using diagnostic tests, including laboratory-based immunologic assays and other techniques/technologies.[12,13]

HBsAg is among the initial markers detectable in serum after infection with HBV. It may be identified in serum as early as 1 to 2 weeks after exposure, before the onset of clinical symptoms and appearance of other serologic/biochemical markers of infection, or up to 11 to 12 weeks after exposure.[14,15] HBsAg may even be transiently detected in serum early after HBV vaccination.[16]

Anti-HBs are detected and/or quantified via immunologic assay. The presence of anti-HBs denotes immunity, whether development occurs as a result of natural infection or vaccination.[17] In some patients, the development of anti-HBs is delayed for weeks or months during a window period in which neither HBsAg nor anti-HBs are detectable.[18] Anti-HBs persist in most patients for life but may fall below detectable levels in some patients.

Hepatitis B Core Antigen and Antibody

HBV core proteins are intracellular antigens that form an icosahedral nucleocapsid containing the partly double-stranded DNA of the HBV virions.[19] HBV core antigen (HBcAg) is detected by immunohistochemical staining of liver biopsy specimens in patients with acute and chronic infection; currently, no commercial assays are available to detect serum HBcAg.[20]

HBcAg-specific antibodies (anti-HBc) develop early in the host immune response to acute HBV infection. Anti-HBc is detected using immunologic assay. During acute HBV infection, anti-HBc appears within 1 to 2 weeks of the detection of HBsAg. Both immunoglobulin (Ig) M class and class-switched IgG anti-HBc are detected during acute infection, with anti-HBc IgM titers generally higher.[17,21] Synchronous detection of HBsAg and anti-HBc IgM is diagnostic for acute HBV infection.[20] Anti-HBc IgM may be detectable for months to years after acute infection and is often observable in patients with exacerbations of chronic HBV.[21] However, anti-HBc IgM titers during chronic HBV exacerbations are lower than that of acute responses, thus differentiating acute from chronic infection.[17,21]

The presence of anti-HBc IgG delineates patients who have recovered from acute infection and is a useful marker of prior HBV exposure and infection. Anti-HBc IgG and HBsAg also persist in those progressing to chronic infection.

The discovery of anti-HBc in the absence of HBsAg and anti-HBs may occur for several reasons:

1. Prior HBV infection, which is the most common reason in populations with increased risk and local prevalence. Most are recovered acute infections whose anti-HBs titers have decreased to undetectable levels, although some patients may have had chronic infection before clearing HBsAg[11];
2. The window period of acute HBV infection, during which case anti-HBc IgM is also reactive[22,23];
3. A false-positive result, particularly in those with no risk factors for HBV in a region of low prevalence (as new, more specific anti-HBc tests are used, this is less common)[24];
4. Mutations in HBsAg leading to false-negative HBsAg results[15]; and
5. HBsAg titer having fallen below the level of detection in those with chronic infection.[25]

Hepatitis B e Antigen and Antibody

Hepatitis B e antigen (HBeAg) is a nonstructural protein coded by the HBV precore gene and secreted by infected hepatocytes. HBeAg is detected early in acute or chronic HBV infection, typically appearing shortly after HBsAg (6–12 weeks after exposure to HBV); HBeAg is not detected in serum without measurable HBsAg, with rare exceptions.[20,26,27] The presence of HBeAg denotes a high level of active viral replication and infectivity and is therefore a strong indicator of active liver disease.[26] During the natural course of HBV infection, seroconversion to HBeAg-specific antibody (anti-HBe) is characteristic of a transition to an inactive infection (along with low levels of HBV DNA), and is associated with reduced morbidity and mortality.[27–29]

HBeAg and anti-HBe are measured by immunologic assays.[27] HBeAg and anti-HBe status help to distinguish the phases of chronic hepatitis B (**Fig. 1**).

ROLE OF SURFACE ANTIGEN

There has been increasing interest in the quantification of the hepatitis B surface antigen (HBsAg). Observations were made that the level of HBsAg could potentially

HBsAg	Anti-HBc Total	Anti-HBc IgM	Anti-HBs	Interpretation
+	+	+	-	Acute infection
+	+	-	-	Chronic infection*
-	+	-	+	Prior HBV infection (resolved)
-	-	-	+	Immune from prior vaccination
-	-	-	-	Non-immune, non-infected
-	+		-	Five possible interpretations**

Fig. 1. Interpretation of screening serologic tests for HBV infection.anti-HBc total: hepatitis B core antibody total (includes IgM and IgG); anti-HBs: hepatitis B surface antibody; HBV: hepatitis B virus; HBsAg: hepatitis B surface antigen; IgM: immunoglobulin M; IgG: immunoglobulin G. *If HBsAg persists $\geq$ six (6) months. **1. Prior HBV infection, but anti-HBs titers have decreased to undetectable levels, 2. Recovering from acute infection (window period), 3. False positive anti-HBc, 4. Mutations in HBsAg leading to false-negative HBsAg results, 5. Chronic infection but HBsAg unable to be detected in serum.

reflect the amount and transcriptional activity of covalently closed circular (ccc) DNA within the hepatocytes.[30,31] Assessment of serum HBsAg kinetics has become incorporated into the standard evaluation of emerging therapeutic agents for the treatment of HBV, as HBsAg seroclearance is considered a functional cure for chronic hepatitis B.[32] Please refer Charatcharoenwitthaya and colleagues's article "Controversies in treating chronic HBV: The role of PEG-interferon-alfa" in this issue, for further discussion on the role of S-antigen and monitoring of patients while on interferon-based therapy.

Virology of HBsAg Production

The HBV encodes the 3 proteins of the HBsAg, which form the viral envelope. These envelope proteins: small (SHBsAg), middle (MHBsAg), and large (LHBsAg) are contained within a membrane that covers the inner shell of the virus, which consists of an icosahedral nucleocapsid. Please see **Fig. 2**. These proteins are translated from 2 mRNA codons: pre-S1 and pre-S2/S in the endoplasmic reticulum. They share the same C-terminal amino acids, named the S domain. The M protein contains an

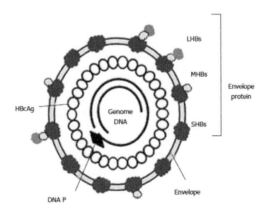

Fig. 2. Hepatitis B surface antigen proteins. (From Yano Y, Azuma T, Hayashi Y. Variations and mutations in the hepatitis B virus genome and their associations with clinical characteristics. *World J Hepatol.* 2015;7(3):583-592. doi:10.4254/wjh.v7.i3.583)

extra domain called the pre-S2 domain compared with the S protein, and the L protein contains two extra domains: pre-S2 and pre-S1. The three proteins have a glycosylated form responsible for the secretion of viral particles. The secreted virion contains majority S proteins and M and L proteins in equal amounts. For the process of envelopment and secretion of HBsAg particles, an excess of S protein over M and L is required.[33] Each protein has a specific role. The S protein exposes a low affinity-binding site for heparan sulfate proteoglycan (HSPG), which is required for infectivity.[33] The L protein with the pre-S1 domain facilitates the envelopment of the core particles and includes the high-affinity attachment site of the HBV, the sodium taurocholate cotransporting polypeptide (NTCP).[34] The M protein is nonessential for infection and morphogenesis.[35]

The covalently closed circular DNA (cccDNA), which is found in the nucleus, drives the production of HBV via reverse transcription.[36] Please refer Loglio and colleagues' article "Novel Therapies That May Cure Chronic Hepatitis B Virus" in this issue for further details.

Reduced secretion of HBsAg occurs as a result of the aforementioned stop codons. Production of HBsAg varies widely in different scenarios. HBsAg levels vary by genotype, with genotypes A and D having higher levels in comparison to genotypes B and C, with the highest levels found in genotype A.[37–39] Interplay between virus and host immune response influences the production of HBsAg; higher immune control of HBV will lower levels of HBsAg.[40,41] Point mutations in the polymerase open reading frame occur under the pressure of nucleos(t)ide analog (NA) therapy for HBV.

Different Stages of HBV and HBsAg

Acute HBV

It was recognized fairly early in the study and understanding of HBV in the 1970s that quantification of HBsAg is useful to monitor and predict the outcome of acute HBV.[42] Please refer Dekker and colleagues' article "Treatment and Prevention of Acute Hepatitis B Virus" in this issue for a detailed outline of acute HBV.

Risk of reactivation of HBV

Screening for HBsAg is useful to identify who are at higher risk for HBV reactivation when exposed to immunosuppressant medications and/or certain chemotherapeutic agents.[43] Patients at the highest risk of reactivation are not just those with anti-HBc status but with HBsAg/anti-HBc. Guidelines have been published to risk stratify patients based on HBV serologies and immunosuppressing agent.[43]

ROLE OF HBV DNA TESTING

HBV DNA is diagnostic of hepatitis B infection, and enables monitoring of infected patients, guidance of therapeutic management, and determination of treatment efficacy. Although qualitative and quantitative serum HBV DNA assays exist, quantitative real-time polymerase chain reaction (qRT-PCR) is used most frequently because of its high sensitivity and specificity, standardized reporting, lower limits of detection, and range of reporting.[27]

HBV DNA is the primary marker of early acute HBV infection, and is detectable within 2 weeks of initial exposure.[26,27] Highly sensitive nucleic acid tests detect HBV DNA 2 to 4 weeks before the appearance of HBsAg.[44] HBV DNA testing is appreciated during the window of HBsAg clearance before the detection of anti-HBs, and to confirm viremia in patients with occult infection.[27]

ROLE OF HBV GENOTYPES

HBV infection is endemic throughout the world, but most notably throughout Asia, Africa, parts of Europe, as well as Latin America.[45] HBV genotypes are uniquely distributed globally and are linked to various predictable clinical outcomes. Various factors such as immune interactions between the host and the virus, specific viral characteristics, and environmental influences play a role in the HBV disease progression: acute hepatitis, chronic hepatitis, liver cirrhosis, and hepatocellular carcinoma.

Global Distribution of HBV Genotypes

Thus far, 10 HBV genotypes (A–J) have been identified with some further classified with subtypes.[46–48] HBV sequence is characterized by a >8% nucleotide differences for genotype, and 4% to 8% nucleotide differences for subtype. A–D and F genotypes are further divided into subtypes, whereas genotypes E, G, and H have no identifiable subtypes.[49–51] Genotype A is endemic in sub-Saharan Africa, Northern Europe, Western Africa, India, and America. Genotypes B and C are most commonly found in Asia, with genotype C primarily observed in Southeast Asia. Genotype D is dominant in Africa, Europe, the Mediterranean region, and India. Thus far, 9 subtypes (D1–D9) have been identified in India. Genotype G is seen in France, Germany, and the United States. Genotype H is seen in Central America and Mexico. Genotype I, which has been recently discovered, is found in isolation in Vietnam and Laos.[52] The other newly identified genotype J is localized to Japan, in particular the Ryukyu Islands. As genotypes B and C are more common in areas of high endemicity because of perinatal/vertical transmission, the global distribution of genotypes is related to routes of exposures. The remaining genotypes are noted to be in regions of horizontal exposure.[45,53–56] Please see **Table 1** for the geographic distribution of HBV genotypes.

Table 1
Geographic distribution of HBV genotypes

Genotypes	Subtypes	Geographic Location
A	A1	Sub-Saharan African, India
	A2	Northern Europe, India
	A3	Western Africa
B	B1	Japan
	B2-5	East Asia, Taiwan, China, Indonesia, Vietnam, The Philippines
	B6	Alaska, Northern Canada, Greenland
C	C1-3	Taiwan, China, Korea, Southeast Asia
	C4	Australia
	C5	The Philippines, Vietnam
	C6-11	Indonesia
D	D1-6	Africa, Europe, Mediterranean region, India, Indonesia
E		West Africa
F	F1-4	Central and South America
G		France, Germany, United States
H		Central America
I		Vietnam, Laos
J		Japan

HBV genotypes and naturally mutant species have a major impact on viral pathogenesis, including the change of host immune recognition, the enhanced virulence with increased HBV replication, promotion of cell attachment or penetration, and association with the development of hepatocellular carcinoma.[57,58] Quasispecies of HBV has emerged, as well as mixed genotypes and intergenotypic recombinations.[59,60] Genotype C has been reported to have a significantly higher HBV serum DNA as compared with genotype B.[61] In addition, those infected with genotype C are more predisposed to the complications of advanced hepatic fibrosis and cirrhosis than genotype B.[62,63] An *in vitro* study demonstrated that intracellular expression of HBV DNA was higher for genotypes C than B and genotypes D than A.[38] Liu and colleagues conducted *in vivo* study that demonstrated that secretion of HBeAg in genotype B was lower than genotype C.

Acute HBV

There have been some differences described regarding various HBV genotypes. Infection with genotype A is the predominant strain in cases of acute HBV in Japan.[64] Of note, genotype A infected acute HBV patients were noted to progress to chronic infection at higher rates. A Japanese nationwide multicenter collaborative demonstrated a persistence of HBsAg positivity for more than 6 months after acute HBV infection was 23.4% in genotype A versus 8.6% ($P = .003$) in genotypes other A.[65] Investigators noted higher peaks level of HBV DNA and lower peak of alanine aminotransferase. In Taiwan, genotype B is most commonly seen in acute HBV infected patients.[66] Data from India indicate that genotype D was the dominant genotype in acute HBV infection; it was also reported that chronicity ratio was relatively higher in patients with genotype D.[67]

HBeAg Seroconversion and HBsAg Seroclearance

Seroconversion of HBeAg and seroclearance of HBsAg have been established as important events in the natural history of HBV infection and reflect the host immuno-control of HBV infection. Data from Taiwan indicate genotype C patients seroconvert HBeAg at a lower rate than genotype B patients (27% vs 47%, $P<.025$).[48] Similar lower rates of lower HBeAg seroconversion were reported by another group investigating Taiwanese patients 7.9% genotype C versus 15.5% genotype B.[68] Genotype C patients are more prone to repeated episodes of acute exacerbation with failure of HBeAg seroconversion[69] and HBeAg seroreversion after HBeAg loss.[70] Chu and colleagues showed that HBeAg seroconversion occurs about 10 years earlier in genotype B as compared with genotype C patients.[71]

Impact of HBV Genotypes and Antiviral Therapy

The impact of the HBV genotype has been characterized for genotypes A–D. Genotypes E–J occur much less frequently, therefore a paucity of data exists regarding response to therapy.

Interferon-Based (IFN) Therapy

HBeAg-positive patients with genotypes A and B had a much better response to standard interferon as compared with genotypes C and D.[72–74] Genotype A patients respond more favorably to IFN than genotype D patients regardless of HBeAg status, and genotype B better than genotype C in HBeAg-positive patients.[75] Larger data sets demonstrated that HBeAg-positive patients with lower HBV DNA levels and higher pretreatment ALT levels and infected with genotypes A–C were more likely to response to IFN as opposed to genotype D patients.[76] It has been noted that

HBeAg-positive patients infected with genotype B demonstrate higher response rates with IFN-based therapies, standard or pegylated (PEG-IFN), yet genotype C infected patients are more likely to respond with PEG-IFN rather than with standard IFN.[77,78]

Genotype and Nucleos(t)ide Analogs

Treatment with the nucleos(t)ide analogs (NUC) is less dependent on host immune responses, so it is no surprise that response does not vary widely among the various genotypes.[46,79–82] A meta-analysis has shown that there was no difference in efficacy between the nucleos(t)ides and HBV genotypes.[75] Genotype B was associated with the development of lamivudine resistance within the first 12 months of therapy compared with genotype C (OR: 8.27; P = .004).[83]

Genotype and Progression to Cirrhosis and Hepatocellular Carcinoma

Observational studies as well as a meta-analysis have shown that genotype C infected patients were at higher risk of developing HCC.[84–86] Genotype C has been demonstrated to carry an increased risk of HCC in the REVEAL-HBV study cohort, with an adjusted hazard ratio of 2.35.[86] Data also suggest that genotype C and high serum DNA were independent predictors of HCC.[61,87,88] Several groups have reported higher hepatitis B viral loads in genotype C patients as compared with genotype B patients.[61,89] Similarly, a prospective study originating from Hong Kong demonstrated that subtypes C1/C2 had a higher risk of HCC compared with genotype B, and higher viral loads were also noted.[90] Furthermore, data from Australia indicate that subtype C4 was associated with more rapid liver disease progression and risk of HCC.[91] Additional data reported that subtype C2 had a high relative risk of HCC.[92,93]

A meta-analysis reported rates of HCC were 25% for genotype C and 12% for genotype B (OR = 2.05, 95% CI: 1.52–2.76, $P<.001$).[94] In addition, genotype C patients were noted to have more severe liver disease. They found no differences between genotypes A and D. Investigators assessed the hepatocarcinogenic potential of genotype A, which is more commonly found in sub-Saharan Africa; it noted to be associated with a higher incidence of HCC than other nongenotype A patients, with a strong contribution of subtype A1 accounting for all cases of HCC in this observational study.[95]

Genotype B may be more likely to be associated with HCC in noncirrhotic patients than genotype C patients.[96] Genotype B has been found to be more prevalent in patients with HCC developing at a younger age compared with age-matched inactive carriers (80% vs 52% in those <50 years and 90% in those <35 years).[97] Genotype A2 is found more in Europe and the United States.[95]

The correlation between other HBV genotypes and HCC is not as pronounced as with genotype C. One study reported higher rates of HCC in genotype D patients than genotype A[98]; yet other studies reported that HCC incidence was higher in genotype F1 patients than genotype A2 and D patients.[99,100] Ghosh and colleagues reported dated from an Indian study that demonstrated a correlation between advanced clinical stage and frequency of mutations in HBeAg-negative genotype D patients. Large number of mutations were localized in regions that regulated transcription (BCP/EnhII/NRE/SP1). The authors noted that deletion at the pre-S region was the most important predictor of cirrhosis.[101] A mutation S183P at the HBV core protein C terminus was noted to be the only clinically relevant mutation, and in fact caused a clinical shift from an inactive carrier state to a chronic stage of infection and progression to cirrhosis.

HBeAg expression and HBV DNA level are closely correlated, and it is well established that HCC risk is increased with higher baseline HBV DNA levels.[102] There is increasing interest in correlating HBV variants and the development of HCC, in particular, basal core promoter (BCP) mutation A1762T/G1764A and the pre-S deletion have also been identified as risk factors for the development of HCC.[48,103–106] A longitudinal cohort study that followed 251 HBeAg spontaneous seroconverters with genotype B and C infection; multivariate analysis showed that BCP mutants were associated with a higher risk of cirrhosis. When investigators set 45% as the cut-off for percentage of mutants, the risk of cirrhosis was higher than cut-offs lower than 45%.[107] A Chinese study identified HBeAg infected patients with C1 subtype, in addition to T1762/A1764 BCP mutations, V1753 and/or A1768 mutations were correlated with HCC.[108] Modifications of HBx protein has been linked to the increased HCC risk in these individuals.[89,109] Additional data from Korea have linked 8 key mutations to HCC in those infected with HBV genotype C2: G1613A, C1653T, T1753V, A1762T, G1764A, A1846T, G1896A, and G1899A.[110,111] Genotype C infected patients are described to have a higher frequency of pre-S deletion than genotype B patients, which may further explain higher rates of HCC.[112]

RELATIONSHIP OF SEROLOGY AND HBV DNA TO DISEASE PROGRESSION

The immune tolerance phase of HBV infection is characterized by high levels of viral replication with hepatitis B viral load up to 10^{12} IU/mL and detectable HBeAg with no histologic evidence of active liver disease and liver normal serum ALT measurement. Most cases of HBV infection occur as a result of perinatal or early childhood horizontal transmission; with transition from the immune tolerance to immune clearance typically occurring during the second and third decades of life. The most important factor influencing prognosis appears to HBV DNA levels greater than 2000 IU/mL. The immune tolerance phase lasts for an extended period usually between 10 and 30 years during which there is a very low rate of spontaneous HBeAg clearance, Lok and colleagues reported only 15% after 20 years of infection.[113]

HBV DNA under 2000 IU/mL has been established as a threshold for clinical significance, whereby levels lower than this are thought to not have a significant impact on a patient's clinical course.[114]

In HBeAg-Positive Patients

HBV DNA levels are typically found to be much higher in HBeAg-positive patients as opposed to HBeAg-negative patients. The immune tolerance phase of HBV infection, one of the earliest stages of HBV infection, is characterized by high HBV DNA in the setting of low ALT. 20,000 IU/mL has been arbitrarily determined to be a major determinant of progression to more advanced stage of hepatic inflammation and fibrosis.[115] Data from the REVEAL-HBV study demonstrated that HBeAg-positive patients with higher HBV DNA showed a linear correlation with presenting with cirrhosis at study entry. In multivariate Cox regression analyses of risk factors including sex, age, habits of cigarette smoking and alcohol drinking, increasing HBV DNA level was the strongest independent predictor.[116] Data from a Korean cohort that stratified noncirrhotic patients into HBV DNA from 4–6 $\log_{10}$, 6–7 $\log_{10}$, 7–8 $\log_{10}$, and greater than 8 $\log_{10}$ IU/mL revealed that modest levels of HBV DNA (6–7 $\log_{10}$ mL) group had the greatest risk of developing HCC, followed by the low level (4–6 $\log_{10}$ IU/mL) group.[117]

HBeAg-Negative

According to newer EASL guidelines from 2017, HBeAg-negative patients are divided into 2 groups, chronic infection and chronic hepatitis, with HBV DNA typically greater than 2000 IU/mL meeting criteria for chronic infection.[118] Previously known as the inactive carrier phase, this phase is characterized as undetectable or low levels of HBV DNA levels less than 2000 IU/mL, normal ALT and minimal hepatic necroinflammatory activity, and low level of hepatic fibrosis. One of the largest studies to date investigating the natural history of CHB HBeAg-negative patients was the first to characterize the proportion of patients to develop immune active hepatitis B phase if subjects had an ALT above the upper limit of normal (ULN) for women $\geq$20 U/L and $\geq$30 U/L for men in the setting of HBV DNA greater than 2000 IU/mL.[119] **(Fig. 3)** Levels of ALT were measured every 6 months, and levels of HBV DNA were measured at study entry and whenever ALT levels exceeded ULN. Liver biopsies were also performed to assess liver histology and degree of inflammation. Only 1 of 16 with low ALT levels and 1 of 19 with HBV DNA between 2000 and 20,000 IU/mL developed moderate or severe hepatitis or fibrosis, whereas 12 of 22 (55%) with ALT greater than twice the ULN and 11 of 18 (61%) with 1 or more HBV DNA greater than 20,000 IU/mL (P<.001) developed significant hepatic findings. The authors did note that HBV DNA levels did fluctuate so assessment at multiple time points was a more reliable assessment. An earlier study from Greece also noted that HBV DNA can fluctuate in HBeAg-negative patients, so serial monitoring is recommended in this cohort of patients.[120] Similar guidance is recommended by the AASLD HBV guidelines.[11]

Regarding the risk of developing HCC, in a community-based, nested case-control study of 44 HBeAg-negative with newly diagnosed HCC and 86 matched controls who were selected from a cohort 1991 male HBeAg-negative HBV carriers from Taiwan, a significant dose-response relationship between serum HBV DNA at study entry and HCC risk was noted.[121] Data from the REVEAL-HBV cohort reveal that high levels of HBV DNA (>2000 IU/mL) were associated with a high risk of HCC and disease progression, regardless of serum ALT levels; the greatest risk for HCC was seen with HBV titers greater than 10^6 copies/mL.[116,122] More recently published data from Korea demonstrated on multivariable analysis that there was a linear relationship with the high risk of developing HCC was in those with the highest HBV DNA (>5 $\log_{10}$ IU/

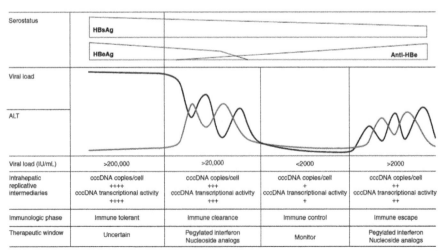

Fig. 3. Natural history of CHB, showing relationships between serology, biochemistry, and molecular virology. (From Burns GS, Thompson AJ. Viral hepatitis B: clinical and epidemiological characteristics. *Cold Spring Harb Perspect Med.* 2014;4(12):a024935. Published 2014 Oct 30. doi:10.1101/cshperspect.a024935)

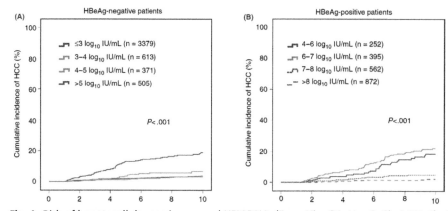

Fig. 4. Risk of hepatocellular carcinoma and HBV DNA. (From Kim GA, Han S, Choi GH, Choi J, Lim YS. Moderate levels of serum hepatitis B virus DNA are associated with the highest risk of hepatocellular carcinoma in chronic hepatitis B patients. *Aliment Pharmacol Ther.* 2020;51(11):1169-1179. doi:10.1111/apt.15725)

mL) in HBeAg-negative noncirrhotic patients.[117] Please see **Fig. 4**. Another observational study from Korea published similar findings of a higher risk of HCC and death in untreated HBeAg-negative patients.[123] The cut-off level for HBV DNA where there was an increased risk of clinical events was identified as 4 $\log_{10}$ IU/mL.

MONITORING ACUTE AND CHRONIC HBV WITH SEROLOGIC TESTING
Acute Infection

The concurrent detection of anti-HBc IgM and HBsAg is the diagnostic hallmark of acute HBV infection.[20] HBV DNA followed by HBsAg and HBeAg are the initial serologic markers detected in the serum of infected individuals.[14] (**Fig. 5**) HBeAg and HBV DNA, indicators of viral replication, present during the initial phase of infection.[15] Anti-HBc IgM appears just before the onset of clinical illness, wherein transaminase levels begin to rise and symptoms develop. Class switch recombination results in a decline in IgM and an increase in detectable anti-HBc IgG.[15] HBeAg wanes early at the peak of clinical

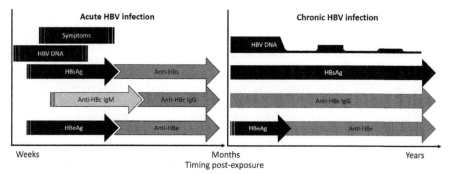

Fig. 5. Serologic markers of acute and chronic hepatitis B virus infection. Clinical presentation of HBV markers during the course of acute infection (left panel) and chronic infection (right panel). anti-HBs: hepatitis B surface antibody; anti-HBc: hepatitis B core antibody; anti-HBe: hepatitis B e antibody; BV: hepatitis B virus; HBsAg: hepatitis B surface antigen; HBeAg: hepatitis B e antigen; IgM immunoglobulin M; IgG: immunoglobulin G.

illness, with anti-HBe appearing shortly thereafter. The collective loss of HBV DNA, HBeAg to anti-HBe seroconversion, and HBsAg to anti-HBs seroconversion signify resolution (recovery). HBsAg typically becomes undetectable in 4 to 6 months, and anti-HBs arise weeks before or after HBsAg clearance during recovery.[15,17,124]

Patients may occasionally present during a window of undetectable HBsAg and anti-HBs, in which case, the anti-HBc IgM alone indicates acute infection.[124] This is seen in patients presenting with fulminant hepatitis (HBsAg and HBV DNA clearance occur rapidly), and in some patients testing negative for HBsAg.[15]

Prior Infection

The presence of anti-HBs and anti-HBc IgG in the absence of detectable HBV DNA is characteristic of those who have recovered from previous HBV infection.[17] Anti-HBs are associated with immunity to HBV; however, not all of those who recover from HBV infection develop detectable anti-HBs.[15,18] In this instance, anti-HBc IgG is the sole marker of prior HBV infection.[15]

Chronic Infection

The presence of HBsAg for at least 6 months defines chronic HBV infection.[11] Chronic HBV infection is a dynamic disease, and individuals may progress through different phases of infection over time. Tracking markers of replication (including HBeAg, HBV DNA, and ALT) temporally elucidates the phase of infection and guides therapeutic decision-making.

Initial infection results in high titers of HBsAg, HBeAg, and HBV DNA, and is associated with elevations in serum aminotransferase levels. Over time, patients may experience continued disease activity with elevated aminotransferases and variable levels of HBV DNA, depending on HBeAg status (immune-active chronic hepatitis B). The disease activity may become senescent, with normal aminotransferases and concurrent high levels of HBeAg and HBV DNA (immune-tolerant chronic hepatitis B), or with a loss of HBeAg and low to undetectable HBV DNA levels (inactive chronic hepatitis B).[11] Occult HBV infection refers to the presence of anti-HBc and HBV DNA in the absence of detectable HBsAg.[125]

Approximately, 0.5% to 0.8% of patients with chronic hepatitis B infection will clear HBsAg annually.[11,23] Those with resolved chronic HBV present with a sustained loss of HBsAg, undetectable HBV DNA, and a lack of clinical evidence of active infection.[11]

MUTATIONS OF HBV AND HOW THIS MAY CONFUSE SEROLOGIC INTERPRETATION
HBV S-Gene Mutants: Pre-S/S Quasispecies

It was reported that the presence of pre-S/S variants correlates negatively with the HBsAg titer.[126] A study from Hong Kong investigating HBsAg-negative patients revealed that a variety of mutations, including deletions in the promoter region, abolition of the pre-S2/S start codon, disruption of the pre-S2S nRNA splice site, nucleotide duplications, and missense mutations in the "a" determinant region, contribute to defects in HBsAg production.[127] Variations in the "a" determinant region cause changes in HBsAg antigenicity and may interfere with detection of HBsAg in HBsAg screening assays.[128,129] It should be highlighted that mutations that cause a conformational change within the "a" determinant could affect the antigenicity of HBsAg, critical for inducing protective antibody, and be responsible for escaping vaccinated induced immunity, escaping anti-HBV immunoglobulin therapy, and causing false-negative results in serologic tests.[130–132]

A Dutch study of 4.4 million blood donations identified 23 HBsAg negative but HBV DNA positive subjects and also reported the presence of multiple escape mutations in the S gene, especially in the Genotype D patients with occult HBV.[133]

PreCore/Core Mutants

The pre-Core/core region contains two regions: Pre-Core (nt 1814–1901) and core (nt 1901–2452). It has been recognized that mutations in the Pre-Core region prevent the expression of HBeAg.[134,135] This mutation typically emerges when HBeAg seroconverts to anti-HBe. The most common is G1896A converting TGG to TAG, a stop codon. In vivo, the G1896A mutation correlates with lower HBeAg levels.[28] Although the function of HBeAg is not completely understood, it may act as an immune "tolerogen," contributing to the establishment of chronic infection.[136]

The core promoter, which drives transcription of Pre-Core RNA and pgRNA, can be divided into BCP and core upstream regulatory sequence. The A1762T/G1746A double mutation is the most common BCP mutation. The BCP mutations reduce but do not completely abolish HBeAg expression.[137,138]

CLINICS CARE POINTS

- The presence of hepatitis B surface antigen (HBsAg) is the hallmark of HBV infection.

- Anti-HBc (core antibody) defines previous exposure to HBV virus, this does not necessarily imply that the patient is chronically actively infected.

- 10 HBV genotypes are uniquely distributed around the world, additionally subtypes are also noted to exist. These can impact treatment decision, primary regarding the use of interferon based therapy.

- HBV genotypes may have an impact on risk of developing HCC.

- HBV DNA is generally found to be higher in patients who are HBeAg- positive.

- Various mutations have been described with HBV, with wide ranging impact on course of disease and interpretation of HBV serologies.

DISCLOSURE

P. J. Zamor: Advisory Board: Gilead Sciences.
A. M. Lane has nothing to disclose.

REFERENCES

1. A L. Eine icterus epidemic. Berl Klin Woschenschr 1885;22:20–3.
2. MacCallum FO. Homologous serum jaundice [An icterus epidemic]. Lancet 1947;2:691–2.
3. Turner RHSJ, Grossman EB, Buchanan RN, et al. Some clinical studies of acute hepatitis occurring in soldiers after inoculation with yellow fever vaccine; with especial consideration of severe attacks. Ann Intern Med 1944;20(2):193–218.
4. Allison AC, Blumberg BS, Ap R. Haptoglobin types in British, Spanish Basque and Nigerian African populations. Nature 1958;181(4612):824–5.
5. Blumberg BS, Allison AC, Garry B. The haptoglobins and haemoglobins of Alaskan Eskimos and Indians. Ann Hum Genet 1959;23:349–56.

6. Blumberg BS, Allison AC, Garry B. The haptoglobins, hemoglobins and serum proteins of the Alaskan Fur seal, ground squirrel and marmot. J Cell Comp Physiol 1960;55:61–71.

7. Dane DS, Cameron CH, Briggs M. Virus-like particles in serum of patients with Australia-antigen-associated hepatitis. Lancet 1970;1(7649):695–8.

8. Almeida JD, Rubenstein D, Stott EJ. New antigen-antibody system in Australia-antigen-positive hepatitis. Lancet 1971;2(7736):1225–7.

9. Kaplan PM, Greenman RL, Gerin JL, et al. DNA polymerase associated with human hepatitis B antigen. J Virol 1973;12(5):995–1005.

10. Robinson WS, Clayton DA, Greenman RL. DNA of a human hepatitis B virus candidate. J Virol 1974;14(2):384–91.

11. Terrault NA, Lok ASF, McMahon BJ, et al. Update on prevention, diagnosis, and treatment of chronic hepatitis B: AASLD 2018 hepatitis B guidance. Hepatology 2018;67(4):1560–99.

12. Liaw YF. Clinical utility of hepatitis B surface antigen quantitation in patients with chronic hepatitis B: a review. Hepatology 2011;53(6):2121–9.

13. Amini A, Varsaneux O, Kelly H, et al. Diagnostic accuracy of tests to detect hepatitis B surface antigen: a systematic review of the literature and meta-analysis. BMC Infect Dis 2017;17(Suppl 1):698.

14. Krugman S, Overby LR, Mushahwar IK, et al. Viral hepatitis, type B. Studies on natural history and prevention re-examined. N Engl J Med 1979;300(3):101–6.

15. Liang TJ. Hepatitis B: the virus and disease. Hepatology 2009;49(5 Suppl): S13–21.

16. Bredberg A, Boe OW, Bredberg J, et al. Detection of hepatitis B surface antigen in blood following vaccination. Vaccine 2018;36(33):4963–5.

17. Trepo C, Chan HL, Lok A. Hepatitis B virus infection. Lancet 2014;384(9959): 2053–63.

18. McMahon BJ, Bender TR, Berquist KR, et al. Delayed development of antibody to hepatitis B surface antigen after symptomatic infection with hepatitis B virus. J Clin Microbiol 1981;14(2):130–4.

19. Tout I, Loureiro D, Mansouri A, et al. Hepatitis B surface antigen seroclearance: immune mechanisms, clinical impact, importance for drug development. J Hepatol 2020;73(2):409–22.

20. Shiffman ML. Management of acute hepatitis B. Clin Liver Dis 2010;14(1):75–91, viii-ix.

21. Maruyama T, Schodel F, Iino S, et al. Distinguishing between acute and symptomatic chronic hepatitis B virus infection. Gastroenterology 1994;106(4): 1006–15.

22. Lok AS, McMahon BJ. Chronic hepatitis B: update 2009. Hepatology 2009; 50(3):661–2.

23. McMahon BJ. The natural history of chronic hepatitis B virus infection. Hepatology 2009;49(5 Suppl):S45–55.

24. McMahon BJ, Parkinson AJ, Helminiak C, et al. Response to hepatitis B vaccine of persons positive for antibody to hepatitis B core antigen. Gastroenterology 1992;103(2):590–4.

25. Liaw YF, Sheen IS, Chen TJ, et al. Incidence, determinants and significance of delayed clearance of serum HBsAg in chronic hepatitis B virus infection: a prospective study. Hepatology 1991;13(4):627–31.

26. Hoofnagle JH, Di Bisceglie AM. Serologic diagnosis of acute and chronic viral hepatitis. Semin Liver Dis 1991;11(2):73–83.

27. Coffin CS, Zhou K, Terrault NA. New and old biomarkers for diagnosis and management of chronic hepatitis B virus infection. Gastroenterology 2019;156(2): 355–68.e3.
28. Thompson AJ, Nguyen T, Iser D, et al. Serum hepatitis B surface antigen and hepatitis B e antigen titers: disease phase influences correlation with viral load and intrahepatic hepatitis B virus markers. Hepatology 2010;51(6): 1933–44.
29. Hoofnagle JH, Dusheiko GM, Seeff LB, et al. Seroconversion from hepatitis B e antigen to antibody in chronic type B hepatitis. Ann Intern Med 1981;94(6): 744–8.
30. Werle-Lapostolle B, Bowden S, Locarnini S, et al. Persistence of cccDNA during the natural history of chronic hepatitis B and decline during adefovir dipivoxil therapy. Gastroenterology 2004;126(7):1750–8.
31. Chan HL, Wong VW, Tse AM, et al. Serum hepatitis B surface antigen quantitation can reflect hepatitis B virus in the liver and predict treatment response. Clin Gastroenterol Hepatol 2007;5(12):1462–8.
32. Locarnini S, Hatzakis A, Chen DS, et al. Strategies to control hepatitis B: Public policy, epidemiology, vaccine and drugs. J Hepatol 2015;62(1 Suppl):S76–86.
33. Bruss V. Hepatitis B virus morphogenesis. World J Gastroenterol 2007;13(1): 65–73.
34. Yan H, Zhong G, Xu G, et al. Sodium taurocholate cotransporting polypeptide is a functional receptor for human hepatitis B and D virus. Elife 2012;3.
35. Gerlich WH. Medical virology of hepatitis B: how it began and where we are now. Virol J 2013;10:239.
36. Bock CT, Schranz P, Schroder CH, et al. Hepatitis B virus genome is organized into nucleosomes in the nucleus of the infected cell. Virus Genes 1994;8(3): 215–29.
37. Jaroszewicz J, Reiberger T, Meyer-Olson D, et al. Hepatitis B surface antigen concentrations in patients with HIV/HBV co-infection. PLoS One 2012;7(8): e43143.
38. Sugiyama M, Tanaka Y, Kato T, et al. Influence of hepatitis B virus genotypes on the intra- and extracellular expression of viral DNA and antigens. Hepatology 2006;44(4):915–24.
39. Brunetto MR, Marcellin P, Cherubini B, et al. Response to peginterferon alfa-2a (40KD) in HBeAg-negative CHB: on-treatment kinetics of HBsAg serum levels vary by HBV genotype. J Hepatol 2013;59(6):1153–9.
40. Jaroszewicz J, Calle Serrano B, Wursthorn K, et al. Hepatitis B surface antigen (HBsAg) levels in the natural history of hepatitis B virus (HBV)-infection: a European perspective. J Hepatol 2010;52(4):514–22.
41. Nguyen T, Thompson AJ, Bowden S, et al. Hepatitis B surface antigen levels during the natural history of chronic hepatitis B: a perspective on Asia. J Hepatol 2010;52(4):508–13.
42. Gerlich W, Stamm B, Thomssen R. Prognostic significance of quantitative HBsAg determination in acute hepatitis B. Partial report of a cooperative clinical study of the DFG-focus of "virus hepatitis". Verh Dtsch Ges Inn Med 1977;83: 554–7. Prognostische Bedeutung des quantitativen HBsAg-Nachweises bei der akuten Hepatitis B. Teilergebnisse einer kooperativen klinischen Studie des DFG-Schwerpunktes "Virushepatitis".
43. Perrillo RP, Gish R, Falck-Ytter YT. American Gastroenterological Association Institute technical review on prevention and treatment of hepatitis B virus

reactivation during immunosuppressive drug therapy. Gastroenterology 2015; 148(1):221–44.e3.

44. Biswas R, Tabor E, Hsia CC, et al. Comparative sensitivity of HBV NATs and HBsAg assays for detection of acute HBV infection. Transfusion 2003;43(6): 788–98.

45. Kao JH, Chen DS. Global control of hepatitis B virus infection. Lancet Infect Dis 2002;2(7):395–403.

46. Kao JH. Hepatitis B viral genotypes: clinical relevance and molecular characteristics. J Gastroenterol Hepatol 2002;17(6):643–50.

47. Kao JH. Hepatitis B virus genotypes and hepatocellular carcinoma in Taiwan. Intervirology 2003;46(6):400–7.

48. Lin CL, Kao JH. The clinical implications of hepatitis B virus genotype: Recent advances. J Gastroenterol Hepatol 2011;26(Suppl 1):123–30.

49. Shi W, Zhang Z, Ling C, et al. Hepatitis B virus subgenotyping: history, effects of recombination, misclassifications, and corrections. Infect Genet Evol 2013;16: 355–61.

50. Cooksley WG. Do we need to determine viral genotype in treating chronic hepatitis B? J Viral Hepat 2010;17(9):601–10.

51. Huang CC, Kuo TM, Yeh CT, et al. One single nucleotide difference alters the differential expression of spliced RNAs between HBV genotypes A and D. Virus Res 2013;174(1–2):18–26.

52. Olinger CM, Jutavijittum P, Hubschen JM, et al. Possible new hepatitis B virus genotype, southeast Asia. Emerg Infect Dis 2008;14(11):1777–80.

53. Liu CJ, Kao JH. Global perspective on the natural history of chronic hepatitis B: role of hepatitis B virus genotypes A to J. Semin Liver Dis 2013;33(2):97–102.

54. Sakamoto T, Tanaka Y, Orito E, et al. Novel subtypes (subgenotypes) of hepatitis B virus genotypes B and C among chronic liver disease patients in the Philippines. J Gen Virol 2006;87(Pt 7):1873–82.

55. Schaefer S. Hepatitis B virus taxonomy and hepatitis B virus genotypes. World J Gastroenterol 2007;13(1):14–21.

56. Allain JP. Epidemiology of Hepatitis B virus and genotype. J Clin Virol 2006; 36(Suppl 1):S12–7.

57. Lin CL, Kao JH. Hepatitis B virus genotypes and variants. Cold Spring Harb Perspect Med 2015;5(5):a021436.

58. Kao JH, Chen PJ, Chen DS. Recent advances in the research of hepatitis B virus-related hepatocellular carcinoma: epidemiologic and molecular biological aspects. Adv Cancer Res 2010;108:21–72.

59. Ngui SL, Teo CG. Hepatitis B virus genomic heterogeneity: variation between quasispecies may confound molecular epidemiological analyses of transmission incidents. J Viral Hepat 1997;4(5):309–15.

60. Locarnini S, Littlejohn M, Aziz MN, et al. Possible origins and evolution of the hepatitis B virus (HBV). Semin Cancer Biol 2013;23(6 Pt B):561–75.

61. Yu MW, Yeh SH, Chen PJ, et al. Hepatitis B virus genotype and DNA level and hepatocellular carcinoma: a prospective study in men. J Natl Cancer Inst 2005; 97(4):265–72.

62. Zhu L, Tse CH, Wong VW, et al. A complete genomic analysis of hepatitis B virus genotypes and mutations in HBeAg-negative chronic hepatitis B in China. J Viral Hepat 2008;15(6):449–58.

63. Chan HL, Tsang SW, Liew CT, et al. Viral genotype and hepatitis B virus DNA levels are correlated with histological liver damage in HBeAg-negative chronic hepatitis B virus infection. Am J Gastroenterol 2002;97(2):406–12.

64. Yotsuyanagi H, Okuse C, Yasuda K, et al. Distinct geographic distributions of hepatitis B virus genotypes in patients with acute infection in Japan. J Med Virol 2005;77(1):39–46.
65. Ito K, Yotsuyanagi H, Yatsuhashi H, et al. Risk factors for long-term persistence of serum hepatitis B surface antigen following acute hepatitis B virus infection in Japanese adults. Hepatology 2014;59(1):89–97.
66. Huang YW, Lin CL, Chen PJ, et al. Hepatitis B viral genotype in Taiwanese patients with acute hepatitis B. Hepatogastroenterology 2008;55(82–83):633–5.
67. Sarkar N, Pal A, Das D, et al. Virological characteristics of acute hepatitis B in Eastern India: critical differences with chronic infection. PLoS One 2015; 10(11):e0141741.
68. Kao JH, Chen PJ, Lai MY, et al. Hepatitis B virus genotypes and spontaneous hepatitis B e antigen seroconversion in Taiwanese hepatitis B carriers. J Med Virol 2004;72(3):363–9.
69. Kao JH, Chen PJ, Lai MY, et al. Genotypes and clinical phenotypes of hepatitis B virus in patients with chronic hepatitis B virus infection. J Clin Microbiol 2002; 40(4):1207–9.
70. Livingston SE, Simonetti JP, Bulkow LR, et al. Clearance of hepatitis B e antigen in patients with chronic hepatitis B and genotypes A, B, C, D, and F. Gastroenterology 2007;133(5):1452–7.
71. Chu CJ, Hussain M, Lok AS. Hepatitis B virus genotype B is associated with earlier HBeAg seroconversion compared with hepatitis B virus genotype C. Gastroenterology 2002;122(7):1756–62.
72. Kao JH, Wu NH, Chen PJ, et al. Hepatitis B genotypes and the response to interferon therapy. J Hepatol 2000;33(6):998–1002.
73. Wai CT, Chu CJ, Hussain M, et al. HBV genotype B is associated with better response to interferon therapy in HBeAg(+) chronic hepatitis than genotype C. Hepatology 2002;36(6):1425–30.
74. Erhardt A, Blondin D, Hauck K, et al. Response to interferon alfa is hepatitis B virus genotype dependent: genotype A is more sensitive to interferon than genotype D. Gut 2005;54(7):1009–13.
75. Wiegand J, Wedemeyer H, Finger A, et al. A decline in hepatitis B virus surface antigen (hbsag) predicts clearance, but does not correlate with quantitative hbeag or HBV DNA levels. Antivir Ther 2008;13(4):547–54.
76. Buster EH, Hansen BE, Lau GK, et al. Factors that predict response of patients with hepatitis B e antigen-positive chronic hepatitis B to peginterferon-alfa. Gastroenterology 2009;137(6):2002–9.
77. Cooksley WG, Piratvisuth T, Lee SD, et al. Peginterferon alpha-2a (40 kDa): an advance in the treatment of hepatitis B e antigen-positive chronic hepatitis B. J Viral Hepat 2003;10(4):298–305.
78. Lau GK, Piratvisuth T, Luo KX, et al. Peginterferon Alfa-2a, lamivudine, and the combination for HBeAg-positive chronic hepatitis B. N Engl J Med 2005; 352(26):2682–95.
79. Chan HL, Wong ML, Hui AY, et al. Hepatitis B virus genotype has no impact on hepatitis B e antigen seroconversion after lamivudine treatment. World J Gastroenterol 2003;9(12):2695–7.
80. Westland C, Delaney WT, Yang H, et al. Hepatitis B virus genotypes and virologic response in 694 patients in phase III studies of adefovir dipivoxil1. Gastroenterology 2003;125(1):107–16.
81. Yuen MF, Wong DK, Sablon E, et al. Hepatitis B virus genotypes B and C do not affect the antiviral response to lamivudine. Antivir Ther 2003;8(6):531–4.

82. Hou J, Yin YK, Xu D, et al. Telbivudine versus lamivudine in Chinese patients with chronic hepatitis B: results at 1 year of a randomized, double-blind trial. Hepatology 2008;47(2):447–54.

83. Hsieh TH, Tseng TC, Liu CJ, et al. Hepatitis B virus genotype B has an earlier emergence of lamivudine resistance than genotype C. Antivir Ther 2009;14(8):1157–63.

84. Fujie H, Moriya K, Shintani Y, et al. Hepatitis B virus genotypes and hepatocellular carcinoma in Japan. Gastroenterology 2001;120(6):1564–5.

85. Ding X, Mizokami M, Yao G, et al. Hepatitis B virus genotype distribution among chronic hepatitis B virus carriers in Shanghai, China. Intervirology 2001;44(1):43–7.

86. Yang HI, Yeh SH, Chen PJ, et al. Associations between hepatitis B virus genotype and mutants and the risk of hepatocellular carcinoma. J Natl Cancer Inst 2008;100(16):1134–43.

87. Chan HL, Hui AY, Wong ML, et al. Genotype C hepatitis B virus infection is associated with an increased risk of hepatocellular carcinoma. Gut 2004;53(10):1494–8.

88. Mahmood S, Niiyama G, Kamei A, et al. Influence of viral load and genotype in the progression of Hepatitis B-associated liver cirrhosis to hepatocellular carcinoma. Liver Int 2005;25(2):220–5.

89. Chen GG, Li MY, Ho RL, et al. Identification of hepatitis B virus X gene mutation in Hong Kong patients with hepatocellular carcinoma. J Clin Virol 2005;34(1):7–12.

90. Chan HL, Tse CH, Mo F, et al. High viral load and hepatitis B virus subgenotype ce are associated with increased risk of hepatocellular carcinoma. J Clin Oncol 2008;26(2):177–82.

91. Littlejohn M, Davies J, Yuen L, et al. Molecular virology of hepatitis B virus, subgenotype C4 in northern Australian Indigenous populations. J Med Virol 2014;86(4):695–706.

92. Shi YH. Correlation between hepatitis B virus genotypes and clinical outcomes. Jpn J Infect Dis 2012;65(6):476–82.

93. Chen Y, Yu D, Zhang W, et al. HBV subgenotype C2 infection, A1762T/G1764A mutations may contribute to hepatocellular carcinoma with cirrhosis in Southeast China. Iran J Public Health 2012;41(11):10–8.

94. Wong GL, Chan HL, Yiu KK, et al. Meta-analysis: the association of hepatitis B virus genotypes and hepatocellular carcinoma. Aliment Pharmacol Ther 2013;37(5):517–26.

95. Kew MC, Kramvis A, Yu MC, et al. Increased hepatocarcinogenic potential of hepatitis B virus genotype A in Bantu-speaking sub-saharan Africans. J Med Virol 2005;75(4):513–21.

96. Lin CL, Chen JD, Liu CJ, et al. Clinicopathological differences between hepatitis B viral genotype B- and C-related resectable hepatocellular carcinoma. J Viral Hepat 2007;14(1):64–9.

97. Kao JH, Chen PJ, Lai MY, et al. Hepatitis B genotypes correlate with clinical outcomes in patients with chronic hepatitis B. Gastroenterology 2000;118(3):554–9.

98. Thakur V, Guptan RC, Kazim SN, et al. Profile, spectrum and significance of HBV genotypes in chronic liver disease patients in the Indian subcontinent. J Gastroenterol Hepatol 2002;17(2):165–70.

99. Livingston SE, Simonetti JP, McMahon BJ, et al. Hepatitis B virus genotypes in Alaska Native people with hepatocellular carcinoma: preponderance of genotype F. J Infect Dis 2007;195(1):5–11.

100. Gounder PP, Bulkow LR, Snowball M, et al. Hepatocellular carcinoma risk in Alaska native children and young adults with hepatitis B virus: Retrospective cohort analysis. J Pediatr 2016;178:206–13.

101. Ghosh S, Mondal RK, Banerjee P, et al. Tracking the naturally occurring mutations across the full-length genome of hepatitis B virus of genotype D in different phases of chronic e-antigen-negative infection. Clin Microbiol Infect 2012; 18(10):E412–8.

102. Lin CL, Kao JH. Review article: the prevention of hepatitis B-related hepatocellular carcinoma. Aliment Pharmacol Ther 2018;48(1):5–14.

103. Lin CL, Liao LY, Wang CS, et al. Basal core-promoter mutant of hepatitis B virus and progression of liver disease in hepatitis B e antigen-negative chronic hepatitis B. Liver Int 2005;25(3):564–70.

104. Liu CJ, Chen BF, Chen PJ, et al. Role of hepatitis B virus precore/core promoter mutations and serum viral load on noncirrhotic hepatocellular carcinoma: a case-control study. J Infect Dis 2006;194(5):594–9.

105. Kao JH, Chen PJ, Lai MY, et al. Basal core promoter mutations of hepatitis B virus increase the risk of hepatocellular carcinoma in hepatitis B carriers. Gastroenterology 2003;124(2):327–34.

106. Fang ZL, Sabin CA, Dong BQ, et al. Hepatitis B virus pre-S deletion mutations are a risk factor for hepatocellular carcinoma: a matched nested case-control study. J Gen Virol 2008;89(Pt 11):2882–90.

107. Tseng TC, Liu CJ, Yang HC, et al. Higher proportion of viral basal core promoter mutant increases the risk of liver cirrhosis in hepatitis B carriers. Gut 2015;64(2): 292–302.

108. Li W, Chen G, Yu X, et al. Accumulation of the mutations in basal core promoter of hepatitis B virus subgenotype C1 increase the risk of hepatocellular carcinoma in Southern China. Int J Clin Exp Pathol 2013;6(6):1076–85.

109. Yeh CT, Shen CH, Tai DI, et al. Identification and characterization of a prevalent hepatitis B virus X protein mutant in Taiwanese patients with hepatocellular carcinoma. Oncogene 2000;19(46):5213–20.

110. Kim JK, Chang HY, Lee JM, et al. Specific mutations in the enhancer II/core promoter/precore regions of hepatitis B virus subgenotype C2 in Korean patients with hepatocellular carcinoma. J Med Virol 2009;81(6):1002–8.

111. Jang JW, Chun JY, Park YM, et al. Mutational complex genotype of the hepatitis B virus X/precore regions as a novel predictive marker for hepatocellular carcinoma. Cancer Sci 2012;103(2):296–304.

112. Lin CL, Liu CH, Chen W, et al. Association of pre-S deletion mutant of hepatitis B virus with risk of hepatocellular carcinoma. J Gastroenterol Hepatol 2007;22(7): 1098–103.

113. Lok AS, Lai CL, Wu PC, et al. Spontaneous hepatitis B e antigen to antibody seroconversion and reversion in Chinese patients with chronic hepatitis B virus infection. Gastroenterology 1987;92(6):1839–43.

114. Lok AS, McMahon BJ. Chronic hepatitis B. Hepatology 2007;45(2):507–39.

115. Hoofnagle JH, Doo E, Liang TJ, et al. Management of hepatitis B: summary of a clinical research workshop. Hepatology 2007;45(4):1056–75.

116. Iloeje UH, Yang HI, Su J, et al. Predicting cirrhosis risk based on the level of circulating hepatitis B viral load. Gastroenterology 2006;130(3):678–86.

117. Kim GA, Han S, Choi GH, et al. Moderate levels of serum hepatitis B virus DNA are associated with the highest risk of hepatocellular carcinoma in chronic hepatitis B patients. Aliment Pharmacol Ther 2020;51(11):1169–79.

118. European Association for the Study of the Liver. Electronic address eee, European association for the study of the L. EASL 2017 clinical Practice guidelines on the management of hepatitis B virus infection. J Hepatol 2017;67(2):370–98.

119. McMahon BJ, Bulkow L, Simons B, et al. Relationship between level of hepatitis B virus DNA and liver disease: a population-based study of hepatitis B e antigen-negative persons with hepatitis B. Clin Gastroenterol Hepatol 2014; 12(4):701–6.e1-3.

120. Zacharakis G, Koskinas J, Kotsiou S, et al. The role of serial measurement of serum HBV DNA levels in patients with chronic HBeAg(-) hepatitis B infection: association with liver disease progression. A prospective cohort study. J Hepatol 2008;49(6):884–91.

121. Yang HI, Lu SN, Liaw YF, et al. Hepatitis B e antigen and the risk of hepatocellular carcinoma. N Engl J Med 2002;347(3):168–74.

122. Chen CJ, Yang HI, Su J, et al. Risk of hepatocellular carcinoma across a biological gradient of serum hepatitis B virus DNA level. JAMA 2006;295(1): 65–73.

123. Choi GH, Kim GA, Choi J, et al. High risk of clinical events in untreated HBeAg-negative chronic hepatitis B patients with high viral load and no significant ALT elevation. Aliment Pharmacol Ther 2019;50(2):215–26.

124. Hatzakis A, Magiorkinis E, Haida C. HBV virological assessment. J Hepatol 2006;44(1 Suppl):S71–6.

125. Kwak MS, Kim YJ. Occult hepatitis B virus infection. World J Hepatol 2014;6(12): 860–9.

126. Pollicino T, Amaddeo G, Restuccia A, et al. Impact of hepatitis B virus (HBV) preS/S genomic variability on HBV surface antigen and HBV DNA serum levels. Hepatology 2012;56(2):434–43.

127. Huang FY, Wong DK, Seto WK, et al. Sequence variations of full-length hepatitis B virus genomes in Chinese patients with HBsAg-negative hepatitis B infection. PLoS One 2014;9(6):e99028.

128. Melegari M, Bruno S, Wands JR. Properties of hepatitis B virus pre-S1 deletion mutants. Virology 1994;199(2):292–300.

129. Carman WF, Mimms LT. Pre-S/S gene variants of hepatitis B virus. Viral hepatitis and liver disease. Edizioni Minerva Med 1997;108–15.

130. Chisari FV. Hepatitis B virus biology and pathogenesis. Mol Genet Med 1992;2: 67–104.

131. Gerlich WH, Glebe D, Schuttler CG. Deficiencies in the standardization and sensitivity of diagnostic tests for hepatitis B virus. J Viral Hepat 2007;14(Suppl 1):16–21.

132. Echevarria JM, Avellon A. Improved detection of natural hepatitis B virus surface antigen (HBsAg) mutants by a new version of the VITROS HBsAg assay. J Med Virol 2008;80(4):598–602.

133. Lieshout-Krikke RW, Molenaar-de Backer MW, van Swieten P, et al. Surface antigen-negative hepatitis B virus infection in Dutch blood donors. Eur J Clin Microbiol Infect Dis 2014;33(1):69–77.

134. Carman WF, Jacyna MR, Hadziyannis S, et al. Mutation preventing formation of hepatitis B e antigen in patients with chronic hepatitis B infection. Lancet 1989; 2(8663):588–91.

135. Brunetto MR, Stemler M, Bonino F, et al. A new hepatitis B virus strain in patients with severe anti-HBe positive chronic hepatitis B. J Hepatol 1990;10(2):258–61.

136. Yang CY, Kuo TH, Ting LP. Human hepatitis B viral e antigen interacts with cellular interleukin-1 receptor accessory protein and triggers interleukin-1 response. J Biol Chem 2006;281(45):34525-36.

137. Buckwold VE, Xu Z, Chen M, et al. Effects of a naturally occurring mutation in the hepatitis B virus basal core promoter on precore gene expression and viral replication. J Virol 1996;70(9):5845-51.

138. Moriyama K, Okamoto H, Tsuda F, et al. Reduced precore transcription and enhanced core-pregenome transcription of hepatitis B virus DNA after replacement of the precore-core promoter with sequences associated with e antigen-seronegative persistent infections. Virology 1996;226(2):269-80.

Treatment and Prevention of Acute Hepatitis B Virus

Simone E. Dekker, MD, PhD[a], Ellen W. Green, MD, PhD[a], Joseph Ahn, MD, MS, MBA[b],*

KEYWORDS

- Acute hepatitis B • Hepatitis B prevention • Hepatitis B in newborns
- Fulminant liver failure • Hepatitis B treatment • Antiviral therapy

KEY POINTS

- The hepatitis B virus (HBV) remains a global health burden despite access and adoption of vaccination with approximately 2 billion people exposed cumulatively.
- Acute HBV is transmitted parenterally, by sexual contact, and via vertical transmission, and manifestations vary from asymptomatic to fulminant liver failure.
- Chronic hepatitis develops in 90% of newborns but less than 5% of infected adults.
- Screening, vaccination, and postexposure prophylaxis are key interventions to reducing acute HBV.
- Antiviral therapy is generally not necessary for uncomplicated symptomatic acute HBV due to spontaneous recovery in 95% of immunocompetent adults and as such antivirals should be used judiciously.

INCIDENCE OF ACUTE HEPATITIS B VIRUS

The hepatitis B virus (HBV) remains a major contributor to the global burden of disease, with more than 2 billion people exposed, of whom an estimated 257 million have chronic infection as of 2013.[1] The highest rates of acute HBV are in sub-Saharan Africa and East Asia, and the lowest rates are reported in North America, Western Europe, and Australia.[1] Remarkably, nearly all countries have experienced a significant decline in acute HBV incidence since 1992, when the World Health Organization (WHO) recommended the hepatitis B vaccine in all infant vaccination programs.[2] Initially, some countries, including some in highly endemic HBV areas, struggled to implement this policy. With the assistance of region-specific collaboratives, areas such as Southeast Asia have been able to work toward a <1% seroprevalence of HBV markers.[3] Globally, regions of low prevalence, such as Scandinavia,

[a] Department of Medicine, Oregon Health & Science University, 3181 Southwest Sam Jackson Park Road, Portland, OR 97239, USA; [b] Division of Gastroenterology and Hepatology, Oregon Health & Science University, 3181 Southwest Sam Jackson Park Road, MNP 4112, Portland, OR 97239, USA
* Corresponding author.
E-mail address: Ahnj@ohsu.edu

Clin Liver Dis 25 (2021) 711–724
https://doi.org/10.1016/j.cld.2021.06.002
1089-3261/21/© 2021 Elsevier Inc. All rights reserved.

liver.theclinics.com

have not found it cost effective and do not have population-wide HBV vaccination efforts.

In the United States, the annual incidence of acute HBV declined by 78%, from approximately 232,000 to 51,000 cases annually, between 1990 and 2005.[4] Since 2006, the overall incidence of acute HBV infection has remained stable in the United States. According to the US Centers for Disease Control and Prevention (CDC), the rate in 2018 was 1.0 case per 100,000 persons.[5] Over half of the more than 21,000 acute HBV cases reported to the CDC were patients aged between 30 and 49 years and 36% of identified exposure risks were due to drug injection.[5] Regarding chronic infection, adults in the 2011 to 2016 National Health and Nutrition Examination Survey had an estimated prevalence of hepatitis B surface antigen (HBsAg) of 0.36% overall and 3.4% in non-Hispanic Asians in the United States.[6] Globally, the incidence of acute HBV cases in Europe has shown a slow but steady decline from 2009 to 2018, with 0.1 to 0.9 cases per 100,000 persons in 2018.[7] Sub-Saharan Africa and Asia have the highest prevalence where 5% to 10% of adults are chronically infected.[8] The changing demographic of HBV and the impact of vaccination on the incidence and prevalence of HBV over the past 50 years is discussed elsewhere in this issue.

CLINICAL COURSE
Transmission and Incubation

Acute HBV is transmitted parenterally, by sexual contact, and via vertical transmission. The incubation period ranges from 28 to 180 days, with most infections exhibiting an intubation between 60 and 110 days.[9] During the incubation period, patients remain asymptomatic and are typically unaware of their exposure to HBV, contributing to further transmission risk. In areas of high HBV prevalence, most infections are through vertical transmission or from horizontal transmission from young children or adolescents within the same household.[10] Vertical transmission via mother to infant is the most frequent mode of HBV infection worldwide. In regions with a low prevalence, acute infection most commonly occurs in nonvaccinated teenagers or adults who have sexual interactions or share items contaminated with infected blood, such as items used for personal hygiene or to prepare or inject drugs. In the vast majority of these cases, the patient is unaware that their partner in these activities has chronic HBV.[2,11]

Symptoms of Acute Hepatitis B Virus

The spectrum of the clinical courses varies from asymptomatic to fulminant liver failure, and likewise the final outcome ranges from complete recovery, chronic hepatitis, or cirrhosis. In most immunocompetent adults, acute HBV infection is self-limited.[12] However, HBV may cause acute hepatitis in the first 6 months after exposure, characterized by liver cell necrosis and periportal inflammation.[9] Acute hepatitis is heralded by nonspecific symptoms shared by other viral hepatitides such as hepatitis A virus (HAV), hepatitis C virus (HCV), or hepatitis E virus: abdominal pain, low-grade fever, nausea, and jaundice. Although these symptoms occur in a minority of patients, only 30% of adults and 10% of children younger than 4 years, they are still at risk of transmitting the virus.

The classic adult presentation of acute HBV involves four phases: incubation, prodrome, icteric, and resolution. The icteric phase occurs in only 30% of infected patients with an average time from infection to the onset of jaundice of 90 days.[13] Most patients with acute icteric hepatitis B recover without residual injury or chronic hepatitis. Clinical symptoms usually abate after 1 to 3 months with the variability as a function of symptom severity during the acute phase.

Many patients do not progress through the afore-described phases, but instead fall into variant presentations, including anicteric acute HBV and acute liver failure (ALF).[2] The anicteric acute HBV is the most common variant and is associated with higher rate of developing chronic HBV when compared with patients who become jaundiced. This variant is often observed in immunocompromised patients, such as patients with human immunodeficiency virus (HIV), diabetes mellitus, and chronic renal failure on dialysis. The acute liver failure variant is described in further detail in later discussion. Some patients show extrahepatic manifestations of HBV infection, such as polyarteritis nodosa, glomerulonephritis, arthritis, peripheral neuropathy, and essential mixed cryoglobulinemia.[9]

The risk of developing chronic infection or carrier state depends on both the age at time of infection and the immune status of the infected patient.[9] Chronic hepatitis develops in 90% of newborns who become infected from perinatal transmission in HBV-infected mothers and in 25% to 50% of infections occurring in young children.[9,14] Conversely, less than 5% of immunocompetent adults progress to chronic hepatitis. Persistent presence of hepatitis B e antigen (HBeAg) and elevated serum HBV DNA levels are associated with adverse clinical outcomes, including an increased risk of cirrhosis and liver-related mortality by 7- and 33-fold, respectively.[15] Older age, male gender, severity of fibrosis, other concurrent viral infections (especially hepatitis delta virus [HDV], more so than HCV), and alcohol intake are additional predictors of adverse clinical outcomes and hepatocellular carcinoma (HCC).[15–18]

Exacerbation in chronic HBV may mimic acute infection. Examples include spontaneous or treatment-induced seroconversion, superinfection with HDV, and reactivation of HBV replication in the setting of immunosuppression. Careful clinical history and examination for features of chronic liver disease will provide clues to differentiate these scenarios. The treatment of chronic HBV infection, chronic HBV infection with HDV or HCV coinfection, and the risk of HCC in patients with chronic HBV are discussed elsewhere in this issue.

Laboratory Findings and Immune Mechanisms of Acute Hepatitis B Virus

When evaluating a patient with concern for hepatitis, in addition to a thorough history and physical examination, laboratory testing should include complete blood cell count, complete metabolic panel (serum alanine aminotransferase [ALT], serum aspartate aminotransferase [AST], total bilirubin, alkaline phosphatase, albumin, and creatinine levels), international normalized ratio (INR), and markers of HBV replication such as IgM antibodies against hepatitis B core (anti-HBc IgM), HBeAg, antibodies against hepatitis B e antigen (anti-HBe), and HBV DNA quantitation. In addition, markers for coinfection with HCV, HDV, and HIV should be obtained along with an assessment of HAV immunity to determine the need for vaccination.[12,19]

Serologic markers in acute HBV are shown in **Fig. 1**. The first detectable viral marker is HBsAg, which becomes detectable in the serum 2 to 8 weeks before any elevation of aminotransferases. Acute HBV is diagnosed by detecting HBsAg and anti-HBc IgM, except during the window period, named for the time between the disappearance of HBsAg and before the presence of antibodies against hepatitis B surface antigen (anti-HBs) in which only anti-HBc IgM is present. In addition, HBV DNA quantitation can be used to detect the presence of HBV viremia in the setting of acute HBV. When liver injury occurs in acute infection, liver enzymes first become elevated at 1 month after infection and last to 6 months, with an average duration of 60 days.

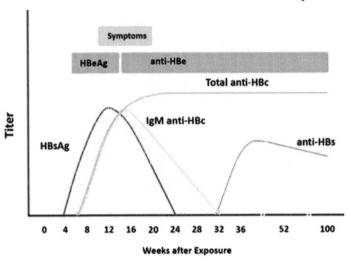

Acute HBV with Recovery

Fig. 1. Serologic markers in acute HBV with recovery.

ALT and AST levels can increase to between 500 and 5000 U/L and decrease after the acute phase of infection. Serum bilirubin levels seldom increase more than 10 mg/dL, the alkaline phosphatase level and prothrombin time are usually normal or mildly elevated, and the serum albumin level is normal or minimally depressed. Peripheral blood counts may show mild leukopenia, with or without relative lymphocytosis. Anti-HBc IgM antibodies are lost within 6 to 12 months from the onset of illness. Loss of HBsAg and the development of anti-HBs signify recovery from the acute infection and the development of immunity.[20] Patients should be monitored for HBsAg and ALT levels to determine whether seroconversion and clearance have occurred.[21] Presence of HBsAg, HBeAg, and high copy numbers of HBV DNA for more than 6 months implies progression to chronic infection.[20]

Immune mechanisms involved in the resolution of acute HBV include both the innate (natural killer cells, macrophages, neutrophils) and adaptive immune system (T lymphocytes). The innate immune response to acute HBV begins during the incubation phase when the patient is still asymptomatic. Resolution of acute HBV is associated with a decline in T lymphocytes and the appearance of anti-HBs. T cells remain responsive to re-exposure to HBV, contributing to the lack of significant disease upon re-exposure.[2]

A detailed review of serologic tests used to detect HBV, the role of HBV genotypes and DNA testing, and monitoring of acute and chronic HBV with serologic testing is detailed elsewhere in this issue. HBV/HCV and HBV/HDV coinfections are also discussed elsewhere in this issue.

PREVENTING ACUTE HEPATITIS B VIRUS IN ADULTS

Chronic HBV typically requires lifelong treatment. As such, prevention should be the primary aim for physicians and public health professionals.[12] Mainstays of prevention are vaccination, as well as avoiding transmission from infected people via blood supply screening, universal health care precautions, and harm reduction education.

Screening

Most international guidelines recommend HBsAg screening for high-risk groups and hepatitis B vaccination (**Table 1**). These populations include those who risk exposure to percutaneous or mucosal exposure to blood, adults and young adults at risk for sexual exposure, international travelers to regions with high or intermediate endemicity for HBV, individuals with chronic liver disease, and those with HIV infection.[10]

Vaccination in Adults

Vaccination is the most important means of reducing the global burden of disease, and recombinant DNA-derived vaccines against HBV have been available in the United States since 1982. HBV vaccination confers long-term protections against

Table 1
High-risk populations recommended for routine hepatitis B screening

AASLD	WHO
Household and sexual contacts of HBsAg-positive persons	Household and sexual contacts of persons with HBV
Persons infected with hepatitis C or/and HIV	Persons infected with HIV
Intravenous drug users	Persons who inject drugs
Men who have sex with men	Men who have sex with men
Inmates of correctional facilities	Persons who are incarcerated
Organ, plasma, blood, tissue, or semen donors	Blood and organ donors
All pregnant women and infants born to HBsAg mothers	Pregnant women
Persons born in regions of high or intermediate HBV endemicity (HBsAg prevalence of $\geq$ 2%) US-born persons not vaccinated as an infant whose parents were born in regions with HBV endemicity $\geq$ 8%	General population screening in countries with high HBV endemicity
Individuals needing immunosuppressive therapy, including chemotherapy, or related to transplantation and various immune-mediated disorders	
Persons with elevated ALT or AST of unknown cause	
Patients with end-stage renal disease needing dialysis	
Persons requesting evaluation/treatment of sexually transmitted disease or have multiple sexual partners	
Health care staff, public safety workers, and staff of facilities for developmentally disabled persons	
Persons traveling to countries with intermediate or high HBV prevalence	
Unvaccinated persons with diabetes aged between 19 and 59 y	

Data from Weinbaum at al.,[53] Vittal et al.,[10] Terrault et al.,[19] the WHO.[54]

HBV, and immunologic memory remains intact for at least 30 years among healthy people who received HBV vaccination after age 6 months. Although the WHO identifies vaccination at birth as a key intervention for infant protection the exact duration of the resultant protection is unknown.[8,22] The American Association for the Study of Liver Diseases (AASLD) and WHO therefore recommend (re)vaccination in high-risk adults (see **Table 1**). The recommended regimen is 3 injections (20 μg Engerix-B or 10 μg Recombivax HB) intramuscularly in the deltoid muscle at 0, 1, and 6 months, or an alternate 4-dose schedule given at 0, 7, and 21 to 30 days, followed by a dose at 12 months for the combination of hepatitis A and B vaccine (Twinrix). Recently, a two-dose vaccination series administered at 0 and 1 month has been approved (Heplisav-B).[23] Vaccine coverage among adults in the United States is low, with an overall prevalence of hepatitis B vaccine-induced immunity of 25% during the period from 2007 to 2012.[24] Verification of vaccine response is unnecessary except in health care workers, patients on long-term hemodialysis or immunocompromised patients, sexual partners of long-term carriers, and infants of HBsAg-positive mothers. Hepatitis B immunity can be determined by measuring anti-HBs titers and HBsAg.

Postexposure Prophylaxis

Once exposure to HBV has occurred in nonimmune persons, prophylaxis should be initiated as soon as possible to prevent the development of HBV infection. Postexposure prophylaxis consists of a single dose of hepatitis B immune globulin (HBIG) injected intramuscularly, immediately followed by HBV vaccination. It is critical to always initiate HBV vaccination in conjunction with HBIG because HBIG can augment protection with passive immunity for 3 to 6 months until a response to vaccination is attained, typically in 1 to 2 months.[25] Specific recommendations for the management of postexposure prophylaxis vary based on occupational settings and vaccination status and are detailed by the CDC.[25]

Hepatitis B Virus Reactivation Prevention in Immunosuppressive Therapy

HBV infection remains present even in people who have demonstrated serologic recovery. As such, immunosuppressive (IS) therapy presents a risk of HBV reactivation that can cause morbidity and mortality related to the hepatitis infection or delays in care for the illness for which IS is indicated. HBV reactivation is defined by changes from baseline serologies and may include increase in HBV DNA titer or seroconversion to HBsAg positive in a previously negative patient. Screening should therefore consist of both HBsAg and anti-HBc studies before IS therapy initiation. The highest rates of reactivation are seen in therapies for malignancy occurring in up to 53% of HBsAg-positive, anti-HBc-positive patients.[19] As such, it is recommended to give HBV prophylaxis in B cell-ablating therapies, such as rituximab, or before treatment start in patients with known chronic disease, using antivirals with low likelihood of resistance development, tenofovir or entecavir (ETV).

PREVENTING ACUTE HEPATITIS B VIRUS IN NEWBORNS
Primary Prevention: Maternal Screening and Treatment

HBV in expecting women and infants remains a public health concern. Between 1998 and 2011, the prevalence of maternal HBV infection was 85.8 cases per 100,000 deliveries in the United States (0.09% of live-born singleton deliveries).[26,27] Increased risk of vertical transmission of 85% to 90% can be seen in mothers with high serum HBV DNA levels (>200,000 IU/mL to 1,000,000 copies/mL), the presence of HBeAg, and with a prior history of vertical transmission, underscoring the importance of prenatal screening.[19] **Fig. 2** illustrates a treatment algorithm for screening and management of pregnant women with HBV.

HBsAg-positive pregnant women should receive counseling on HBV-specific perinatal care, and HBV treatment options as indications for treatment in HBV-infected pregnant women are the same as for other adults.[28] The AASLD recommends antiviral therapy, preferably with tenofovir disoproxil fumarate (TDF) in the third trimester of pregnancy to women with HBV DNA levels > 200,000 IU/mL until 4 weeks postpartum (see **Table 1**). Data from the Antiretroviral Pregnancy Registry in pregnant HIV-positive women showed that TDF has the most extensive safety data in pregnant HBV-positive women and a favorable resistance profile.[29] Whether the use of ETV is safe during pregnancy remains unknown, and interferon-based therapy is contraindicated during pregnancy.[28] Tenofovir alafenamide (TAF) has been found to have a better safety profile in the general public, and clinical trials are ongoing to determine the effect on end points such as vertical transmission (NCT04237376).

Pregnant women who go untreated or discontinue anti-HBV therapy during or shortly after pregnancy require close monitoring, because they are at increased risk of hepatic flares especially after delivery.[28] HBV is not transmitted through breastmilk, and breastfeeding is not contraindicated in HBV-infected mothers on antiviral therapy;

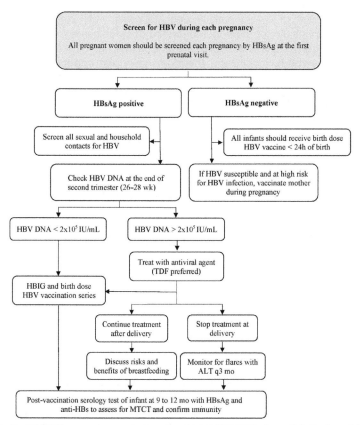

Fig. 2. Perinatal HBV screening and management. HBV DNA, hepatitis B virus DNA level; MTCT, mother-to-child transmission. (*Adapted from* Rajbhandari et al.,[12] Tang et al.,[30] Apuzzio et al.,[51] Owens et al.,[52] and WHO.[29])

however, drug metabolites may appear in breast milk. HBV vaccination and HBIG will protect against transmission from blood exposure such as through cracked nipples.[30] Specifics regarding the management of labor and delivery are beyond the scope of this article.

Primary Prevention: Newborn Vaccination

The importance of primary prevention via universal newborn vaccination cannot be understated. The HBV vaccine is included in the universal immunization program for newborns in the United States. HBV vaccination has been promoted by the WHO as routine care since 1997. Engerix-B and Recombivax HB are the 2 recombinant hepatitis B vaccines that are approved for vaccination starting at birth. Use of Heplisav-B is not recommended at this time because of insufficient data in this population.[21] The primary hepatitis B immunization series consists of 3 vaccine doses. All infants should receive their first dose as soon as possible after birth, preferably within 24 hours, followed by 2 or 3 doses separated by 4 weeks.[21] Low-birth-weight (<2000 g) and premature infants should receive 3 additional doses to complete the vaccination schedule.[21] This vaccination series is 90% to 95% effective in preventing HBV infection, as well as decreasing vulnerability to future HBV transmission if the subsequent doses are administered.[12,28] Adherence to this vaccine schedule is particularly important in countries with high endemicity, where HBV is mainly spread at birth or during childhood.[31] In areas of low endemicity, perinatal or early childhood transmission of HBV may be responsible for more than one-third of chronic infections.[32]

Transmission early in life is associated with a higher risk of developing a chronic infection, and newborn vaccination therefore has great impact on reducing the burden of chronic infection.[10,33] Countries that have implemented universal HBV infant vaccination programs have experienced a dramatic decrease in prevalence of HBV and HCC in children.[34] However, HBV infant vaccination programs are not widespread. In 2014, 49% of 194 countries provided the hepatitis birth dose vaccination as part of their national immunization program. That same year, less than 38% of infants born worldwide received the hepatitis B vaccine within 24 hours of delivery.[10] About 5% to 10% of vaccinated children have a poor response to vaccination and will be at risk of HBV infection as adults.[28] More work remains to be done in preventing HBV in newborns and young children through universal HBV vaccination implementation.

FULMINANT LIVER FAILURE FROM ACUTE HEPATITIS B VIRUS

As described earlier, between 0.1% and 1% of patients with acute HBV develop acute liver failure, a life-threatening sequelae of infection.[35] Characteristics include evidence of acute liver injury (although a protracted course can yield persistent symptoms for longer than 4 weeks and is a poor prognostic indicator), coagulopathy (INR > 1.5), and hepatic encephalopathy.[15,35,36]

HBV accounts for 5% to 10% of the cases of acute liver failure and is the most common viral cause of severe acute liver failure and acute liver injury. Acute HBV is the second most common cause for acute liver failure worldwide, after toxicity from medications.[2,37,38] The pathophysiology is thought to involve massive immune-mediated lysis of infected hepatocytes, which may explain the lack of evidence of HBV replication in patients presenting with fulminant hepatitis B.[39] Fulminant liver failure can be the result of either de novo infection, reactivation in a patient with previous HBV infection, or HDV superinfection.[35,40] The risk of developing acute liver failure in patients with acute HBV infections is higher in patients with HDV or HCV coinfections. The risk of acute liver failure and mortality is higher in reactivation of HBV in long-term carriers during immunosuppression, compared with the de novo HBV infections.[41,42]

Wai and colleagues studied the clinical outcome and virologic characteristics of hepatitis B-related acute liver failure in the United States and found that the rates of overall survival and spontaneous recovery for patients with HBV-ALF were 67% and 25%, respectively.[42] The investigators did not find a relationship between virological factors and overall survival or spontaneous recovery; this suggests that host factors such as age, comorbidities, concurrent drug use, and race/ethnicity may be more important than virological factors in determining outcomes in HBV-ALF.[43] However, HBV genotype D was more frequently found in patients with HBV-related acute liver failure compared with chronic HBV infection in the United States.[42] Liver transplantation should be considered in fulminant or advanced liver disease, as mortality from a fulminant course approaches 80% without liver transplantation and 20% with transplantation.[9] Patients fortunate to have a more indolent course should be educated on prevention of further liver damage, such as limiting alcohol intake and avoiding medications or supplements that could be hepatotoxic.[12]

INDICATIONS FOR ORAL ANTIVIRAL AGENTS IN ACUTE HEPATITIS B VIRUS

Antiviral therapy is generally not necessary for uncomplicated symptomatic acute HBV due to spontaneous recovery in 95% of immunocompetent adults, and the likelihood of fulminant hepatitis B is less than 1%.[44] There is no clear evidence that early therapy with antiviral agents for uncomplicated acute hepatitis B decreases the risk of chronicity or speeds recovery.

Indications for treatment include fulminant liver disease and those with protracted, acute severe hepatitis persisting for more than 4 weeks.[12,45,46] The AASLD recommends treatment with a nucleos(t)ide analogue (NA) to reduce the risk of recurrent hepatitis B and improve survival. Multicenter double-blind randomized controlled trials are lacking, but several cohort studies suggest that the early antiviral therapy with highly potent NAs can prevent progression to acute liver failure and subsequent liver transplantation or mortality.[15,47] This protective effect is not seen if treatment is initiated when patients have already manifested acute liver failure and advanced hepatic encephalopathy, suggesting that consideration of prompt and timely antiviral therapy is crucial.[12,48]

Table 2 describes treatment strategies and end points of treatment of acute HBV. Large case series support that lamivudine (LAM), TDF, and ETV can be safely used in acute severe HBV.[47,49] TAF is a prodrug related to TDF that has been demonstrated as noninferior in trials regardless of HBeAg status and is noted for its reduced renal toxicity and osteomalacia, when compared with TDF.[19] However, there have been limited studies in the use of TAF in acute HBV. Owing to their antiviral potency, ETV or TDF are the preferred agents for the treatment of acute or fulminant hepatitis B, for the treatment of decompensated cirrhosis, and in patients undergoing immunosuppressive treatment.[12] If it is unclear if the patient has acute HBV or an acute exacerbation of chronic HBV, ETV or TDF are preferred because these agents have higher barrier to resistance. LAM, adefovir, and telbivudine are not recommended because of their low barrier to resistance, low potency, and high adverse event profile. Treatment should be continued until HBsAg clearance is confirmed, or indefinitely in patients who undergo liver transplantation.[12]

There is no added benefit from de novo combination of 2 NAs. The combination of pegylated-interferon (peg-IFN) and NAs is also not recommended by the AASLD.

Table 2
Treatment strategies and end points for acute hepatitis B virus

Indication	Treatment	End points
Acute/symptomatic hepatitis B or fulminant hepatitis B	TDF or ETV	Treatment should be continued until HBsAg clearance is confirmed or indefinitely in those who undergo liver transplant
Presence of compensated cirrhosis, plus HBV DNA levels >2000 IU/mL or persistent ALT level elevation	TDF, TAF, or ETV	Lifelong therapy
Presence of decompensated cirrhosis	TDF or ETV	Lifelong therapy
Pregnant mothers with high viral load	TDF preferred	Initiate therapy at 28–30 wk gestation and monitor for flares if therapy is ceased after delivery
HBV/HIV coinfection	TDF + emtricitabine or LAM or ETV + ARV regimen	Lifelong unless the patient has achieved HBeAg seroconversion and has completed an adequate course of consolidation treatment
HBsAg-positive, anti-HBc-positive patients who will receive malignancy or IS therapy	TDF, TAF, or ETV	6–12 mo beyond malignancy or IS therapy, >12 mo in anti-CD20 antibody therapy

Adapted from Rajbhandari et al.[12] Indications for treatment and treatment strategies of chronic HBV are discussed elsewhere in this issue.
Abbreviations: ARV, antiretroviral; LAM, lamivudine.

Interferon treatment failed to be effective in severe acute HBV and is not recommended in acute liver failure or decompensated cirrhosis.[46]

IS THERE HARM IN USING ANTIVIRAL THERAPY IN EARLY HEPATITIS B VIRUS INFECTION?

Use of antiviral agents is not recommended in early HBV infection because most adult patients with an acute HBV monoinfection will clear HBsAg without medical therapy. Antiviral therapy should be used judiciously given the risks of adverse effects (nephrotoxicity, lactic acidosis, resistance, and withdrawal flare), particularly in pregnant women, the elderly, and patients with renal impairment.[50] In the absence of ALF or cirrhosis, the risks (albeit low) start to become more relevant. In these situations, the benefit of treating acute HBV with NAs is unclear. In addition, treatment may cloud the clinical picture of whether the patient has suppressed HBV on their own or because of the addition of the NA. Thus, in these cases, careful monitoring of the patient and their laboratory tests is an acceptable alternative to initiation of antiviral therapy.

Patients with compensated cirrhosis and HBV DNA levels >2000 IU/ml or persistent ALT level elevation require lifelong therapy. Patients with decompensated cirrhosis require treatment regardless of HBV DNA, HBeAg status, and ALT levels (see

Table 2).[19] In these situations, treatment with ETV or TDF is preferred. As described earlier, peg-IFN is contraindicated.[19] Treatment should be continued until HBsAg clearance is confirmed or indefinitely in those who undergo liver transplantation.

SUMMARY

The HBV remains a major contributor to the global burden of disease, despite the availability of highly effective vaccines and antiviral therapies. As vertical transmission is one of the most prominent sources of new infections worldwide, it is prudent to seek opportunities to use routine maternal care interactions for counseling, screening, and treatment of HBV infections; this coupled with newborn vaccination strategies and ongoing counseling of groups vulnerable to HBV exposure may reduce the suffering of downstream sequelae including cirrhosis, liver failure, and death related to HBV.

CLINICS CARE POINTS

- Newborn vaccination is a cornerstone of reducing the burden of chronic HBV infection.
- HBV screening:
  - Utilize HBsAg to screen high risk-groups. AASLD highlights individuals on immunosuppression, immune-mediated disorders, and health care exposure in addition to the WHO screening guidelines.
  - More extensive HBV screening serologies (including HBsAg and anti-HBc) is warranted prior to initiation of immunosuppressive therapies.
  - All pregnant women should be screened each pregnancy by HBsAg at the first prenatal visit.
- After HBV exposure, HBV labs should be drawn and HBIG and HBV vaccination series should be administered.
- Antiviral therapy is generally not necessary for uncomplicated symptomatic acute HBV due to spontaneous recovery in 95% of immunocompetent adults and the likelihood of fulminant hepatitis B is less than 1%. As such antivirals should be used judiciously given the risks of adverse effects (nephrotoxicity, lactic acidosis, resistance, and withdrawal flare), particularly in pregnant women, the elderly, and patients with renal impairment.
- Treatment is indicated for fulminant liver disease and those with protracted (> 4 weeks), acute severe hepatitis (total bilirubin >3 mg/dL, (or direct bilirubin >1.5 mg/dL), INR >1.5, encephalopathy, or ascites).
- ETV or TDF are the preferred agents for the treatment of acute or fulminant hepatitis B and continues until HBsAg clearance.

DISCLOSURE

The authors have nothing to disclose.

REFERENCES

1. Schweitzer A, Horn J, Mikolajczyk RT, et al. Estimations of worldwide prevalence of chronic hepatitis B virus infection: a systematic review of data published between 1965 and 2013. Lancet 2015;386(10003):1546–55.
2. Shiffman ML. Management of acute hepatitis B. Clin Liver Dis 2010;14(1):75–91, viii-ix.

3. Sandhu H, Roesel S, Sharifuzzaman M, et al. Progress toward hepatitis B control — South-East Asia region, 2016–2019. MMWR Morb Mortal Wkly Rep 2020;69: 988–92.

4. Centers for Disease Control and Prevention. A comprehensive immunization strategy to eliminate transmission of hepatitis B virus infection in the United States. MMWR Morb Mortal Wkly Rep 2006;55(No. RR-16):1–33.

5. Centers for Disease Control and Prevention. Viral hepatitis surveillance — United States, 2018. Atlanta (GA): Centers for Disease Control and Prevention; 2020.

6. Patel EU, Thio CL, Boon D, et al. Prevalence of hepatitis B and hepatitis D virus infections in the United States, 2011-2016. Clin Infect Dis 2019;69(4):709–12.

7. European Centre for Disease Prevention and Control. Hepatitis B. In: ECDC, editor. Annual epidemiological report for 2018. Solna (Sweden): ECDC; 2020.

8. World Health Organization. Global health sector strategy on viral hepatitis 2016–2021. Geneva: WHO; 2016.

9. Juszczyk J. Clinical course and consequences of hepatitis B infection. Vaccine 2000;18:S23–5.

10. Vittal A, Ghany MG. WHO guidelines for prevention, care and treatment of individuals infected with HBV: a US perspective. Clin Liver Dis 2019;23(3):417–32.

11. Alter MJ. Epidemiology and prevention of hepatitis B. Semin Liver Dis 2003;23(1): 39–46.

12. Rajbhandari R, Chung RT. Treatment of hepatitis B: a concise review. Clin Transl Gastroenterol 2016;7(9):e190.

13. Krugman S, Overby LR, Mushahwar IK, et al. Viral hepatitis, type B. N Engl J Med 1979;300(3):101–6.

14. McMahon BJ. Natural history of chronic hepatitis B. Clin Liver Dis 2010;14(3): 381–96.

15. Lampertico P, Maini M, Papatheodoridis G. Optimal management of hepatitis B virus infection - EASL special conference. J Hepatol 2015;63(5):1238–53.

16. Chen YC, Chu CM, Liaw YF. Age-specific prognosis following spontaneous hepatitis B e antigen seroconversion in chronic hepatitis B. Hepatology 2010;51(2): 435–44.

17. Iloeje UH, Yang HI, Su J, et al. Predicting cirrhosis risk based on the level of circulating hepatitis B viral load. Gastroenterology 2006;130(3):678–86.

18. Liaw YF, Chen YC, Sheen IS, et al. Impact of acute hepatitis C virus superinfection in patients with chronic hepatitis B virus infection. Gastroenterology 2004;126(4): 1024–9.

19. Terrault NA, Lok ASF, McMahon BJ, et al. Update on prevention, diagnosis, and treatment of chronic hepatitis B: AASLD 2018 hepatitis B guidance. Hepatology 2018;67(4):1560–99.

20. Pan CQ, Zhang JX. Natural history and clinical consequences of hepatitis B virus infection. Int J Med Sci 2005;2(1):36–40.

21. World Health Organization. Hepatitis B vaccines: WHO position paper—recommendations. Vaccine 2010;28(3):589–90.

22. Bruce MG, Bruden D, Hurlburt D, et al. Antibody levels and protection after hepatitis B vaccine: results of a 30-year follow-up study and response to a booster dose. J Infect Dis 2016;214(1):16–22.

23. Cooper C, Mackie D. Hepatitis B surface antigen-1018 ISS adjuvant-containing vaccine: a review of HEPLISAV safety and efficacy. Expert Rev Vaccin 2011; 10(4):417–27.

24. Harris AM, Iqbal K, Schillie S, et al. Increases in acute hepatitis B virus infections - Kentucky, Tennessee, and West Virginia, 2006-2013. MMWR Morb Mortal Wkly Rep 2016;65(3):47–50.

25. Schillie S, Vellozzi C, Reingold A, et al. Prevention of hepatitis B virus infection in the United States: recommendations of the advisory committee on immunization practices. MMWR Recomm Rep 2018;67(1):1–31.

26. Salemi JL, Spooner KK, Mejia de Grubb MC, et al. National trends of hepatitis B and C during pregnancy across sociodemographic, behavioral, and clinical factors, United States, 1998-2011. J Med Virol 2017;89(6):1025–32.

27. Henderson JT, Webber EM, Bean SI. Screening for hepatitis B infection in pregnant women: updated evidence report and systematic review for the US preventive services task force. JAMA 2019;322(4):360–2.

28. World Health Organization. Guidelines for the prevention, care and treatment of persons with chronic hepatitis B infection. Geneva: WHO; 2015.

29. World Health Organization. Consolidated guidelines on the use of antiretroviral drugs for treating and preventing HIV infection: recommendations for a public health approach. Geneva: WHO; 2013.

30. Tang AS, Thornton K, and HBV Primary Care Workgroup. Hepatitis B Management: Guidance for the Primary Care Provider. Available at: https://www.hepatitisB.uw.edu/hbv-pcw/guidance.

31. Goldstein ST, Zhou F, Hadler SC, et al. A mathematical model to estimate global hepatitis B disease burden and vaccination impact. Int J Epidemiol 2005;34(6):1329–39.

32. Margolis HS, Coleman PJ, Brown RE, et al. Prevention of hepatitis B virus transmission by immunization. An economic analysis of current recommendations. JAMA 1995;274(15):1201–8.

33. Beasley RP, Hwang LY, Lee GC, et al. Prevention of perinatally transmitted hepatitis B virus infections with hepatitis B immune globulin and hepatitis B vaccine. Lancet 1983;2(8359):1099–102.

34. Chen DS. Hepatitis B vaccination: the key towards elimination and eradication of hepatitis B. J Hepatol 2009;50(4):805–16.

35. European Association for the Study of the Liver, Clinical Practice Guidelines Panel, Wendon J, et al. EASL Clinical Practical Guidelines on the management of acute (fulminant) liver failure. J Hepatol 2017;66(5):1047–81.

36. European Association for the Study of the Liver. EASL 2017 clinical practice guidelines on the management of hepatitis B virus infection. J Hepatol 2017;67(2):370–98.

37. Lee WM. Etiologies of acute liver failure. Semin Liver Dis 2008;28(2):142–52.

38. Dong V, Nanchal R, Karvellas CJ. Pathophysiology of acute liver failure. Nutr Clin Pract 2020;35(1):24–9.

39. Wright TL, Mamish D, Combs C, et al. Hepatitis B virus and apparent fulminant non-A, non-B hepatitis. Lancet 1992;339(8799):952–5.

40. Chang ML, Liaw YF. Hepatitis B flares in chronic hepatitis B: pathogenesis, natural course, and management. J Hepatol 2014;61(6):1407–17.

41. Yeo W, Zee B, Zhong S, et al. Comprehensive analysis of risk factors associating with Hepatitis B virus (HBV) reactivation in cancer patients undergoing cytotoxic chemotherapy. Br J Cancer 2004;90(7):1306–11.

42. Wai CT, Fontana RJ, Polson J, et al. Clinical outcome and virological characteristics of hepatitis B-related acute liver failure in the United States. J Viral Hepat 2005;12(2):192–8.

43. Garfein RS, Bower WA, Loney CM, et al. Factors associated with fulminant liver failure during an outbreak among injection drug users with acute hepatitis B. Hepatology 2004;40(4):865–73.
44. Tassopoulos NC, Papaevangelou GJ, Sjogren MH, et al. Natural history of acute hepatitis B surface antigen-positive hepatitis in Greek adults. Gastroenterology 1987;92(6):1844–50.
45. Tillmann HL, Hadem J, Leifeld L, et al. Safety and efficacy of lamivudine in patients with severe acute or fulminant hepatitis B, a multicenter experience. J Viral Hepat 2006;13(4):256–63.
46. Tillmann HL, Zachou K, Dalekos GN. Management of severe acute to fulminant hepatitis B: to treat or not to treat or when to treat? Liver Int 2012;32(4):544–53.
47. Jochum C, Maischack F, Anastasiou OE, et al. Treatment of fulminant acute hepatitis B with nucles(t)id analogues is safe and does not lead to secondary chronification of hepatitis B. Z Gastroenterol 2016;54(12):1306–11.
48. Wang CY, Zhao P, Liu WW, Acute Liver Failure Study Team. Acute liver failure caused by severe acute hepatitis B: a case series from a multi-center investigation. Ann Clin Microbiol Antimicrob 2014;13:23.
49. Streinu-Cercel A, Sandulescu O, Stefan M, et al. Treatment with lamivudine and entecavir in severe acute hepatitis B. Indian J Med Microbiol 2016;34(2):166–72.
50. Fontana RJ. Side effects of long-term oral antiviral therapy for hepatitis B. Hepatology 2009;49(5 Suppl):S185–95.
51. Apuzzio J, Block JM, Cullison S, et al. Chronic hepatitis B in pregnancy: a workshop consensus statement on screening, evaluation, and management, part 1. Female Patient 2012;37:22–34.
52. Owens DK, Davidson KW, Krist AH, et al. Screening for hepatitis B virus infection in pregnant women: US preventive services task force reaffirmation recommendation statement. JAMA 2019;322(4):349–54.
53. Weinbaum CM, Williams I, Mast EE, et al. Recommendations for identification and public health management of persons with chronic hepatitis B virus infection. MMWR Recomm Rep 2008;57(Rr-8):1–20.
54. World Health Organization. Hepatitis B vaccines: WHO position paper, July 2017 - recommendations. Vaccine 2019;37(2):223–5.

Treatment of Chronic Hepatitis B Virus with Oral Anti-Viral Therapy

Maria Buti, MD[a,b,*], Mar Riveiro-Barciela, MD, PhD[a,b], Rafael Esteban, MD[a,b]

KEYWORDS

- Hepatitis B • Tenofovir alafenomide (TAF) • Therapy

KEY POINTS

- Hepatitis B e antigen status play an important role for the identification of patients with indication of therapy, monitoring and the potential of therapy discontinuation.
- Real-world studies confirmed the efficacy and safety of entecavir, tenofovir disoproxil fumarate, and tenofovir alafenamide across a broad range of patients reflective of routine clinical practice.
- In patients with persistent low levels of viremia under nucleoside analogue or with multi-drug resistance new data suggest that switching to tenofovir disoproxil fumarate achieves a similar efficacy in terms of virologic response than the combination of tenofovir and entecavir.

Nucleoside analogues (NAs) are the drugs most commonly used in the treatment of chronic hepatitis B (CHB). These agents mainly act by inhibiting viral replication, and they have a minimal impact on hepatitis B surface antigen (HBsAg) loss. NAs are indicated in patients with chronic hepatitis, cirrhosis, decompensated cirrhosis, or hepatocellular carcinoma (HCC), as well as in those with extrahepatic manifestations. Real-world experience with NAs has been ongoing for more than 10 years, and the efficacy and safety results obtained are similar to those reported in clinical trials. Prolonged NA use is needed to maintain the suppression of viral replication, to prevent the development of liver cirrhosis and decompensated cirrhosis, and to decrease the risk of HCC. In patients with low viremia levels despite treatment with potent NAs, such as tenofovir disoproxil fumarate (TDF), tenofovir alafenamide (TAF), and entecavir (ETV), switching to combination therapy has not proven to be superior to maintaining monotherapy.

[a] Liver Unit, Internal Medicine Department, Hospital Universitari Vall d'Hebron, Passeig Vall d'Hebron 119-129, General Hospital, 5th floor, Barcelona 08035, Spain; [b] Centro de Investigación Biomédica en Red de Enfermedades Hepáticas y Digestivas (CIBERehd), Instituto de Salud Carlos III, Madrid, Spain
* Corresponding author. Liver Unit, Internal Medicine Department, Hospital Universitari Vall d'Hebron, Vall d'Hebron Barcelona Hospital Campus, Barcelona 08035, Spain.
E-mail address: mbuti@vhebron.net

Clin Liver Dis 25 (2021) 725–740
https://doi.org/10.1016/j.cld.2021.06.003
1089-3261/21/© 2021 Elsevier Inc. All rights reserved.

INDICATIONS FOR ANTIVIRAL THERAPY

The suppression of viral replication by NAs improves survival and the quality of life of patients with hepatitis B virus (HBV).[1] NAs with high barriers to resistance, such as ETV, TDF, and TAF, remain as the first-line treatments in clinical practice,[2,3] because all of them are highly effective at controlling HBV replication, are well-tolerated, and have a favorable safety profile.[4]

Achievement of HBsAg loss and, therefore, functional cure of chronic HBV infection is rare with NAs. The main aim of this therapy is prevention of disease progression and HCC development.[2,3] These goals usually require long-term treatment maintenance; hence, the indications for NA withdrawal are limited.[2,3] Additional aims of antiviral therapy include prevention of vertical HBV transmission from mothers to newborns, HBV reactivation in immunosuppressed patients, acute hepatitis B in cases of acute liver injury (international normalized ratio of >1.5) or acute liver failure (international normalized ratio of >1.5 plus hepatic encephalopathy), and treatment of HBV-associated extrahepatic manifestations.[2,5] The following are the main indications for antiviral therapy in patients chronically infected by HBV.

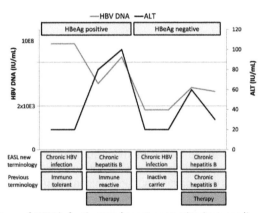

Fig. 1. Natural history of HBV infection and treatment criteria according to the HBV phase.

Liver Cirrhosis

Patients with HBV-related cirrhosis and detectable HBV DNA must be considered for antiviral therapy, regardless of their alanine aminotransferase (ALT) levels. This point is especially urgent in cases of decompensated cirrhosis, because NA treatment with the suppression of viral replication leads to a significant clinical improvement.[6] In compensated liver cirrhosis, NAs can achieve regression of cirrhosis, as was seen in the TDF registry study: 74% of patients with baseline liver cirrhosis were no longer cirrhotic after 5 years of TDF treatment.[7] NA therapy also decreases the risk of developing HCC, although studies in both Asian and Caucasian populations have reported that the risk persists despite long-term antiviral treatment.[8] A multicenter cohort study in the United States that included 841 patients treated with ETV for a median of 4 years—36% hepatitis B e antigen (HBeAg) positive and 9.3% cirrhotic—reported an HCC rate of 2.7%.[9] In Europe, a 10-center cohort study with 1951 adult Caucasian patients with CHB showed a decrease in the HCC incidence rate from 1.22% in the first year of NAs to 0.73% after the fifth year, a decrease that was particularly significant in individuals with underlying cirrhosis (3.22% vs 1.57%; $P = .039$).[10] Although some recent reports have indicated a higher risk of HCC among Asian patients with CHB treated with ETV than those receiving TDF,[11,12] a recent meta-analysis including 31 studies with 119,053 patients found no significant difference between the 2 drugs in their association with incident HCC.[13] Similarly, a recent multicenter study including 1935 Caucasians with CHB found no differences HCC incidence between those treated with ETV (5.4%) or TDF (6.0%).[14]

Hepatitis B e Antigen–Positive Chronic Hepatitis B

After a variable period of HBeAg-positive chronic infection, depending on the age at acquisition and HBV genotype, the HBeAg-positive chronic hepatitis phase emerges (**Fig. 1**). This stage is characterized by fluctuating and progressively decreasing HBV DNA values (although usually >20,000 IU/mL), elevated ALT concentration, and hepatic necroinflammation.[15] The ALT increases and flares are attributable to the host's immune response against the virus, with higher ALT values indicating a more vigorous response and more extensive hepatocyte damage.[16] These flares are associated with the development of liver cirrhosis, but they can also lead to hepatic decompensation and an 0.5% overall occurrence of liver failure.[17] Moreover, HBeAg-positive status is a well-recognized risk factor for developing HCC,[18,19] with an estimated incidence rate of 1169 cases per 100,000 person-years.[20] In the REACH-B cohort, which included 3584 untreated Taiwanese patients without cirrhosis and a validation group of 1505 patients from Hong Kong and South Korea, HBeAg-positive individuals had a 2.3-fold higher risk of developing HCC than HBeAg-negative participants.[18]

Periodic follow-up every 3 to 6 months is recommended for untreated HBeAg-positive individuals with a normal ALT and, if the patient's profile persists, a biopsy should be considered. Management decisions should be individualized, taking into account age, family history, health status, and socioeconomic factors.[21]

Hepatitis B e Antigen–Negative Chronic Hepatitis B

HBeAg-negative chronic hepatitis is the most common form of CHB worldwide, especially in European countries (**Fig. 2**).[22] In contrast with HBeAg-positive individuals, those with HBeAg-negative CHB are usually older and more likely to have cirrhosis at the time of the diagnosis.[22,23] This phase of the infection is characterized by HBV DNA of more than 2000 IU/mL plus increased ALT values, although these patients can show considerable fluctuations in serum ALT. Indeed, 20% to 30% of individuals with histologic evidence of significant liver fibrosis or necroinflammation have normal ALT values.[23] For this reason, the assessment of liver fibrosis is recommended in patients with a normal ALT and HBV DNA persistently of greater than 2000 IU/mL, because the presence of significant liver fibrosis or necroinflammation would be an indication for antiviral therapy.[2,3] Liver disease severity can be determined by biopsy findings or noninvasive tests such as elastography. In patients with normal ALT levels, liver stiffness values of greater than 9 kPa indicate significant liver damage with a specificity of 93%, whereas liver stiffness of less tan 6 kPa confirms the absence of significant fibrosis with a sensitivity of 94%.[24,25] Long-term longitudinal studies have reported that 15% to 24% of patients with HBeAg-negative chronic infection develop CHB over follow-up.[26,27] These data emphasize the need for close follow-up in HBeAg-negative patients with fluctuating HBV DNA levels, despite a normal ALT. Overall, for HBeAg-negative untreated patients with persistently normal ALT under close follow-up, the guidelines recommend ALT and HBV DNA monitoring every 6 months if HBV DNA is less than 2000 IU/mL. The follow-up intervals should be shortened when HBV DNA is 2000 to 20,000 IU/mL and liver biopsy is recommended when it reaches greater than 20,000 IU/mL.[21]

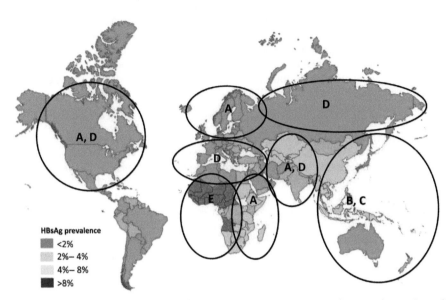

Fig. 2. HBsAg prevalence and most frequent HBV genotypes according to the region of origin.

Hepatocellular Carcinoma

Older age, male sex and the presence of cirrhosis are the most commonly accepted risk factors for developing HCC in patients with CHB,[28,29] and, as was mentioned elsewhere in this article, one of the main aims of NA therapy is to decrease the risk of HCC. However, NA treatment is also important in patients with established HBV-induced HCC; first, to suppress HBV replication with the aim of compensating the liver disease and, second, to decrease to the risk of HCC recurrence after potentially curative HCC treatment.[30]

Special mention should be made of patients with a family history of HCC. These individuals can receive antiviral therapy regardless of the previously mentioned criteria.[2,3] This recommendation lies in the synergistic effect between an HCC family history and HBV infection, regardless of the HBeAg or HBV DNA status.[31,32] A study performed in Taiwan including 374 cases of incident HCC over 362,268 person-years of follow-up reported a 15.8% cumulative risk of HCC in patients with a family history and 7.5% in those without ($P < .001$).[32]

Extrahepatic Manifestations of Hepatitis B Infection

Several extrahepatic immune-mediated disorders have been associated with chronic HBV infection, secondary to circulating immune complexes that activate serum complement.[33] The most common are glomerulonephritis, vasculitis such as polyarteritis nodosa, and reactive arthritis.[34] Although the available data on antiviral therapy in these disorders are limited and heterogeneous, NAs are recommended because of the potential prognostic improvement related to suppression of viral replication and possible seroconversion to an HBeAg-negative state.[35]

ROLE OF HEPATITIS B HBV DNA AS THE INDICATION FOR ANTIVIRAL THERAPY

HBV replication with subsequent immune-mediated liver injury is the main driver of the 2 main complications of CHB: cirrhosis and HCC. Data from large population-based studies, mainly including HBeAg-negative individuals, have shown that the risk of HCC, cirrhosis, and death increases proportionally with increasing HBV DNA values. In a prospective study from Taiwan with 3653 HBsAg-positive participants, the incidence of HCC increased with serum HBV DNA level in a dose–response relationship ranging from 1.3% in patients with HBV DNA less than 300 copies/mL to 14.9% in those with HBV 1 million or more copies/mL.[36] Interestingly, the risk of HCC associated with higher HBV DNA values remained significant after adjusting for classical HCC risk factors, such as sex, age, HBeAg status, ALT concentration, and the presence of liver cirrhosis at inclusion.[36] In this same cohort, the cumulative incidence of cirrhosis increased along with the HBV-DNA level, ranging from 4.5% in patients with a viral load of less than 300 copies/mL to 36.2% in those with 1 million or more copies/mL (P<.001).[37] Similar results have been reported in European studies. For example, Papatheodoridis and colleagues[38] evaluated liver disease severity in 399 HBeAg-negative patients with increased ALT values and found that the higher the HBV DNA level, the greater the percentage of patients with significant fibrosis or necroinflammation, ranging from 62% at HBV DNA less than 2000 IU/mL to 91% at more than 200,000 IU/mL.

Finally, special mention is due to the possible impact of HBV DNA level in HBeAg-positive patients. Although individuals in the immune-tolerant or HBeAg-positive infection phase are believed to have a good prognosis, recent data from a study conducted in Taiwan showed a non-negligible rate of both cirrhosis and HCC. In a cohort of 413 untreated HBeAg-positive patients with normal ALT (women, <19 IU/mL; men, <30 IU/mL) and HBV DNA of more than 20,000 IU/mL, the estimated 10-year cumulative incidence of HCC and death or transplantation was 12.7% and 9.7%, respectively, statistically higher rates than in HBeAg-positive patients with CHB receiving NAs (6.1% and 3.4%, respectively).[39]

ROLE OF E ANTIGEN STATUS IN THERAPY

HBeAg status has an important contribution in the indication for NA therapy, monitoring, and the possibility of stopping therapy. The indication for therapy in both HBeAg-positive and HBeAg-negative CHB is based on ALT and HBV DNA levels, and the presence of some degree of fibrosis. There are some slight differences in the indications between the international guidelines. The European Association for the Study of the Liver (EASL) and Asian Pacific Association for the Study of the Liver hepatitis B guidelines apply the same criteria for HBeAg-positive and HBeAg-negative patients to indicate initiation of therapy, whereas American Association for Study of Liver Disease requires an HBV DNA level of 20,000 IU/mL or greater in HBeAg-positive and 2000 IU/mL or greater in HBeAg-negative patients.[2,3]

A specific end point during antiviral therapy only in HBeAg-positive individuals is a serologic response, defined by HBeAg loss and HBeAg seroconversion. These events are associated with the induction of partial immune control and transition to a low replicative phase of CHB. However, HBeAg loss is not always stable and HBeAg seroreversion can occur after stopping therapy. A more persistent serologic response is seen when 12 months of NA consolidation therapy is used after HBeAg seroconversion, as reported in a systematic review in which most patients (90%) remained anti-HBe positive at 1 year after therapy discontinuation.[40]

Patients who achieve HBeAg loss and seroconversion to anti-HBe during the first 24 weeks of NA therapy have the highest likelihood of HBsAg loss and development of anti-HBs.[41] For this reason, some clinicians continue oral antiviral therapy regardless of the HBeAg response until HBsAg loss. However, scientific evidence supporting this strategy is still weak.

Long-term NA therapy is recommended in HBeAg-negative CHB until HBsAg loss is achieved, if there are no safety issues. The EASL guidelines state that NA therapy can be discontinued in selected noncirrhotic HBeAg-negative patients who remain HBsAg positive despite persistent NA viral suppression.[2] Two important requisites for NA discontinuation are the patient's desire to stop therapy and the guarantee of close post-NA follow-up. Several retrospective studies have been performed in this setting, but very few have a randomized, prospective design. In these reports, there is a trend to achieving HBsAg loss more often in Caucasian than in Asian HBeAg-negative patients. In a large prospective study, 159 virally suppressed HBeAg-negative patients without cirrhosis were randomized to stop therapy or continue TDF for 96 weeks. After this period, HBsAg loss was achieved in 10% of patients in the group that stopped and in none of those that continued with TDF ($P = .006$). HBV DNA levels were 20 IU/mL or less in 31% of patients who stopped TDF and in all patients who continued ($P<.001$). These results indicate the potential of discontinuing long-term NA treatment to induce durable immune control and HBsAg clearance in HBeAg-negative patients with CHB.[42]

In addition, several studies have shown that low HBsAg concentration (<100 IU/mL) at the time of NA discontinuation is associated with a higher likelihood of HBsAg loss.

In summary, HBeAg status is important for identifying patients with an indication for therapy, for monitoring purposes, and for determining the potential of therapy discontinuation.

RESULTS OF ORAL ANTIVIRAL THERAPY: A COMPARISON OF EFFICACY AND SIDE EFFECTS

Oral antivirals are the drugs most often used in the treatment of CHB. Three drugs—ETV, TDF, and TAF—are the first-line recommended treatments for CHB in adults. All these agents act by blocking the reverse transcriptase and inhibiting reverse transcription of pregenomic RNA to HBV DNA, thereby preventing HBV from multiplying. TDF and TAF are both prodrugs of tenofovir. TAF is more stable than TDF in plasma and it provides a more efficient delivery of tenofovir to liver cells. In addition, TAF can be given in lower doses than TDF, which implies less associated renal and bone toxicity.

ETV was approved by the US Food and Drug Administration for treating CHB in 2005, TDF in 2008 (although it had been approved for HIV in 2001), and TAF in 2018. Therefore, the real-world clinical experience is more extensive and longer for ETV and TDF than for TAF. All 3 drugs are potent antivirals with a high genetic barrier to resistance in naïve patients. In patients previously treated with lamivudine (LAM); however, ETV has been associated with a high risk of genotypic resistance (50% after 5 years). Regarding renal function, dosing of both ETV and TDF must be adjusted to the estimated glomerular filtration rate (eGFR) in patients with values of less than 50. TAF is given in a fixed dosed and can be administered without dose adjustment in patients with an eGFR less than 50. Adverse effects on renal function and bone mineral density have been associated with TDF, whereas TAF has a potentially better renal and bone profile. Finally, ETV is not indicated in patients with HIV receiving antiretroviral therapy because of the risk of HIV resistance, and it is contraindicated in pregnancy. The indications and management of these 3 drugs in patients with CHB are summarized in **Table 1**.[2,3]

In the related registration studies, the efficacy and safety of ETV and TDF were not compared in a head-to-head design, whereas TDF and TAF were evaluated in a randomized double-blind study. Overall, the serum ALT normalization rates, viral suppression assessed by HBV DNA of less than 60 IU/mL, HBeAg loss with or without

Table 1
Summary of the indications and management of recommended drugs for patients with CHB

	ETV	TDF	TAF
Efficacy	Potent antiviral activity	Potent antiviral activity	Potent antiviral activity
Drug resistance	High barrier to resistance Genotypic resistance rates are higher (51% at 5 y) in ETV-treated patients with preexisting LAM-resistant CHB	High barrier to resistance	High barrier to resistance
Renal Considerations	Dose adjustment in patients with $eGFR_{CG}$ of <50 mL/min Can be used in hemodialysis patients	Dose adjustment in patients with $eGFR_{CG}$ of <50 mL/min Renal events reported	Can be used in patients with $eGFR_{CG}$ of <50 mL/min without dose adjustment Less progression to CKD compared with TDF
Bone Considerations		Greater bone toxicity compared with TAF	Less bone toxicity compared with TDF
General Considerations	Not used in patients with HIV without HAART Not used in pregnancy		

Abbreviations: CKD, chronic kidney disease; $eGFR_{CG}$, Estimated glomerular filtration rate by Cockcroft-Gault; HAART, highly active antiretroviral therapy; HIV, human immunodeficiency virus.

anti-HBe detection, HBsAg loss, and improvements in liver histology were very similar between ETV- and TDF-treated patients. After 3 years of TDF or ETV therapy, HBV DNA suppression (<60 IU/mL) occurred in 61% to 71% of HBeAg-positive patients and 90% to 93% of HBeAg-negative patients. In most cases, HBV DNA suppression was associated with normalization of ALT levels. In addition, very few patients cleared HBsAg: 4% to 8% of HBeAg-positive and 0% to 1% of HBeAg-negative patients. Hence, the majority needed long-term therapy. A recent study performed in China compared the efficacy and safety of ETV and TDF in 320 treatment-naïve HBeAg-positive patients with CHB who randomly received either ETV or TDF for 144 weeks. After this period, there were no differences in viral suppression (HBV DNA levels with ETV vs TDF, $-6.6485 \log_{10}$ IU/mL vs $-6.692 \log_{10}$ IU/mL; $P = .807$), ALT normalization, or serologic response. The safety profile was comparable between the 2 drugs and there were no obvious fluctuations in the eGFR.[43]

TDF and TAF were compared in 425 HBeAg-negative and 873 HBeAg-positive patients included in 2 identically designed double-blind, phase III studies. Patients were randomized to receive TAF or TDF in a 2:1 ratio for 3 years. The antiviral efficacy of TAF was noninferior to that of TDF, with superior renal and bone safety. After completing up to 3 years of double-blind treatment, patients entered an open-label TAF phase through year 8. Currently, results are available to year 5. Of 1298 randomized and treated patients, 1157 (89%; 775 TAF, 382 TDF) entered the open-label phase, including 180 and 202 TDF-treated patients, beginning TAF at week 96 (TDF-OLTAF

3y) and week 144 (TDF- OLTAF 2y), respectively, before a protocol amendment. At year 5, the majority of patients remained on treatment, and virologic suppression (HBV DNA of <29 IU/mL) occurred in 93% of those receiving TAF and 92% to 96% of those who switched from TDF to TAF at year 2 or 3. ALT normalization was achieved in 74% to 76% of cases and HBsAg loss in only 1% to 3%, independent of the therapeutic group. No genotypic resistance to TAF was observed. Rates of grade 3 and 4 adverse events and adverse events leading to discontinuation were low and similar between the groups. After experiencing decreases in the eGFR and in hip and spine bone mineral density over 2 or 3 years of TDF treatment, the patients' renal and bone outcomes improved after the switch to open-label TAF.[44]

ETV, TDF, and TAF have been widely used in real-world practice, particularly TDF and ETV. The efficacy and safety of ETV in previously untreated patients is similar to the performance reported in registration studies. Retrospective analysis of ETV in a real-world study in 841 treatment-naïve patients with CHB in the United States showed undetectable HBV DNA rates at 1, 3, and 5 years of 34.6%, 64.7%, and 84.6% in HBeAg-positive patients, and 81.9%, 90.3%, and 96.2% in HBeAg-negative patients. ALT had normalized at 1, 3, and 5 years in 37.2%, 48.7%, and 56.2% of HBeAg-positive and 39.6%, 46.8%, and 55.6% of HBeAg-negative patients, respectively. HBsAg loss was reported at 4.6%. ETV was discontinued in 1.2% of patients owing to adverse events. The study showed that ETV treatment was safe in a large cohort of patients, but ALT normalization was lower than previously reported in clinical trials.[9] Another real-world study with ETV is a 5-year prospective trial that enrolled 3408 patients with CHB in China. Among them, 1807 and 628 received ETV- and LAM-based therapy, respectively. The virologic response rate at week 240 was 73% in both treatment groups. Compared with LAM-based therapy, ETV was associated with a significantly lower incidence of viral breakthrough (12.6% vs 2.1%) and genotypic resistance (10.1% vs 1.2%) (P<.0001 for both), as well as lower rates of progression to decompensated cirrhosis (9.6% vs 6.4%) and HCC (1.9% vs 0.8%).[45]

Real-world data on TDF have also confirmed the results of registration studies. TDF was evaluated in 440 consecutive patients with CHB in an observational multicenter study in France. After 36 months, 96% of the overall cohort achieved virologic response (HBV DNA <69 IU/mL) and 77% had normal ALT levels. TDF was well tolerated over the 36-month study, even in the 14 women who became pregnant during the study. The median eGFR did not change markedly from baseline, regardless of the prior treatment history.[46]

In Spain, the effectiveness and safety of ETV and TDF was analyzed in 187 patients receiving ETV and 424 TDF for more than 4 years. Viral suppression (HBV DNA <69 IU/mL) and ALT normalization were achieved in 90% of patients by month 36. HBeAg clearance occurred in 33% of cases, whereas only 4 patients lost HBsAg. Renal function remained stable on long-term follow-up.[47] In all these studies, TDF demonstrated a potent virologic and biochemical response across a broad range of patients, such as those encountered in routine clinical practice. The safety profile was consistent with results from pivotal trials.

However, the long-term effects of TDF on renal function in CHB are still controversial. In a cohort of 640 treatment-naïve patients with CHB who received TDF for 5 years, the serum creatinine increased from 0.77 ± 0.01 mg/dL to 0.85 ± 0.02 mg/dL (P<.001), and the eGFR decreased from 102.6 ± 0.6 mL/min/1.73 m^2 to 93.4 ± 1.4 mL/min/1.73 m^2 (P<.001). The eGFR decrease was more evident in patients with a baseline eGFR of less than 60 mL/min/1.73 m^2 and in those taking diuretics.[48]

One retrospective study included experienced patients with moderate-to-severe renal failure who received either ETV or TDF for a median follow-up of 3.1 years. The effectiveness was similar between treatments. Only 1.9% of TDF-treated patients experienced renal tubular dysfunction.[49] Another retrospective study investigated 4983 treatment-naïve and risk factor-matched adult patients with CHB who received either TDF (n = 1790) or ETV (n = 3193) for more than 12 months. Among those with an eGFR of greater than 60 mL/min/1.73 m^2, the 5-year cumulative incidence of renal impairment was 45% for ETV and 49.8% for TDF (P = .0039). Factors associated with worsening renal function on Cox regression analysis were TDF therapy (hazard ratio [HR], 1.41), older age (HR, 1.02), male sex (HR, 2.16), the presence of diabetes or hypertension (HR, 1.4), and a higher Fibrosis-4 score (HR, 1.02). These results suggest that TDF should be used with caution in patients with a high risk of renal impairment.[50]

TAF has been evaluated in a multicenter phase III study in which 489 patients receiving TDF were randomly assigned (1:1) to receive TAF 25 mg/d or continue with TDF up to week 48; thereafter, all patients received open-label TAF up to week 96. Virologic suppression (HBV DNA of <20 IU/mL) was similar in the 2 groups (95% vs 94%). The increases in spine and hip bone mineral density at week 96 were also similar in patients switched to TAF at baseline and those switched at week 48. In the TDF group, the eGFR decrease seen at week 48 (−2.7 mL/min) had improved at week 96 after switching to TAF (−0.39 mL/min). These findings suggest that TAF can be substituted for TDF in patients with HBV infection to improve safety without a loss of efficacy.[51]

Patients with CHB and renal impartment require periodic dose adjustment of ETV and TDF. In this setting, TAF has the advantage that it can be given to patients with an eGFR of less than 50 without dose adjustment. In 93 renally impaired (moderate/severe impairment 78, end-stage renal disease 15) patients with CHB, virally suppressed with TDF or another NA, switching to TAF was associated with maintenance of viral suppression in nearly all patients and a high percentage had normal ALT levels. In addition, it resulted in stable hip and spine bone mineral density and slight improvements in the eGFR and markers of renal tubular function in moderate to severely impaired patients, with no changes in those with end-stage renal disease at week 48.[52]

The TRIO HBV network analyzed the real-world efficacy and safety of TAF in 270 patients with CHB. After a mean follow-up of 508 days in patients previously receiving TDF (81%), ETV (8%), or other drugs, switching to TAF was associated with statistically significant improvements in ALT levels, HBV DNA suppression, and stabilization of renal function.[53] In elderly patients, a pooled analysis of 124 patients aged 65 years or older treated with TAF in large trials showed that older patients had a lower eGFR and hip and spine bone mineral density than younger ones. During TAF treatment, the rates of virologic suppression, adverse events, and serious adverse events were similar between older and younger patients. However, eGFR increases were greater in younger patients receiving TAF, whereas changes in hip and spine bone mineral density were similar. TDF treatment resulted in decreases in bone mineral density and eGFR. Small improvements in renal and bone parameters were seen in older patients switched from TDF to TAF.[54] TAF was analyzed retrospectively in 409 patients with CHB switched from ETV. Suppression of viral replication increased from 91.0% to 97.8% (P = .001) at 18 months after switching and there were no changes in the distribution of chronic kidney disease stages during this period. All these studies confirm that TAF is a better option than TDF for patients with risk factors for renal or bone changes, as recommended in the EASL guidelines.[2,55]

WHAT TO DO WHEN ORAL ANTIVIRAL THERAPY FAILS TO DECREASE HEPATITIS B DNA TO UNDETECTABLE: IS THERE A ROLE FOR COMBINATION THERAPY?

Most patients receiving oral antiviral therapy achieve a decrease in HBV DNA. However, in some cases, low HBV DNA levels or virologic blips emerge after viremia becomes undetectable during therapy. Virologic blips are usually attributable to low adherence to the medication. Low viremia levels or a slow virologic response are generally seen in HBeAg-positive patients with high pretreatment HBV DNA levels, usually greater than 10^7 IU/mL. HBeAg positive high pretreatment levels represents 10% to 30% of HBeAg-positive patients during the first 2 years of therapy. Virologic response takes more time in HBeAg-positive patients with low HBV DNA levels than in negative patients, and the low viremia levels detected are not related to poor effectiveness or drug resistance.[56] In ETV-, TDF- or TAF-treated patients with persistently detectable HBV DNA after week 48, it is important to determine HBV DNA levels and kinetics and to ascertain adherence to medication. If there is a continuous decline in HBV DNA regardless of adherence, the patient can continue with the same drug. A complete virologic response is expected by extending therapy. If there is low adherence to medication, the recommendation is to reinforce compliance.

The impact of low viremia levels during antiviral therapy on liver-related outcomes was evaluated by Jang and colleagues.[57] The study compared long-term follow-up findings between patients who achieved and maintained a virologic response (HBV DNA <20 IU/mL) and patients who did not achieve this response or had intermittently or persistently detectable HBV DNA after it had become undetectable. The cumulative 10-year survival rates were 71.6% in those with a maintained virologic response compared with only 18.8% in those without and 57.2% in those with intermittent viremia. However, the authors reported that the type of previous virologic response did not have a significant influence on the risk of incident HCC, with rates of 37% to 48%, depending on the type of response. In contrast, a study performed in patients with compensated CHB found that persistent or intermittent low-level viremia (HBV DNA of <2000 IU/mL) was associated with a significantly higher HCC risk than in those who maintained a virologic response.[58]

The current recommendation for patients with persistent viremia is to continue with the same drug if there is a continuous decline in viremia levels.[2] If viremia remains stable or increases under ETV, TDF, or TAF, combination therapy is usually not recommended. Resistance to these drugs is minimal and results from several studies have shown that TDF monotherapy suffices when adherence to therapy is adequate.

Patients who present virologic blips during therapy after undetectable viremia represent another situation. In this case, it is always important to check for therapy adherence. If patients are receiving drugs with a low barrier to resistance such as LAM, adefovir (ADV), or telbivudine, a change is recommended to a more potent antiviral with a high barrier to resistance and no cross-resistance. In cases of partial response to LAM or ETV, TDF or TAF can be used, and in cases of partial response to ADV, the recommended switch is to ETV (if LAM has not been used previously) or to TDF or TAF.

SWITCHING TO TENOFOVIR DISOPROXIL FUMARATE VERSUS COMBINATION THERAPY

In an open-label, randomized controlled trial including 45 patients with CHB who had a partial virologic response and no resistance to ETV after 12 months, 22 patients were randomly switched to TDF and 23 continued with ETV. The suppression of viral replication (HBV DNA of <20 IU/mL) per protocol analysis was significantly higher in the TDF than the ETV group (55% vs 20%; P = .022) at 12 months after the switch, showing that this strategy is more effective than continuing with ETV.[59]

In patients with CHB who have developed multidrug resistance, several studies show that TDF is an excellent rescue therapy (**Table 2**). One prospective, multicenter, real-world cohort study included 174 patients receiving rescue monotherapy with TDF and 249 receiving TDF-based combination therapy (LAM or telbivudine or ETV). Cumulative virologic response rates did not differ significantly between patients receiving TDF monotherapy or combination therapy at 48 weeks (71.7% vs 68.9%), 96 weeks (85.1% vs 84.2%), 144 weeks (92.1% vs 92.7%), 192 weeks (93.4% vs 95.7%), or 240 weeks (97.7% vs 97.2%). There were no significant differences in the virologic response according to age, sex, presence of cirrhosis, HBeAg status, or renal function (all, P>.05).[60]

Another study evaluated the outcome of TDF monotherapy versus ETV plus TDF combination therapy in 90 patients with CHB with ETV resistance and 102 with ADV resistance. Patients were randomized 1:1 to receive TDF or TDF plus ETV for 48 weeks, and thereafter, TDF monotherapy up to week 240. The percentage of patients at week 240 with undetectable serum HBV DNA (<15 IU/mL) did not differ significantly between the ETV and ADV resistance groups in the full analysis set (84.4% vs 73.5%; P = .07). Few patients presented HBV DNA blips, and these events were associated with suboptimal adherence to medication. None developed additional HBV resistance mutations. However, significant decreases from baseline in the eGFR (-3.21 mL/min/ 1.73 m^2, P<.001) and bone mineral density (P<.001) were observed at week 240; hence, safety was the main concern.[61]

SWITCHING TO TENOFOVIR ALAFENAMIDE

To improve the safety profile of TDF, the efficacy and safety of TAF switching in patients with CHB with advanced fibrosis and a partial response to other NAs was investigated in 80 patients (fibrosis stage 3 and cirrhosis) with detectable HBV DNA receiving NAs. The preliminary results in 24 patients previously treated with ETV

Table 2
Studies comparing the efficacy of monotherapy versus combination therapy in patients with CHB with persistent, low HBV DNA or multidrug resistance to first-line oral antiviral

Previous Drug	Response in Patients with Chronic Liver Disease	Author, Year
ETV partial virologic response	Switch to TDF vs continue ETV TDF (n = 22) HBV DNA undetectable, 55% at month 12 ETV (n = 23) HBV DNA undetectable, 20% at month 12	Yim et al,[59] 2018
Multidrug resistance	Multicenter, prospective, real-world study TDF (n = 174) virologic response, 97.7% at week 240 TDF combination with NA (LAM or telbivudine), or ETV (n = 249) 97.2% at week 24	Lee et al,[60] 2019
ADV resistance ETV resistance	Randomized TDF or TDF + ETV (1:1) for 48 weeks, and TDF thereafter up to week 240 ETV resistance group (n = 90), viral response 84.4% ADV resistance group (n = 102), viral response 73.5%	Lim et al,[61] 2019

(n = 14) or TDF (n = 9) and LAM (n = 1) showed a decrease in HBV DNA, which became undetectable in 75% at week 24 after switching. There were no significant changes in the serum creatinine or eGFR levels from enrollment to week 24. TAF has the advantage of a better renal and bone safety profile for patients with multidrug resistance requiring long-term therapy.[62]

SUMMARY

In patients with low levels of viremia while receiving NAs and in those with multidrug resistance, new data suggest that switching to TDF will achieve a virologic response similar to that of combination therapy with TDF and an NA. Control of viral replication will further improve the outcome of chronic HBV infection.

CLINICS CARE POINTS

- Oral nucleoside analogues therapies improve survival and quality of life of patients with chronic hepatitis B.
- Nucleoside analogues are highly effective in suppressing HBV replication though rarely achieve HBsAg lost or functional cure.
- Long-term nucleoside analogues prevent progression of HBV-related fibrosis and reduce the risk of hepatocellular cacinoma development.
- Real-world experience with nucleoside analogues has confirmed the high efficacy and safety results observed in clinical trials.

DISCLOSURE

M. Buti has received research grants from Gilead and has served as advisors for Gilead, Bristol-Myers Squibb, and Novartis. M. Riveiro-Barciela has received research grants from Gilead and served as speaker for Gilead and Grifols. R. Esteban has received research grants from Gilead and has served as advisors for Gilead, Bristol-Myers Squibb, and Novartis.

REFERENCES

1. Lok AS, McMahon BJ, Brown RS Jr, et al. Antiviral therapy for chronic hepatitis B viral infection in adults: a systematic review and meta-analysis. Hepatology 2016; 63(1):284–306.
2. EASL 2017 Clinical Practice Guidelines on the management of hepatitis B virus infection. J Hepatol 2017;67(2):370–98.
3. Terrault NA, Lok ASF, McMahon BJ, et al. Update on prevention, diagnosis, and treatment of chronic hepatitis B: AASLD 2018 hepatitis B guidance. Hepatology 2018;67(4):1560–99.
4. Roade R, Riveiro-Barciela R, Esteban R, et al. Long-term efficacy and safety of nucleos(t)ides analogues in patients with chronic hepatitis B. Ther Adv Infect Dis 2021;8:1–13.
5. Wendon J, Cordoba J, Dhawan A, et al. EASL Clinical Practical Guidelines on the management of acute (fulminant) liver failure. J Hepatol 2017;66(5):1047–81.
6. Shim JH, Lee HC, Kim KM, et al. Efficacy of entecavir in treatment-naïve patients with hepatitis B virus-related decompensated cirrhosis. J Hepatol 2010;52(2): 176–82.

7. Marcellin P, Gane E, Buti M, et al. Regression of cirrhosis during treatment with tenofovir disoproxil fumarate for chronic hepatitis B: a 5-year open-label follow-up study. Lancet 2013;381(9865):468–75.

8. Papatheodoridis GV, Chan HL, Hansen BE, et al. Risk of hepatocellular carcinoma in chronic hepatitis B: assessment and modification with current antiviral therapy. J Hepatol 2015;62(4):956–67.

9. Ahn J, Lee HM, Lim JK, et al. Entecavir safety and effectiveness in a national cohort of treatment-naïve chronic hepatitis B patients in the US - the ENUMERATE study. Aliment Pharmacol Ther 2016;43(1):134–44.

10. Papatheodoridis GV, Idilman R, Dalekos GN, et al. The risk of hepatocellular carcinoma decreases after the first 5 years of entecavir or tenofovir in Caucasians with chronic hepatitis B. Hepatology 2017;66(5):1444–53.

11. Choi J, Kim HJ, Lee J, et al. Risk of hepatocellular carcinoma in patients treated with entecavir vs tenofovir for chronic hepatitis B: a Korean nationwide cohort study. JAMA Oncol 2019;5(1):30–6.

12. Yip TC, Wong VW, Chan HL, et al. Tenofovir is associated with lower risk of hepatocellular carcinoma than entecavir in patients with chronic HBV infection in China. Gastroenterology 2020;158(1):215–25.e216.

13. Tseng CH, Hsu YC, Chen TH, et al. Hepatocellular carcinoma incidence with tenofovir versus entecavir in chronic hepatitis B: a systematic review and meta-analysis. Lancet Gastroenterol Hepatol 2020;5(12):1039–52.

14. Papatheodoridis GV, Dalekos GN, Idilman R, et al. Similar risk of hepatocellular carcinoma during long-term entecavir or tenofovir therapy in Caucasian patients with chronic hepatitis B. J Hepatol 2020;73(5):1037–45.

15. Fattovich G, Bortolotti F, Donato F. Natural history of chronic hepatitis B: special emphasis on disease progression and prognostic factors. J Hepatol 2008; 48(2):335–52.

16. Liaw YF. Hepatitis flares and hepatitis B e antigen seroconversion: implication in anti-hepatitis B virus therapy. J Gastroenterol Hepatol 2003;18(3):246–52.

17. Chu CM, Liaw YF. Increased incidence of fulminant hepatic failure in previously unrecognized HBsAg carriers with acute hepatitis independent of etiology. Infection 2005;33(3):136–9.

18. Yang HI, Yuen MF, Chan HL, et al. Risk estimation for hepatocellular carcinoma in chronic hepatitis B (REACH-B): development and validation of a predictive score. Lancet Oncol 2011;12(6):568–74.

19. Jung KS, Kim SU, Ahn SH, et al. Risk assessment of hepatitis B virus-related hepatocellular carcinoma development using liver stiffness measurement (FibroScan). Hepatology 2011;53(3):885–94.

20. Yang HI, Lu SN, Liaw YF, et al. Hepatitis B e antigen and the risk of hepatocellular carcinoma. N Engl J Med 2002;347(3):168–74.

21. Lampertico P, Maini M, Papatheodoridis G. Optimal management of hepatitis B virus infection - EASL Special Conference. J Hepatol 2015;63(5):1238–53.

22. Zarski JP, Marcellin P, Leroy V, et al. Characteristics of patients with chronic hepatitis B in France: predominant frequency of HBe antigen negative cases. J Hepatol 2006;45(3):355–60.

23. Hadziyannis SJ, Papatheodoridis GV. Hepatitis B e antigen-negative chronic hepatitis B: natural history and treatment. Semin Liver Dis 2006;26(2):130–41.

24. Viganò M, Paggi S, Lampertico P, et al. Dual cut-off transient elastography to assess liver fibrosis in chronic hepatitis B: a cohort study with internal validation. Aliment Pharmacol Ther 2011;34(3):353–62.

25. EASL-ALEH Clinical Practice Guidelines. Non-invasive tests for evaluation of liver disease severity and prognosis. J Hepatol 2015;63(1):237–64.

26. Fattovich G, Olivari N, Pasino M, et al. Long-term outcome of chronic hepatitis B in Caucasian patients: mortality after 25 years. Gut 2008;57(1):84–90.

27. McMahon BJ, Holck P, Bulkow L, et al. Serologic and clinical outcomes of 1536 Alaska Natives chronically infected with hepatitis B virus. Ann Intern Med 2001; 135(9):759–68.

28. Papatheodoridis G, Dalekos G, Sypsa V, et al. PAGE-B predicts the risk of developing hepatocellular carcinoma in Caucasians with chronic hepatitis B on 5-year antiviral therapy. J Hepatol 2016;64(4):800–6.

29. Voulgaris T, Papatheodoridi M, Lampertico P, et al. Clinical utility of hepatocellular carcinoma risk scores in chronic hepatitis B. Liver Int 2020;40(3):484–95.

30. EASL-EORTC clinical practice guidelines: management of hepatocellular carcinoma. J Hepatol 2012;56(4):908–43.

31. Varbobitis I, Papatheodoridis GV. The assessment of hepatocellular carcinoma risk in patients with chronic hepatitis B under antiviral therapy. Clin Mol Hepatol 2016;22(3):319–26.

32. Loomba R, Liu J, Yang HI, et al. Synergistic effects of family history of hepatocellular carcinoma and hepatitis B virus infection on risk for incident hepatocellular carcinoma. Clin Gastroenterol Hepatol 2013;11(12):1636, 1645.e1631-1633.

33. Shah AS, Amarapurkar DN. Spectrum of hepatitis B and renal involvement. Liver Int 2018;38(1):23–32.

34. Seto WK, Lo YR, Pawlotsky JM, et al. Chronic hepatitis B virus infection. Lancet 2018;392(10161):2313–24.

35. Han SH. Extrahepatic manifestations of chronic hepatitis B. Clin Liver Dis 2004; 8(2):403–18.

36. Chen CJ, Yang HI, Su J, et al. Risk of hepatocellular carcinoma across a biological gradient of serum hepatitis B virus DNA level. JAMA 2006;295(1):65–73.

37. Iloeje UH, Yang HI, Su J, et al. Predicting cirrhosis risk based on the level of circulating hepatitis B viral load. Gastroenterology 2006;130(3):678–86.

38. Papatheodoridis GV, Manesis EK, Manolakopoulos S, et al. Is there a meaningful serum hepatitis B virus DNA cutoff level for therapeutic decisions in hepatitis B e antigen-negative chronic hepatitis B virus infection? Hepatology 2008;48(5): 1451–9.

39. Kim GA, Lim YS, Han S, et al. High risk of hepatocellular carcinoma and death in patients with immune-tolerant-phase chronic hepatitis B. Gut 2018;67(5):945–52.

40. Papatheodoridis G, Vlachogiannakos I, Cholongitas E, et al. Discontinuation of oral antivirals in chronic hepatitis B: a systematic review. Hepatology 2016; 63(5):1481–92.

41. Marcellin P, Buti M, Krastev Z, et al. Kinetics of hepatitis B surface antigen loss in patients with HBeAg-positive chronic hepatitis B treated with tenofovir disoproxil fumarate. J Hepatol 2014;61(6):1228–37.

42. van Bömmel F, Stein K, Heyne R, et al. Response to discontinuation of long-term nucleos(t)ide analogue treatment in HBeAg negative patients: results of the Stop-NUC trial. J Hepatol 2020;73:S118.

43. Cai D, Pan C, Yu W, et al. Comparison of the long-term efficacy of tenofovir and entecavir in nucleos(t)ide analogue-naïve HBeAg-positive patients with chronic hepatitis B: a large, multicentre, randomized controlled trials. Medicine 2019; 98(1):e13983.

44. Chan H, Buti M, Agarwal K, et al. Maintenance of high levels of viral suppression and improved safety profile of tenofovir alafenamide (TAF) relative to tenofovir

disoproxil fumarate (TDF) in chronic hepatitis B patients treated for 5 years in 2 ongoing phase 3 studies. Hepatology 2020;72(S1):490A.

45. Jia J, Shang J, Tang H, et al. Long-term outcomes in Chinese patients with chronic hepatitis B receiving nucleoside/nucleotide analogue therapy in real-world clinical practice: 5-year results from the EVOLVE study. Antivir Ther 2020; 25(6):293–304.

46. Marcellin P, Zoulim F, Hézode C, et al. Effectiveness and safety of tenofovir disoproxil fumarate in chronic hepatitis B: a 3-year, prospective, real-world study in France. Dig Dis Sci 2016;61(10):3072–83.

47. Riveiro-Barciela M, Tabernero D, Calleja JL, et al. Effectiveness and safety of entecavir or tenofovir in a Spanish cohort of chronic hepatitis B patients: validation of the page-B score to predict hepatocellular carcinoma. Dig Dis Sci 2017;62(3): 784–93.

48. Lim TS, Lee JS, Kim BK, et al. An observational study on long-term renal outcome in patients with chronic hepatitis B treated with tenofovir disoproxil fumarate. J viral Hepat 2020;27(3):316–22.

49. Lampertico P, Berg T, Buti M, et al. Treatment with tenofovir disoproxil fumarate or entecavir in chronic hepatitis B virus-infected patients with renal impairment: results from a 7-year, multicentre retrospective cohort study. Aliment Pharmacol Ther 2020;52(3):500–12.

50. Mak L, Hoang J, Jun D, et al. Longitudinal real-world study on estimated glomerular filtration rate (eGFR) changes in entecavir (ETV) versus tenofovir disoproxil fumarate (TDF)-treated chronic hepatitis B (CHB) patients: a REAL-B study. Hepatology 2020;72(S1):17A.

51. Lampertico P, Buti M, Ramji A, et al. A phase 3 study comparing switching from tenofovir disoproxil fumarate (TDF) to tenofovir alafenamide (TAF) with continued TDF treatment in virologically-suppressed patients with chronic hepatitis B (CHB): final week 96 efficacy and safety results. J Hepatol 2020;73:S67.

52. Janssen H, Lampertico P, Chen C, et al. Safety and efficacy of switching to tenofovir alafenamide (TAF) in virally suppressed chronic hepatitis B (CHB) patients with renal impairment: week 48 results from a phase 2 open label study. J Hepatol 2020;72:S866–7.

53. Reddy R, Curry M, Bae H, et al. Longer-term experience with tenofovir alafenamide (TAF) in HBV infected patients; changes in EGFR, FIB4, ALT, and DNA suppression. J Hepatol 2020;73:S881–2.

54. Fung S, Brunetto S, Buti M, et al. Safety and efficacy of tenofovir alafenamide in geriatric patients with chronic hepatitis B: experience from four ongoing phase 2 and phase 3 clinical trials. J Hepatol 2020;73:S883–4.

55. Nguyen M, Atsukawa M, Ishikawa T, et al. Increased viral suppression rate in real-world chronic hepatitis B (CHB) patients after switch from long-term entecavir therapy to tenofovir alafenamide (TAF): a multicenter study. Hepatology 2020; 72(Suppl 1):486A.

56. Gordon SC, Krastev Z, Horban A, et al. Efficacy of tenofovir disoproxil fumarate at 240 weeks in patients with chronic hepatitis B with high baseline viral load. Hepatology 2013;58(2):505–13.

57. Jang JW, Choi JY, Kim YS, et al. Effects of virologic response to treatment on short- and long-term outcomes of patients with chronic hepatitis B virus infection and decompensated cirrhosis. Clin Gastroenterol Hepatol 2018;16(12): 1954–63.e1953.

58. Kim JH, Sinn DH, Kang W, et al. Low-level viremia and the increased risk of hepatocellular carcinoma in patients receiving entecavir treatment. Hepatology 2017;66(2):335–43.

59. Yim HJ, Kim IH, Suh SJ, et al. Switching to tenofovir vs continuing entecavir for hepatitis B virus with partial virologic response to entecavir: a randomized controlled trial. J viral Hepat 2018;25(11):1321–30.

60. Lee HW, Park JY, Lee JW, et al. Long-term efficacy of tenofovir disoproxil fumarate monotherapy for multidrug-resistant chronic HBV infection. Clin Gastroenterol Hepatol 2019;17(7):1348–55.e1342.

61. Lim YS, Gwak GY, Choi J, et al. Monotherapy with tenofovir disoproxil fumarate for adefovir-resistant vs. entecavir-resistant chronic hepatitis B: a 5-year clinical trial. J Hepatol 2019;71(1):35–44.

62. Yeh M, Chen C, Cheng P, et al. Efficacy and safety of switching to tenofovir alafenamide for chronic hepatitis B patients with advanced fibrosis and partial virologic response to oral nucleos(t)ide analogues (ESTAB-AFPVR) - an interim report. J Hepatol 2020;73(Suppl 1):S878.

Controversies in Treating Chronic HBV

The Role of PEG-interferon-alfa

Phunchai Charatcharoenwitthaya, MD, Msc[a],
Apichat Kaewdech, MD[b], Teerha Piratvisuth, MD[b,c],*

KEYWORDS:

- Chronic hepatitis B • Hepatitis B surface antigen • Peginterferon • Nucleo(s) tide analogs

KEY POINTS

- Pegylated interferon is a first-line treatment for chronic hepatitis B.
- Finite treatment duration, absence of drug resistance, delayed response, and higher hepatitis B surface antigen loss than nucleos(t)ides analog therapy are the advantages of pegylated interferon-alpha treatment.
- Response-guided therapy using hepatitis B surface antigen level can optimize treatment outcomes.
- Combination with nucleos(t)ides analog therapy may improve outcomes, but remains controversial.

INTRODUCTION

Chronic hepatitis B virus (HBV) infection remains a global public health problem.[1] Two classes of approved antiviral agents, including interferon (IFN) and nucleos(t)ide analogs (NA), can efficiently keep the HBV infection under control. However, relapse of viremia is frequent after treatment cessation.[2–4] The HBV elimination during treatment is difficult owing to the conversion of the viral genome into the covalently closed circular DNA (cccDNA) in the nucleus of the infected hepatocytes.[5] Thus, the ultimate

The authors thank the Faculty of Medicine, Prince of Songkla University, Songkhla, Thailand for the support in this review. The work is that of the authors only.

[a] Gastroenterology Division, Department of Internal Medicine, Faculty of Medicine, Siriraj Hospital, Mahidol University, Wang-Lang Road, Bangkok 10700, Thailand; [b] Gastroenterology and Hepatology Unit, Department of Internal Medicine, Faculty of Medicine, Prince of Songkla University, Kanchanawanich Road, Songkhla 90110, Thailand; [c] NKC Institute of Gastroenterology and Hepatology, Songklanagarind Hospital, Prince of Songkla University, Kanchanawanich Road, Songkhla 90110, Thailand
* Corresponding author. Gastroenterology and Hepatology Unit, Department of Medicine, Faculty of Medicine, Prince of Songkla University, Kanchanawanich Road, Songkhla 90110, Thailand.
E-mail address: teerha.p@psu.ac.th

Clin Liver Dis 25 (2021) 741–762
https://doi.org/10.1016/j.cld.2021.06.004
1089-3261/21/© 2021 Elsevier Inc. All rights reserved.

liver.theclinics.com

treatment end point of a functional cure defined by the loss of hepatitis B surface antigen (HBsAg) and undetectable HBV DNA levels in serum is rarely achieved with existing antiviral therapy.[6]

Currently, recombinant IFN is the only therapeutic agent with the possibility of achieving a functional cure and has the strength of a finite treatment duration without the risk of drug resistance. Therefore, the role of IFN should remain in chronic hepatitis B (CHB) treatment, either in mono or combination therapy in some specific population. However, the main challenge of IFN therapy in clinical practice is identifying patients with CHB who mostly respond to treatment. This article reviews the mechanisms of action, efficacy, predictors of response, and clinical use of IFN therapy for patients with CHB.

INTERFERON AND PEGYLATED INTERFERON FOR THE TREATMENT OF CHRONIC HEPATITIS B VIRUS
Antiviral Mechanisms of Interferon

The antiviral IFN-α effect is speculated to act on various parts of the HBV life cycle and enhance cell-mediated immunity.[6] The effector pathways independently block viral transcription, degrade viral RNA, inhibit translation, and modify protein function to control all steps of viral replication.[6–9] Additional IFN-α activity is mediated by the epigenetic modifications of the HBV cccDNA and can induce the degradation of minichromosome by the activation of APOBEC3s in infected cells.[10,11] This effect is believed to be an important mechanism of IFN-α in promoting clearance of HBV-infected hepatocytes.

E-ANTIGEN AND S-ANTIGEN SEROCONVERSION WITH PEGYLATED INTERFERON VERSUS ORAL ANTIVIRAL THERAPY
Efficacy of Pegylated Interferon for Chronic Hepatitis B

Patients with hepatitis B e antigen-positive disease
A meta-analysis of 15 randomized, controlled studies involving 837 patients with hepatitis B e antigen (HBeAg)-positive treated with IFN-α confirmed the beneficial effect of conventional IFN-α therapy.[12] Overall, patients receiving IFN-α for at least 3 months had higher rates of undetectable HBV DNA (37% vs 17%), HBeAg loss (33% vs 12%), and HBsAg loss (7.8% vs 1.8%) than the untreated controls.[12]

In the pegylated interferon (PEG-IFN)-α-2a licensing trial, 814 patients with HBeAg-positive CHB were randomly assigned to receive either PEG-IFN-α-2a (180 µg once weekly) monotherapy or in combination with lamivudine (LAM; 100 mg/d) or LAM monotherapy for 48 weeks.[13] Patients treated with PEG-IFN-α-2a mono or combination therapy significantly achieved the end points of interest compared with those treated with LAM monotherapy when assessed 24 weeks after completion of treatment: HBeAg seroconversion (32% and 27% vs 19%), HBV DNA less than 20,000 IU/mL (32% and 34% vs 22%), and HBsAg loss (3% vs 0%).

The appropriate PEG-IFN-α-2a dose and duration were evaluated in a randomized trial of 544 patients with HBeAg-positive compared with PEG-IFN-α-2a at a dose of 90 µg weekly versus 180 for 24 or 48 weeks.[14] According to the primary treatment end point of the noninferiority study, the HBeAg seroconversion rate was highest in the 48-week 180 µg group (36%) compared with 26% for the 48-week 90 µg group, 23% in the 24-week 180 µg group, and 14% in the 24-week 90 µg group. The licensed PEG-IFN-α-2a at a dosage of 180 µg for 48 weeks was the most efficacious and beneficial for patients with HBeAg-positive disease predominantly infected with HBV genotypes B or C.

The use of PEG-IFN-α-2b has been evaluated for the treatment of patients with HBeAg-positive. In a randomized, controlled trial of 266 patients with HBeAg-positive CHB, PEG-IFN-α-2b (100 μg weekly) alone or in combination with LAM (100 mg/d) for 52 weeks resulted in HBeAg loss in 35% to 36% of patients when assessed 26 weeks after treatment cessation.[15] The combination with LAM in the regimen is not superior to monotherapy. Moreover, HBV genotype is an important predictor of treatment response. In another trial, 100 patients with HBeAg-positive CHB were randomly assigned to either PEG-IFN-α-2b (1.5 μm/kg weekly; maximum, 100 μg) for 32 weeks plus LAM (100 mg/d) or LAM monotherapy for 52 weeks.[16] The rate of sustained virologic response defined as HBeAg seroconversion and an HBV DNA level of less than 100,000 IU/mL at least 24 weeks after the end of the treatment was significantly higher in the combination therapy group (36% vs 14%).

Responses to PEG-IFN-α-2b therapy assessed at a mean of 3.0 ± 0.8 years after treatment completion found the loss of HBeAg and HBsAg in 37% and 11%, respectively.[17] The durability of HBeAg seroclearance and HBsAg loss was observed in 81% and 30%, respectively, among the initial responders. In another cohort study, 85 patients with HBeAg-positive receiving PEG-IFN-α-2b (1.5 μg/kg/wk) for 32 weeks and LAM (100 mg/d) for 52 or 104 weeks were prospectively followed for 6.1 ± 1.7 years after treatment.[18] The HBeAg seroconversion rates increased progressively from 37% at the end of treatment to 60% at 5 years. The follow-up data also showed that 77% of the initial responders had sustained HBeAg seroconversion and alanine aminotransferase (ALT) normalization at 5 years. However, only 2 patients had lost HBsAg.

Patients with hepatitis B e antigen-negative disease

Treatment with standard IFN-α in patients with HBeAg-negative disease usually leads to a decrease in the serum HBV DNA and ALT levels. However, relapse after cessation of therapy is common.[19,20] A longer treatment course (24 months) may be more effective in inducing a sustained response (ALT normalization and undetectable HBV DNA) with rates of up to 33%.[21,22]

The approval of PEG-IFN-α treatment for HBeAg-negative CHB was based on a randomized controlled trial of 537 patients randomly assigned to receive PEG-IFN-α-2a (180 μg weekly) monotherapy, in combination with LAM (100 mg/d) or LAM monotherapy for 48 weeks.[23] After 24 weeks of follow-up, patients treated with PEG-IFN-α-2a monotherapy or combination therapy significantly achieved the end points of interest (normalization of serum ALT levels or HBV DNA levels of less than approximately 4000 IU/mL) compared with those treated with LAM monotherapy. The rates of sustained viral suppression to below approximately 80 IU/mL were also significantly higher in the PEG-IFN mono or combination therapy groups than LAM monotherapy (19% and 20% vs 7%, respectively). The loss of HBsAg occurred in 7 and 5 patients in the PEG-IFN monotherapy and the combination therapy groups, respectively, compared with none in the LAM group. A subsequent post-treatment observational study reported that HBeAg-negative patients treated with PEG-IFN-α-2a with or without LAM had higher rates of HBV DNA levels of less than 2000 IU/mL (28% vs 15%) and HBsAg seroclearance (8.7% vs 0%) compared with those treated with LAM monotherapy 3 years after treatment.[24] The 48-week course of PEG-IFN-α-2a has been shown to induce sustained biochemical and virologic responses 3 years after treatment in approximately 25% of patients with HBeAg-negative disease.

The benefit of extending the PEG-IFN treatment duration has been explored in patients with HBeAg-negative CHB. In a trial, 128 patients with HBeAg-negative, mainly genotype D, were randomized to receive PEG-IFN-α-2a (180 μg weekly) for 48 weeks followed by 135 µg weekly for an additional 48 weeks or a combination of PEG-IFN-α-2a (180 µg weekly) and LAM (100 mg/d) for 48 weeks followed by PEG-IFN-α-2a (135 mg weekly) for 48 weeks.[25] At the 48-week post-treatment follow-up, a greater proportion of patients receiving PEG-IFN monotherapy for 96 weeks achieved HBV DNA of less than 2000 IU/mL (29% vs 12%) compared with those treated with PEG-IFN for only 48 weeks. Combination treatment was not associated with a higher virologic response as compared with PEG-IFN monotherapy. Although PEG-IFN treatment for 96 weeks was well-tolerated, given the higher costs, the benefits of extended therapy with PEG-IFN-α-2a need to be validated in more extensive studies.

ROLE OF S-ANTIGEN TITER IN MONITORING PEGYLATED INTERFERON TREATMENT

The HBV encodes 3 proteins of HBsAg to form the viral envelope; small HBsAg, middle HBsAg, and large HBsAg (**Fig. 1**).[26] The surface proteins can assemble to produce noninfectious subviral particles. The production of subviral particles can be found up to 10,000- to 100,000-fold than the virions.[27–29] HBsAg level or quantification during PEG-IFN treatment has been reported as useful markers for monitoring and predicting treatment response in both HBeAg-positive and -negative CHB.[30–36]

Hepatitis B surface antigen level in the prediction of pegylated interferon treatment response in hepatitis B e antigen-positive chronic hepatitis B

Prediction of response
This study reported lower HBsAg level at weeks 12 or 24 of PEG-IFN treatment was associated with higher treatment response at 24-week after treatment. Patients with HBsAg level less than 1500 IU/mL at week 12 of PEG-IFN treatment have an HBeAg seroconversion rate of 54.7% and HBsAg loss of 11% at 24 weeks after treatment. Similar to the 12-week HBsAg level, HBeAg seroconversion and HBsAg losses were 54.4% and 11.8%, respectively, in patients with HBsAg level less than 1500 IU/mL at 24 weeks of PEG-IFN treatment.[37] Moreover, on-treatment HBsAg level has been confirmed in predicting responses in both Caucasian and Asian patients.[13,38–40]

Stopping rule
Almost all patients in genotypes B and C will not achieve HBeAg seroconversion if HBsAg level is greater than 20,000 IU/mL at weeks 12 or 24 of PEG-IFN treatment

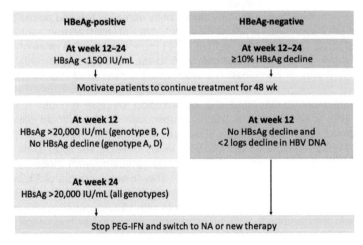

Fig. 1. Response-guided therapy by using HBsAg level during PEG-IFN treatment.

(negative predictive value [NPV], 97%–100%).[37,41] In all genotypes, an HBsAg level of greater than 20,000 IU/mL at 24 weeks of treatment is associated with a less than 3% HBeAg loss and HBV DNA of less than 2000 IU/mL at 24-week after treatment (NPV, 97%–100%).[42,43] Therefore, an HBsAg level of greater than 20,000 IU/mL at week 24 of PEG-IFN treatment can be used as a stopping rule in HBeAg-positive CHB regardless of HBV genotype. No decrease in the HBsAg level at week 12 of PEG-IFN treatment in the CHB genotype D could also be used as a stopping rule with NPV of 97%.[44]

Hepatitis B Surface Antigen Level or Decline in Predicting Pegylated Interferon Treatment Response in Hepatitis B e Antigen-Negative Chronic Hepatitis B

Prediction of response
A greater HBsAg decrease at weeks 12 or 24 of PEG-IFN treatment is associated with higher rates of post-treatment sustained response.[45–49] Patients with at least a 10% decrease in HBsAg at week 12 had sustained HBV DNA of less than 2000 IU/mL of 47% and 43% at 1 and 5 years after 48 weeks of PEG-IFN treatment, respectively.[49] At least a 10% decrease in HBsAg at week 12 of treatment was associated with an HBsAg loss of 9.4% and 22.6% at 1 and 5 years after treatment, respectively.[49] A lower HBsAg level at the end of the 48-week PEG-IFN treatment was associated with a sustained HBV DNA of less than 2000 IU/mL at 24 weeks after treatment (sustained responses were 80%, 20%, and 0% in HBsAg levels at the end of treatment of <10, 101–1000, and >5000, respectively).[50] The HBsAg level at the end of PEG-IFN treatment also predicts sustained virologic response at 1 year after treatment (75% in patients with HBsAg level <1000 IU/mL vs 17% in HBsAg level ≥1000 IU/mL).[46]

Stopping rule
In genotype D, HBeAg-negative CHB without any decrease in the HBsAg level and having a less than 2 log decrease in HBV DNA at week 12 of PEG-IFN treatment failed to achieve sustained response after 48 weeks of PEG-IFN treatment with a NPV of 100%.[48,51] However, using this HBsAg and HBV DNA decrease in Asian patients with predominant HBV genotypes B and C could predict nonresponders with an NPV of 83% to 100%.[52] Thus, future studies with large numbers of patients are required for HBV genotypes B and C.

Using Hepatitis B surface Antigen level for response-guided therapy to optimize pegylated interferon treatment in Chronic Hepatitis B

Patients with hepatitis B e antigen chronic hepatitis B

- Motivate patients to continue treatment for 48 weeks in those with an HBsAg level at week 12 of PEG-IFN treatment of less than 1500 IU/mL because they are as good responders with positive predictive value of 45% to 57%.[14,37,48]
- Stop treatment and switch to NA treatment in patients with an HBsAg level greater than of 20,000 IU/mL (HBV genotypes B and C) or no decrease in the HBsAg level (genotypes A and D) at week 12 of PEG-IFN treatment with NPV response of 97% to 100%.[14,37,43,44] Moreover, approximately 20% of patients can stop treatment a week 12, which allows them to avoid the side effects of PEG-IFN with a minimal chance of achieving response.

Patients with hepatitis B e antigen-negative chronic hepatitis B

- Motivate patients to continue PEG-IFN treatment for 48 weeks in those who achieve an HBsAg decrease of at least 10% at week 12 of treatment.[48] The positive predictive value of sustained response with an HBV of less than 2000 IU/mL at 24 weeks after treatment is 47% to 59%.

- Stop PEG-IFN treatment and switch to NA therapy in patients without a decrease in the HBsAg level and achieving a less than 2 log decrease in HBV DNA at week 12 of PEG-IFN therapy.[47,51]
- Stop PEG-IFN treatment and switch treatment to NA or new therapy in patients with an HBsAg level of greater than 20,000 IU/mL at week 24 of treatment, regardless of HBV genotype.[43] They are unlikely to achieve treatment response with an NPV of 97%.

Using on-treatment HBsAg levels for response-guided PEG-IFN treatment has been validated in a recent meta-analysis.[32,33] The novel biomarkers (eg, hepatitis B core-related antigen and HBV RNA during PEG-IFN treatment) have been reported as the new markers for predicting PEG-IFN treatment response.[53–55]

COMBINING PEGYLATED INTERFERON AND ORAL ANTIVIRAL THERAPY

Several strategies have been devised to cure HBV, including novel drugs,[56] stop NA strategies,[57] or combination therapy with NA and PEG-IFN,[58,59] although HBsAg loss is difficult to be desired. Combination therapy with an oral NA and PEG-IFN is an interesting modality to accelerate HBsAg clearance. Moreover, PEG-IFN can enhance the immune system in patients with CHB as well as a reduction of HBV replication from NA effects, consequently eliminating the cccDNA from the liver.[13,23,60] Several treatment strategies of combination therapy including de novo strategy, add-on combination, or switch-to therapy.

De Novo Strategy

Patients with hepatitis B e antigen-positive chronic hepatitis B. A multicenter, randomized controlled study including 814 patients with HBeAg-positive CHB, mostly from Asia, reported that the HBeAg seroconversion rate 24 weeks after treatment was significantly higher in the PEG-IFN-α-2a with or without the LAM group compared with the LAM alone group (32%, 27%, and 19%, respectively).[13] Moreover, the combination group showed that the PEG-IFN-α-2a plus LAM combination had the highest virologic response at the end of treatment. Furthermore, HBsAg seroconversion occurred in 16 patients among the PEG-IFN-α-2a with or without the LAM group compared with no HBsAg loss in the LAM group. However, the combination therapy did not add the additional benefits in terms of HBeAg seroconversion and HBsAg clearance at week 72. Another multicenter study with 74% Caucasian participants showed that, at the end of the treatment at 52 weeks, the HBeAg loss, virologic response, and ALT normalization were significantly higher in the combination than the monotherapy group (44% vs 29%, 74% vs 29%, and 51% vs 34%, respectively).[15] Nevertheless, the HBsAg clearance was comparable between the 2 groups (7% and 5% in the combination and monotherapy groups, respectively). At the end of the follow-up at 26 weeks after treatment, the HBeAg loss, HBeAg seroconversion, HBV DNA response, and ALT normalization were comparable between the 2 groups, indicating that an additional LAM to PEG-IFN-α-2b did not provide any advantages.

Patients with hepatitis B e antigen-negative chronic hepatitis B. A large, multicenter, randomized study investigated the efficacy of a 48-week PEG-IFN-α-2a combined with LAM or PEG-IFN-α-2a alone or LAM alone.[23] Notably, at week 72 of the follow-up period, the biochemical and virologic response in PEG-IFN-α-2a with or without LAM was significantly higher than the LAM alone group. Consequently, 5 and 7 patients in the combination therapy and PEG-IFN-α-2a alone groups developed subsequent HBsAg loss. However, adding LAM to the PEG-IFN-α-2a regimen demonstrated the failure to achieve a better clinical end point.

Patients with both hepatitis B e antigen-positive and -negative chronic hepatitis B. A large randomized 4-arm study with three-quarters Asian patients with CHB investigated the efficacy of PEG-IFN-α-2a with tenofovir disoproxil fumarate (TDF, 48 weeks) or PEG-IFN-α-2a (16 weeks) followed by TDF (32 weeks) or monotherapy with PEG-IFN-α-2a or TDF (48 weeks).[61] The highest HBsAg clearance rate was 9.1% in patients receiving a 48-week combination of PEG-IFN-α-2a plus TDF compared with 2.8%, 0%, and 2.8% in a shorter duration of PEG-IFN-α-2a treatment with TDF, TDF alone, and PEG-IFN-α-2a alone, respectively. Unfortunately, the result was not uniform across all genotypes, particularly in genotype A. Moreover, Patients with CHB had the highest HBsAg loss and tended toward the patients with HBeAg-positive. A post hoc analysis study at week 120 of follow-up indicated that HBsAg loss in 48-week combination therapy was the highest (10.36%) compared with 3.49% and 3.51% in 16 weeks of PEG-IFN-α-2a followed by 32 weeks of TDF therapy, respectively.[62] Over the course of 120 weeks, no patient in the TDF group developed HBsAg clearance.

More recently, a real-world experience study from China investigated the efficacy of de novo combined TDF to PEG-IFN-α-2a for 48 weeks compared with monotherapy either in PEG-IFN-α-2a or TDF.[63] The authors reported that in 395 patients with 78% HBeAg-positive CHB, the rate of HBsAg loss at week 72 was observed in 11%, 5.7%, and 0% in the combination, PEG-IFN-α-2a, and TDF groups, respectively. Another interesting finding was that the HBsAg level decrease of more than 1.5 $\log_{10}$ IU/mL at week 24 from the baseline can predict the 72-week HBsAg loss with an area under the receiving operating characteristic curve of 0.846. A summary of the studies is shown in **Table 1**.

In conclusion, the de novo combination of PEG-IFN and low-potency NA in naïve patients with CHB had no additional advantages over PEG-IFN monotherapy after the follow-up period. Interestingly, a combination of PEG-IFN with high-potency NA such as TDF had a better response compared with the PEG-IFN monotherapy.

Add-on Strategy

The add-on therapy with immunomodulators may increase the chance of HBsAg loss. **Table 2** demonstrates the studies that address the add-on strategy of PEG-IFN to NA.

Early add-on pegylated interferon to nucleos(t)ides analogs (defined as starting nucleos(t)ides analogs before pegylated interferon <1 year)

The ARES study, which included 175 patients with CHB, demonstrated that the primary end point was HBeAg loss and HBV DNA less than 200 IU/mL at week 48.[64] The primary end point in the add-on therapy was greater, but not statistically (19% vs 10%), than the entecavir (ETV) monotherapy. Furthermore, a long-term follow-up study with a median duration of 226 weeks demonstrated that a combination end point was not different between the add-on PEG-IFN-α-2a and ETV (27% vs 23%) group.[65] However, the add-on therapy group had a reduction of HBsAg level of greater than 1 log, which was significantly higher than the ETV group (59% vs 28%).

Late add-on pegylated interferon to nucleos(t)ides analog (defined as starting nucleos(t)ides analog before pegylated interferon >1 year)

Patients with hepatitis B e antigen-positive chronic hepatitis B. The PEGON study from China and Netherlands investigated the efficacy of the add-on a 48-week PEG-IFN-α-2b who received ETV or TDF for at least 1 year.[66] The primary end point

Table 1
Summarized studies of de novo strategy

Author, Year	HBeAg Status	n	Regimen	End of Treatment			Follow-up Duration (weeks)	End of Follow-up		
				HBV DNA Response (HBV DNA <400 Copies/mL) (%)	HBeAg Seroconversion (%)	HBsAg Loss (n)		HBV DNA Response (HBV DNA <400 Copies/mL) (%)	HBeAg Seroconversion (%)	HBsAg Loss (n)
Marcellin, 2004[23]	Negative	177	PEG-IFN-α 2a 48 wk	63	-	NR	72	19	-	7
		179	PEG-IFN-α 2a 48 wk plus LAM	87	-	NR		20	-	5
		181	LAM	73	-	NR		7	-	0
Lau, 2005[13]	Positive	271	PEG-IFN-α 2a 48 wk	25	27	NR	72	14[a]	32[a]	8
		271	PEG-IFN-α 2a 48 wk plus LAM	69	24	NR		14[a]	27[a]	8
		272	LAM	40	20	NR		5[a]	19[a]	0
Janssen, 2005[15]	Positive	130	PEG-IFN-α 2b 52 wk plus LAM	33[a]	25	9	78	9	29	9
		136	PEG-IFN-α 2b 52 wk	10[a]	22	7		7	29	9
Wursthorn, 2006[83]	Both	26	PEG-IFN-α 2b 48 wk plus ADV	54[b]	33	4 (HBsAg seroconversion)	-	NR	NR	NR

Study	HBeAg	N	Regimen							
Marcellin, 2016[61]	Positive	186	PEG-IFN-α 2a 48 wk plus TDF	68.8[c]	23.1	7.3%	72	9.1[ac]	25[a]	9.1%[a]
		184	PEG-IFN-α 2a 48 wk plus TDF 16 wk then TDF 32 wk	71.2[c]	19	2.8%		6.5[ac]	23.8	2.8%
		185	TDF 120 wk	60.5[c]	8.3	0		71.9[c]	12.8	0
		185	PEG-IFN-α 2a 48 wk	21.3[c]	12.3	2.8%		9.2[c]	24.5	2.8%
Tangkijvanich, 2016[36]	Negative	63	PEG-IFN-α 2b 48 wk plus ETV	87.3[ad]	-	2	96	6.3	-	3
		63	PEG-IFN-α 2b 48 wk	41.3[ad]	-	6		11.1	-	6
de Niet, 2017[84]	Both, low viral load patients, ALT < 5× ULN	52	PEG-IFN-α 2a 48 wk plus ADV	NR	NR	1	72	NR	NR	2
		51	PEG-IFN-α 2a 48 wk plus ADV	NR	NR	3		NR	NR	2
		48	No treatment	NR	NR	0		NR	NR	0
Hagiwara, 2018[85]	Both	26	PEG-IFN 48 wk plus ETV	96	33 (HBeAg-positive)	NR	72	62	60 (HBeAg-positive)	NR
Zheng, 2019[86]	Positive	77	PEG-IFN-α 2a 48 wk plus TDF	33.8[a]	Approximately 30	10[a]	NR	NR	NR	NR
		66	TDF	16.7[a]	Approximately 25	2[a]		NR	NR	NR

Abbreviations: ADV, adefovir; ETV, entecavir; NR, not reported; TDF, tenofovir disoproxil fumarate; ULN, upper limit of normal.

[a] $P < .05$.
[b] HBV DNA less than 100 copies/mL.
[c] HBV DNA less than 15 IU/mL.
[d] HBV DNA less than 10 IU/mL.

Table 2
Summarized studies of add-on IFN to NA

Author, Year	HBeAg Status	Duration of NA before PEG-IFN (mo)	n	Regimen	End of Treatment					End of Follow-up			
					HBV DNA Response (%)	HBeAg Seroconversion (%)	HBsAg Level Decrease of >0.5 log10 IU/mL (%)	HBsAg Loss (n)	Follow-up Duration (wk)	HBV DNA Response (%)	HBeAg Seroconversion (%)	HBsAg Level Reduction > 0.5 log10 IU/mL (%)	HBsAg Loss (n)
Li, 2015[87]	Positive	>24	81	PEG-IFN-α 2a 48 wk plus ETV	NR	44[a]	NR	2	96	NR	NR	NR	NR
			116	ETV	NR	6[a]	NR	0		NR	NR	NR	NR
Brouwer, 2015 (ARES)[64]	Positive	6	85	PEG-IFN week 24–48 plus ETV	61	44	NR	1	96	57	26[a]	NR	1
			90	ETV	50	6	NR	0		54	13[a]	NR	0
Chi, 2017 (PEGON)[66]	Positive	> 12	39	PEG-IFN-α 2a 48 wk plus ETV or TDF	85	15	33[a]	0	96	77	21	13	0
			38	ETV or TDF	84	5	3[a]	0		84	8	13	0
van Campenhout, 2019 (ARES long-term follow-up)[65]	Positive	6	48	PEG-IFN week 24–48 plus ETV	61	44	NR	1	226	69	29	59 (>1 og10 IU/mL)[a]	1
			48	ETV	50	6	NR	0		67	21	28 (>1 og10 IU/mL)[a]	0
Liem, 2019 (ARES and PEGON)[67]	Positive	> 6–12	118	PEG-IFN week 24–48 plus ETV	32	16[a]	26[a]	1	96	31	24[a]	23[a]	1
			116	ETV	35	1.7[a]	1.7[a]	0		35	9.6[a]	9.6[a]	0
Lampertico, 2018 (HERMES)[81]	Negative	27	70	PEG-IFN-α 2a 48 wk plus NA	NR	-	NR	1	96	NR	-	14	1

Study	Population	Duration	N	Treatment									
Bourlière, 2017 (ANRS HB06 PEGAN)[69]	Negative	2.7–3.3 y	90	PEG-IFN-α 2a 48 wk plus NA	NR	NR	–	NR	7[a]	96	NR	–	NR	7
			93	NA	NR	NR	–	NR	0[a]	96	NR	–	NR	3
Matsumoto, 2020[70]	Both HBsAg level >800 IU/mL	3.4–4.1 y	32	PEG-IFN-α 2a 48 wk plus TDF	NR	13	–	NR	0	96	NR	–	NR	0
			51	TDF	NR	0	–	NR	0	NR	NR	–	NR	0

Abbreviations: ETV, entecavir; NR, not reported; TDF, tenofovir disoproxil fumarate.
[a] $P < .05$.

with HBeAg seroconversion and HBV DNA of less than 200 IU/mL at week 96 was not statistically significant (18% in the add-on group vs 8% in the NA monotherapy group). The HBeAg seroconversion rate was significantly higher in the PEG-IFN-α-2b add-on therapy (30% vs 7%, respectively). Another post hoc analysis from the ARES and PEGON studies assessed the efficacy of the add-on PEG-IFN therapy for 6 to 12 months compared with ETV monotherapy.[67] The end point of HBeAg loss combined with HBV DNA of less than 200 IU/mL reached 33% and 20% in the add-on and monotherapy ($P = .03$) groups, respectively. Moreover, the baseline HBsAg level of less than 4000 IU/mL plus the baseline HBV DNA of less than 50 IU/mL could be the best response predictor in the add-on strategy.

Patients with hepatitis B e antigen-negative chronic hepatitis N. Allocated to receive an add-on of 48 weeks of PEG-IFN-α-2a with NA except telbivudine were 70 Caucasians patients with genotype D CHB.[68] The participants had an undetectable HBV DNA for more than 1 year at baseline. The primary end point was defined as a 50% decrease in the HBsAg level at the end of treatment and was achieved in 62.5% of the patients. However, this study had no comparison group. Another randomized controlled French study investigated the efficacy of the add-on PEG-IFN-α-2a regimen compared with NA alone.[69] The median duration of NA treatment was longer at 2.7 and 3.3 years in the add-on and NA monotherapy groups, respectively. HBsAg loss occurred 7.8% in the add-on group compared with 3.2% in the NA monotherapy group at 96 weeks ($P = .15$). Furthermore, the baseline HBsAg level at week 0 was less than 3 $\log_{10}$ IU/mL, which correlated with HBsAg clearance.

Patients with both hepatitis B e antigen-positive and -negative chronic hepatitis B. More recently, a Japanese pilot study including 83 Patients with CHB was assigned to receive PEG-IFN-α-2a and TDF or TDF alone.[70] Interestingly, 41% of the patients had a significant steep decline in the HBsAg level compared with 2% in the TDF monotherapy group at the end of the follow-up at week 96.

Finally, most studies on the add-on strategy provide the benefit of HBsAg level decline. However, the HBsAg clearance rate is still low in the short-term follow-up. Thus, further follow-up studies may be needed.

Switch-to Strategy

Switch nucleos(t)ides analog to pegylated interferon

Table 3 illustrates the previous studies of the switch-to strategy, including patient characteristics, regimen, and end points. The OSST trial including 197 Chinese patients who received ETV for 9 to 36 months with an HBV DNA level of less than 200 IU/mL plus an HBeAg level of less than 100 PEIU/mL were allocated to 48 weeks of PEG-IFN-α-2a or ETV.[71] The switch to the PEG-IFN arm had a significant increase in HBeAg seroconversion of 14.9% compared with 6.1% in the ETV arm at week 48. Moreover, an 8.5% HBsAg clearance was observed in the switch arm, whereas there was none in the patient in the ETV arm. Another important finding in ETV-treated patients with HBeAg loss at the time of switching therapy and with an HBsAg level of less than 1500 IU/mL could be the switch to PEG-IFN because of a high chance of HBsAg loss (22.2%) and HBeAg seroconversion (33.3%). Moreover, HBsAg levels of less than 200 IU/mL at 12 weeks after switch therapy predicted a great chance of treatment success in contrast with am HBsAg level of 1500 IU/mL or greater, which predicts a poor response after switch therapy. A 1-year of follow-up, the OSST study reported a significant increase in HBeAg seroconversion to 38.7% at 1 year after treatment. Another multicenter Chinese study (new switch study) recruited the patients on NA therapy for a median duration of 2.1 to 2.2 years with

Table 3
Summarized studies of the switch-to strategy

Author, Year	HBeAg Status	Duration of NA before PEG-IFN (mo)	n	Regimen	End of Treatment		
					HBV DNA Response (%)	HBeAg Sero-conversion (%)	HBsAg Loss (n)
Ning, 2014 (OSST)[71]	Positive	19.9–20.5	94	PEG-IFN-α 2a 48 wk	72[a]	14.9[a]	8[a]
			98	ETV	97.8[a]	6.1[a]	0[a]
Xie, 2014[88]	Positive	-	72	PEG-IFN-α 2a 48 wk	52.8	19	3
		-	73	PEG-IFN-α 2a 48 wk plus ETV add on week 13 (24 wk)	72.6	18	5
		21	73	PEG-IFN-α 2a start at week 21 of ETV (24 wk)	47.9	21	2
Han, 2016 (OSST 1 y follow-up)[89]	Positive	19.9–20.5	62	PEG-IFN-α 2a 48 wk	51.6[b]	38.7[b]	6[b]
Huang, 2017[90]	Positive	3.44–3.64 y	43	PEG-IFN-α 2b 48 wk (continue NA in first 4 wk)	NR	23[a]	11[a]
			45	ETV	NR	8[a]	0[a]
Tamaki, 2017[91]		4 y	49	PEG-IFN-α 2a 48 wk	NR	44[a]	2[a]
			147	NA	NR	8[a]	0[a]
Hu, 2018 (New switch)[92]	Positive	2.1–2.2 y	153	PEG-IFN-α 2a 48 wk	76.5	54.9	22
			150	PEG-IFN-α 2a 96 wk	74	60.7	31
Zhou, 2019[93]	Positive	3.81–4.65 y	24	PEG-IFN-α 2a 48 wk	NR	NR	6
			24	NA	NR	NR	0

Abbreviations: ETV, entecavir; NR, not reported; TDF, tenofovir disoproxil fumarate.
[a] $P < .05$.
[b] At 1 year of follow-up.

HBeAg loss plus HBV DNA less than 200 IU/mL. To assess the efficacy of a 48- or 96-week PEG-IFN-α-2a, the HBsAg loss at the end of the treatment and 96 after treatment was not different between the durations of PEG-IFN-α-2a (14.4 vs 20.7% and 9.8% vs 15.3%, respectively). Furthermore, safety issues, particularly serious adverse events, observed in 96 weeks of PEG-IFN-α-2a is more in the shorter duration.

In conclusion, the switch-to strategy had benefits in the finite treatment duration and may potentiate HBeAg seroconversion and HBsAg loss. However, a good candidate predicting the best response may be required, including a low HBsAg level at the time of switching therapy or a low on-treatment HBsAg level. The major drawback of HBV flare after treatment cessation should be focused on particularly in those who have advanced fibrosis or cirrhotic liver.

PATIENTS WHO ARE THE BEST CANDIDATES FOR PEGYLATED INTERFERON THERAPY CONSIDERATION

Identifying patients who have a high treatment response chance would allow the optimization of the PEG-IFN therapy. Using baseline the predictors of response are reasonable before considering PEG-IFN therapy. Several response predictors are shown in **Table 4**. Caucasians are more likely to achieve HBeAg seroconversion or

Table 4
Baseline predictors of response to PEG-IFN therapy in chronic hepatitis B

Characters	Favorable Response
Ethnicity	Caucasian
Serum ALT	Higher ALT
HBV DNA	Lower HBV DNA
HBV genotype	A > D
	B > C
HBsAg level	Lower HBsAg level

sustained response than Asians.[55,72] Moreover, a higher baseline serum ALT and a lower baseline HBV DNA level are associated with higher rates of PEG-IFN treatment response.[13,15,73,74] HBV genotypes A and B have a better response to PEG-IFN treatment than genotypes D and C, respectively.[13,15,75] Consequently, a lower serum HBsAg level is associated with a higher sustained response after 48 weeks of PEG-IFN therapy.[76–78] A baseline HBsAg level of less than 20,000 IU/mL is associated with lower response rates (<10% HBeAg loss and HBV DNA <2000 IU/mL in patients with HBeAg-positive disease; <40% HBV DNA <2000 IU/mL in HBeAg-negative disease at 24 weeks after treatment).[49]

Baseline quantitative anti-HBc level was shown to be associated with HBeAg seroconversion at 24 weeks of PEG-IFN treatment. Moreover, 52.6% of patients with baseline anti-HBc level of greater than 50,000 IU/mL achieved HBeAg seroconversion at 24 weeks after treatment.[79]

Table 5
Scoring system for prediction response to PEG-IFN in HBeAg-positive chronic hepatitis B

Characteristic	Score
Age (y)	
≥40	0
<40	1
Gender	
Male	0
Female	1
Serum ALT, × ULN	
≤4	0
>4	1
HBV DNA $\log_{10}$ IU/mL	
>7.7	0
>6.0–7.7	1
≤6.0	2
HBsAg IU/mL	
>25,000	0
≤25,000	1

Abbreviation: ULN, upper limit of normal.

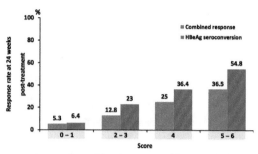

Fig. 2. HBeAg seroconversion and combined response (HBeAg seroconversion and HBV DNA <2000 IU/mL) at 24 weeks after treatment.

This study developed an easy-to-use baseline prediction score to identify patients with HBeAg-positive CHB who are likely to respond to the PEG-IFN therapy depicted (**Table 5**).[80] The response rates are predicted by using this scoring system in HBV genotypes B and C (**Fig 2**).[80] The baseline prediction scoring of HBeAg-negative CHB treated with 48 weeks of PEG-IFN in HBV genotypes B and C are shown in **Table 6** and **Fig. 3**.[81]

In summary, the 48-week PEG-IFN therapy is one of the first-line CHB treatments.[55,78,82] Finite treatment duration, absence of drug resistance, delayed response, and higher HBsAg loss than NA therapy are the advantages of the PEG-IFN treatment. However, common side effects and subcutaneous injection requirements limit the use of PEG-IFN. Thus, identifying patients who likely to respond to PEG-IFN is very reasonable. Furthermore, HBsAg monitoring during PEG-IFN treatment can optimize treatment. The patients are motivated to complete the 48-week treatment in those who achieve HBsAg less than 1500 IU/mL or a HBsAg decrease of 10 IU/mL or greater at week 12 of treatment, because they are likely to respond to treatment, stopping PEG-IFN treatment, or switching to other treatment strategies in patients with the stopping rule criteria (HBsAg level of >20,000 IU/mL or lack of any HBsAg decrease at week 12 of treatment in HBeAg-positive and -negative CHB,

Table 6 Scoring for predictive baseline characteristics	
Characteristic	**Score**
Age (y)	
>45	0
<30–≤45	1
≤30	2
ALT × ULN	
<5	0
≥5	1
HBV genotype	
B	0
C	1
HBsAg levels (IU/mL)	
≥1250	0
<1250	1

Abbreviation: ULN, upper limit of normal.

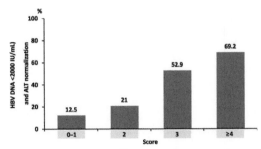

Fig. 3. Sustained response 48 weeks after 48 weeks of PEG-IFN therapy in HBeAg-negative CHB, genotype B/C.

respectively). Identifying nonresponders could allow the patients to withdraw early from treatment and avoid the side effects with early switching to other treatment strategies.

CLINICS CARE POINTS

- Baseline predictors of response to PEG-IFN therapy are used in selecting the patients who are likely to respond to treatment.
- On-treatment HBsAg levels can predict the treatment response and are used as respond-guided therapy.
- NA and PEG-IFN Combination may improve treatment response, but requires further study before applying in clinical practice.
- Monitoring side effects and prompt rescue strategy are recommended during PEG-IFN therapy.

DISCLOSURE

T. Piratvisuth has received research grants from Gilead Sciences, Roche Diagnostic, Janssen, Fibrogen and VIR, and speaker honoraria from Bristol-Myers Squibb, Gilead Sciences, Bayer, Abbott, Esai, Mylan, Ferring, and MSD. P. Charatcharoenwitthaya and A. Kaewdech have no conflicts of interest to declare.

REFERENCES

1. Schweitzer A, Horn J, Mikolajczyk RT, et al. Estimations of worldwide prevalence of chronic hepatitis B virus infection: a systematic review of data published between 1965 and 2013. Lancet 2015;386(10003):1546–55.
2. European Association for the Study of the Liver. EASL 2017 Clinical Practice Guidelines on the management of hepatitis B virus infection. J Hepatol 2017; 67(2):370–98.
3. Terrault NA, Lok ASF, McMahon BJ, et al. Update on prevention, diagnosis, and treatment of chronic hepatitis B: AASLD 2018 hepatitis B guidance. Hepatology 2018;67(4):1560–99.
4. Sarin SK, Kumar M, Lau GK, et al. Asian-Pacific clinical practice guidelines on the management of hepatitis B: a 2015 update. Hepatol Int 2016;10(1):1–98.

5. Gish RG, Given BD, Lai C-L, et al. Chronic hepatitis B: virology, natural history, current management and a glimpse at future opportunities. Antiviral Res 2015; 121:47–58.

6. Sadler AJ, Williams BRG. Interferon-inducible antiviral effectors. Nat Rev Immunol 2008;8(7):559–68.

7. Wieland SF, Guidotti LG, Chisari FV. Intrahepatic induction of alpha/beta interferon eliminates viral RNA-containing capsids in hepatitis B virus transgenic mice. J Virol 2000;74(9):4165–73.

8. Xu C, Guo H, Pan X-B, et al. Interferons accelerate decay of replication-competent nucleocapsids of hepatitis B virus. J Virol 2010;84(18):9332–40.

9. Li J, Lin S, Chen Q, et al. Inhibition of hepatitis B virus replication by MyD88 involves accelerated degradation of pregenomic RNA and nuclear retention of pre-S/S RNAs. J Virol 2010;84(13):6387–99.

10. Dandri M, Petersen J. Mechanism of hepatitis B virus persistence in hepatocytes and its carcinogenic potential. Clin Infect Dis 2016;62(Suppl 4):S281–8.

11. Belloni L, Allweiss L, Guerrieri F, et al. IFN-α inhibits HBV transcription and replication in cell culture and in humanized mice by targeting the epigenetic regulation of the nuclear cccDNA minichromosome. J Clin Invest 2012;122(2):529–37.

12. Wong DK, Cheung AM, O'Rourke K, et al. Effect of alpha-interferon treatment in patients with hepatitis B e antigen-positive chronic hepatitis B. A meta-analysis. Ann Intern Med 1993;119(4):312–23.

13. Lau GKK, Piratvisuth T, Luo KX, et al. Peginterferon Alfa-2a, lamivudine, and the combination for HBeAg-positive chronic hepatitis B. N Engl J Med 2005;352(26): 2682–95.

14. Liaw Y-F, Jia J-D, Chan HLY, et al. Shorter durations and lower doses of peginterferon alfa-2a are associated with inferior hepatitis B e antigen seroconversion rates in hepatitis B virus genotypes B or C. Hepatology 2011;54(5):1591–9.

15. Janssen HLA, van Zonneveld M, Senturk H, et al. Pegylated interferon alfa-2b alone or in combination with lamivudine for HBeAg-positive chronic hepatitis B: a randomised trial. Lancet 2005;365(9454):123–9.

16. Chan HL-Y, Leung NW-Y, Hui AY, et al. A randomized, controlled trial of combination therapy for chronic hepatitis B: comparing pegylated interferon-alpha2b and lamivudine with lamivudine alone. Ann Intern Med 2005;142(4):240–50.

17. Buster EHCJ, Flink HJ, Cakaloglu Y, et al. Sustained HBeAg and HBsAg loss after long-term follow-up of HBeAg-positive patients treated with peginterferon alpha-2b. Gastroenterology 2008;135(2):459–67.

18. Wong VW-S, Wong GL-H, Yan KK-L, et al. Durability of peginterferon alfa-2b treatment at 5 years in patients with hepatitis B e antigen–positive chronic hepatitis B. Hepatology 2010;51(6):1945–53.

19. Brunetto MR, Giarin M, Saracco G, et al. Hepatitis B virus unable to secrete e antigen and response to interferon in chronic hepatitis B. Gastroenterology 1993; 105(3):845–50.

20. Fattovich G, Farci P, Rugge M, et al. A randomized controlled trial of lymphoblastoid interferon-alpha in patients with chronic hepatitis B lacking HBeAg. Hepatology 1992;15(4):584–9.

21. Lampertico P, Del Ninno E, Viganò M, et al. Long-term suppression of hepatitis B e antigen-negative chronic hepatitis B by 24-month interferon therapy. Hepatology 2003;37(4):756–63.

22. Lampertico P, Ninno ED, Manzin A, et al. A randomized, controlled trial of a 24-month course of interferon alfa 2b in patients with chronic hepatitis B who had

hepatitis B virus DNA without hepatitis B e antigen in serum. Hepatology (Baltimore, Md) 1997;26(6):1621–5.

23. Marcellin P, Lau GKK, Bonino F, et al. Peginterferon alfa-2a alone, lamivudine alone, and the two in combination in patients with HBeAg-negative chronic hepatitis B. N Engl J Med 2004;351(12):1206–17.

24. Marcellin P, Bonino F, Lau GKK, et al. Sustained response of hepatitis B e antigen-negative patients 3 years after treatment with peginterferon alpha-2a. Gastroenterology 2009;136(7):2169–79, e1-4.

25. Lampertico P, Viganò M, Di Costanzo GG, et al. Randomised study comparing 48 and 96 weeks peginterferon α-2a therapy in genotype D HBeAg-negative chronic hepatitis B. Gut 2013;62(2):290–8.

26. Heermann KH, Goldmann U, Schwartz W, et al. Large surface proteins of hepatitis B virus containing the pre-s sequence. J Virol 1984;52(2):396–402.

27. Hu J, Liu K. Complete and incomplete hepatitis B virus particles: formation, function, and application. Viruses 2017;9(3):56.

28. Ho JK-T, Jeevan-Raj B, Netter H-J. Hepatitis B virus (HBV) subviral particles as protective vaccines and vaccine platforms. Viruses 2020;12(2):126.

29. Bruss V. Hepatitis B virus morphogenesis. World J Gastroenterol 2007;13(1):65–73.

30. Martinot-Peignoux M, Lapalus M, Asselah T, et al. HBsAg quantification: useful for monitoring natural history and treatment outcome. Liver Int 2014;34(Suppl 1):97–107.

31. Hadziyannis E, Hadziyannis SJ. Hepatitis B surface antigen quantification in chronic hepatitis B and its clinical utility. Expert Rev Gastroenterol Hepatol 2014;8(2):185–95.

32. Peng H, Wei F, Liu J-Y, et al. Response-guided therapy of regimens based on PEG-interferon for chronic hepatitis B using on-treatment hepatitis B surface antigen quantification: a meta-analysis. Hepatol Int 2015;9(4):543–57.

33. Pavlovic V, Yang L, Chan HL-Y, et al. Peginterferon alfa-2a (40 kD) stopping rules in chronic hepatitis B: a systematic review and meta-analysis of individual participant data. Antivir Ther 2019;24(2):133–40.

34. Sonneveld MJ, Zoutendijk R, Flink HJ, et al. Close monitoring of hepatitis B surface antigen levels helps classify flares during peginterferon therapy and predicts treatment response. Clin Infect Dis 2013;56(1):100–5.

35. Martinot-Peignoux M, Marcellin P. Virological and serological tools to optimize the management of patients with chronic hepatitis B. Liver Int 2016;36(Suppl 1):78–84.

36. Tangkijvanich P, Chittmittraprap S, Poovorawan K, et al. A randomized clinical trial of peginterferon alpha-2b with or without entecavir in patients with HBeAg-negative chronic hepatitis B: role of host and viral factors associated with treatment response. J Viral Hepat 2016;23(6):427–38.

37. Piratvisuth T, Marcellin P, Popescu M, et al. Hepatitis B surface antigen: association with sustained response to peginterferon alfa-2a in hepatitis B e antigen-positive patients. Hepatol Int 2013;7(2):429–36.

38. Buster EHCJ, Hansen BE, Lau GKK, et al. Factors that predict response of patients with hepatitis B e antigen-positive chronic hepatitis B to peginterferon-alfa. Gastroenterology 2009;137(6):2002–9.

39. Chan HL-Y, Wong VW-S, Chim AM-L, et al. Serum HBsAg quantification to predict response to peginterferon therapy of e antigen positive chronic hepatitis B. Aliment Pharmacol Ther 2010;32(11–12):1323–31.

40. Chen G-Y, Zhu M-F, Zheng D-L, et al. Baseline HBsAg predicts response to pegylated interferon-α2b in HBeAg-positive chronic hepatitis B patients. World J Gastroenterol 2014;20(25):8195–200.

41. Liaw Y-F. Clinical utility of hepatitis B surface antigen quantitation in patients with chronic hepatitis B: a review. Hepatology 2011;54(2):E1–9.

42. Sonneveld MJ, Rijckborst V, Cakaloglu Y, et al. Durable hepatitis B surface antigen decline in hepatitis B e antigen-positive chronic hepatitis B patients treated with pegylated interferon-α2b: relation to response and HBV genotype. Antivir Ther 2011;17(1):9–17.

43. Sonneveld MJ, Hansen BE, Piratvisuth T, et al. Response-guided peginterferon therapy in hepatitis B e antigen-positive chronic hepatitis B using serum hepatitis B surface antigen levels. Hepatology 2013;58(3):872–80.

44. Sonneveld MJ, Rijckborst V, Boucher CAB, et al. Prediction of sustained response to peginterferon alfa-2b for hepatitis B e antigen-positive chronic hepatitis B using on-treatment hepatitis B surface antigen decline. Hepatology 2010;52(4): 1251–7.

45. Moucari R, Martinot-Peignoux M, Mackiewicz V, et al. Influence of genotype on hepatitis B surface antigen kinetics in hepatitis B e antigen-negative patients treated with pegylated interferon-alpha2a. Antivir Ther 2009;14(8):1183–8.

46. Brunetto MR, Marcellin P, Cherubini B, et al. Response to peginterferon alfa-2a (40KD) in HBeAg-negative CHB: on-treatment kinetics of HBsAg serum levels vary by HBV genotype. J Hepatol 2013;59(6):1153–9.

47. Papatheodoridis GV, Manesis EK, Manolakopoulos S, et al. Is there a meaningful serum hepatitis B virus DNA cutoff level for therapeutic decisions in hepatitis B e antigen-negative chronic hepatitis B virus infection? Hepatology 2008;48(5): 1451–9.

48. Rijckborst V, Hansen BE, Cakaloglu Y, et al. Early on-treatment prediction of response to peginterferon alfa-2a for HBeAg-negative chronic hepatitis B using HBsAg and HBV DNA levels. Hepatology 2010;52(2):454–61.

49. Marcellin P, Bonino F, Yurdaydin C, et al. Hepatitis B surface antigen levels: association with 5-year response to peginterferon alfa-2a in hepatitis B e-antigennegative patients. Hepatol Int 2013;7(1):88–97.

50. Brunetto MR, Moriconi F, Bonino F, et al. Hepatitis B virus surface antigen levels: a guide to sustained response to peginterferon alfa-2a in HBeAg-negative chronic hepatitis B. Hepatology 2009;49(4):1141–50.

51. Rijckborst V, Hansen BE, Ferenci P, et al. Validation of a stopping rule at week 12 using HBsAg and HBV DNA for HBeAg-negative patients treated with peginterferon alfa-2a. J Hepatol 2012;56(5):1006–11.

52. Tangkijvanich P, Komolmit P, Mahachai V, et al. Low pretreatment serum HBsAg level and viral mutations as predictors of response to PEG-interferon alpha-2b therapy in chronic hepatitis B. J Clin Virol 2009;46(2):117–23.

53. Chuaypen N, Posuwan N, Payungporn S, et al. Serum hepatitis B core-related antigen as a treatment predictor of pegylated interferon in patients with HBeAg-positive chronic hepatitis B. Liver Int 2016;36(6):827–36.

54. Chuaypen N, Posuwan N, Chittmittraprap S, et al. Predictive role of serum HBsAg and HBcrAg kinetics in patients with HBeAg-negative chronic hepatitis B receiving pegylated interferon-based therapy. Clin Microbiol Infect 2018;24(3): 306.e7–13.

55. Marcellin P, Heathcote EJ, Buti M, et al. TDF disoproxil fumarate versus adefovir Dipivoxil for chronic hepatitis B. N Engl J Med 2008;359(23):2442–55.

56. Fanning GC, Zoulim F, Hou J, et al. Therapeutic strategies for hepatitis B virus infection: towards a cure. Nat Rev Drug Discov 2019;18(11):827–44.

57. Kaewdech A, Tangkijvanich P, Sripongpun P, et al. Hepatitis B surface antigen, core-related antigen and HBV RNA: predicting clinical relapse after NA therapy discontinuation. Liver Int 2020;40(12):2961–71.

58. Viganò M, Invernizzi F, Grossi G, et al. Review article: the potential of interferon and nucleos(t)ide analogue combination therapy in chronic hepatitis B infection. Aliment Pharmacol Ther 2016;44(7):653–61.

59. Yoshida K, Enomoto M, Tamori A, et al. Combination of entecavir or TDF with pegylated interferon-α for long-term reduction in hepatitis B surface antigen levels: simultaneous, sequential, or add-on combination therapy. Int J Mol Sci 2021; 22(3):1456.

60. Ahn J, Lee HM, Lim JK, et al. Entecavir safety and effectiveness in a national cohort of treatment-naïve chronic hepatitis B patients in the US – the ENUMERATE study. Aliment Pharmacol Ther 2016;43(1):134–44.

61. Marcellin P, Ahn SH, Ma X, et al. Combination of TDF disoproxil fumarate and peginterferon α-2a increases loss of hepatitis B surface antigen in patients with chronic hepatitis B. Gastroenterology 2016;150(1):134–44.e10.

62. Ahn SH, Marcellin P, Ma X, et al. Hepatitis B surface antigen loss with TDF disoproxil fumarate plus peginterferon alfa-2a: week 120 analysis. Dig Dis Sci 2018; 63(12):3487–97.

63. Hu C, Song Y, Tang C, et al. Effect of pegylated interferon plus TDF combination on higher hepatitis B surface antigen loss in treatment-naive patients with hepatitis B e antigen -positive chronic hepatitis B: a real-world experience. Clin Ther 2021;43(3):572–81.

64. Brouwer WP, Xie Q, Sonneveld MJ, et al. Adding pegylated interferon to entecavir for hepatitis B e antigen-positive chronic hepatitis B: a multicenter randomized trial (ARES study). Hepatology 2015;61(5):1512–22.

65. van Campenhout MJH, Brouwer WP, Xie Q, et al. Long-term follow-up of patients treated with entecavir and peginterferon add-on therapy for HBeAg-positive chronic hepatitis B infection: ARES long-term follow-up. J Viral Hepat 2019; 26(1):109–17.

66. Chi H, Hansen BE, Guo S, et al. Pegylated interferon alfa-2b add-on treatment in hepatitis B virus envelope antigen-positive chronic hepatitis B patients treated with nucleos(t)ide analogue: a randomized, controlled trial (PEGON). J Infect Dis 2017;215(7):1085–93.

67. Liem KS, van Campenhout MJH, Xie Q, et al. Low hepatitis B surface antigen and HBV DNA levels predict response to the addition of pegylated interferon to entecavir in hepatitis B e antigen positive chronic hepatitis B. Aliment Pharmacol Ther 2019;49(4):448–56.

68. Lampertico P, Brunetto MR, Craxì A, et al. Add-on peginterferon alfa-2a to nucleos(t)ide analogue therapy for Caucasian patients with hepatitis B 'e' antigen-negative chronic hepatitis B genotype D. J Viral Hepat 2019;26(1):118–25.

69. Bourlière M, Rabiega P, Ganne-Carrie N, et al. Effect on HBs antigen clearance of addition of pegylated interferon alfa-2a to nucleos(t)ide analogue therapy versus nucleos(t)ide analogue therapy alone in patients with HBe antigen-negative chronic hepatitis B and sustained undetectable plasma hepatitis B virus DNA: a randomised, controlled, open-label trial. Lancet Gastroenterol Hepatol 2017; 2(3):177–88.

70. Matsumoto A, Nishiguchi S, Enomoto H, et al. Pilot study of TDF disoproxil fumarate and pegylated interferon-alpha 2a add-on therapy in Japanese patients with chronic hepatitis B. J Gastroenterol 2020;55(10):977–89.

71. Ning Q, Han M, Sun Y, et al. Switching from entecavir to PegIFN alfa-2a in patients with HBeAg-positive chronic hepatitis B: a randomised open-label trial (OSST trial). J Hepatol 2014;61(4):777–84.

72. Chan HL-Y, Wong GL-H, Wong VW-S. A review of the natural history of chronic hepatitis B in the era of transient elastography. Antivir Ther 2009;14(4):489–99.

73. Lok AS, Wu PC, Lai CL, et al. A controlled trial of interferon with or without prednisone priming for chronic hepatitis B. Gastroenterology 1992;102(6):2091–7.

74. Perrillo RP, Schiff ER, Davis GL, et al. A randomized, controlled trial of interferon alfa-2b alone and after prednisone withdrawal for the treatment of chronic hepatitis B. The Hepatitis Interventional Therapy Group. N Engl J Med 1990;323(5):295–301.

75. Erhardt A, Blondin D, Hauck K, et al. Response to interferon alfa is hepatitis B virus genotype dependent: genotype A is more sensitive to interferon than genotype D. Gut 2005;54(7):1009–13.

76. Zeuzem S, Gane E, Liaw Y-F, et al. Baseline characteristics and early on-treatment response predict the outcomes of 2 years of telbivudine treatment of chronic hepatitis B. J Hepatol 2009;51(1):11–20.

77. Chan HL-Y, Wong VW-S, Tse AM-L, et al. Serum hepatitis B surface antigen quantitation can reflect hepatitis B virus in the liver and predict treatment response. Clin Gastroenterol Hepatol 2007;5(12):1462–8.

78. Takkenberg RB, Jansen L, de Niet A, et al. Baseline hepatitis B surface antigen (HBsAg) as predictor of sustained HBsAg loss in chronic hepatitis B patients treated with pegylated interferon-α2a and adefovir. Antivir Ther 2013;18(7):895–904.

79. Hou F-Q, Song L-W, Yuan Q, et al. Quantitative hepatitis B core antibody level is a new predictor for treatment response in HBeAg-positive chronic hepatitis B patients receiving peginterferon. Theranostics 2015;5(3):218–26.

80. Chan HLY, Messinger D, Papatheodoridis GV, et al. A baseline tool for predicting response to peginterferon alfa-2a in HBeAg-positive patients with chronic hepatitis B. Aliment Pharmacol Ther 2018;48(5):547–55.

81. Lampertico P, Messinger D, Oladipupo H, et al. An easy-to-use baseline scoring system to predict response to peginterferon alfa-2a in patients with chronic hepatitis B in resource-limited settings. Antivir Ther 2018;23(8):655–63.

82. Lok ASF, McMahon BJ. Chronic hepatitis B. Hepatology 2007;45(2):507–39.

83. Wursthorn K, Lutgehetmann M, Dandri M, et al. Peginterferon alpha-2b plus adefovir induce strong cccDNA decline and HBsAg reduction in patients with chronic hepatitis B. Hepatology 2006;44(3):675–84.

84. de Niet A, Jansen L, Stelma F, et al. Peg-interferon plus nucleotide analogue treatment versus no treatment in patients with chronic hepatitis B with a low viral load: a randomised controlled, open-label trial. Lancet Gastroenterol Hepatol 2017;2(8):576–84.

85. Hagiwara S, Nishida N, Watanabe T, et al. Sustained antiviral effects and clearance of hepatitis surface antigen after combination therapy with entecavir and pegylated interferon in chronic hepatitis B. Antivir Ther 2018;23(6):513–21.

86. Zheng C, Yan H, Zeng J, et al. Comparison of pegylated interferon monotherapy and de novo pegylated interferon plus TDF combination therapy in patients with chronic hepatitis B. Infect Drug Resist 2019;12:845–54.

87. Li G-J, Yu Y-Q, Chen S-L, et al. Sequential combination therapy with pegylated interferon leads to loss of hepatitis B surface antigen and hepatitis B e antigen (HBeAg) seroconversion in HBeAg-positive chronic hepatitis B patients receiving long-term entecavir treatment. Antimicrob Agents Chemother 2015;59(7):4121–8.
88. Xie Q, Zhou H, Bai X, et al. A randomized, open-label clinical study of combined pegylated interferon Alfa-2a (40KD) and entecavir treatment for hepatitis B "e" antigen-positive chronic hepatitis B. Clin Infect Dis 2014;59(12):1714–23.
89. Han M, Jiang J, Hou J, et al. Sustained immune control in HBeAg-positive patients who switched from entecavir therapy to pegylated interferon-α2a: 1 year follow-up of the OSST study. Antivir Ther 2016;21(4):337–44.
90. Huang J, Zhang K, Chen W, et al. Switching to PegIFNα-2b leads to HBsAg loss in patients with low HBsAg levels and HBV DNA suppressed by NAs. Sci Rep 2017;7(1):13383.
91. Tamaki N, Kurosaki M, Kusakabe A, et al. Hepatitis B surface antigen reduction by switching from long-term nucleoside/nucleotide analogue administration to pegylated interferon. J Viral Hepat 2017;24(8):672–8.
92. Hu P, Shang J, Zhang W, et al. HBsAg loss with peg-interferon alfa-2a in hepatitis B patients with partial response to nucleos(t)ide analog: new switch study. J Clin Translational Hepatol 2018;6(1):25–34.
93. Zhou Y, Yan R, Ru GQ, et al. Pegylated-interferon consolidation treatment versus nucleos(t)ide analogue consolidation treatment in non-cirrhotic hepatitis B patients with hepatitis B e antigen seroconversion: an open-label pilot trial. Hepatol Int 2019;13(4):422–30.

Controversies in Treating Chronic Hepatitis B virus

The Role of Hepatitis B Virus DNA and Surface Antigen Titer

Daniel Q. Huang, MBBS, MRCP[a,b], Guan Sen Kew, MBBS, MRCP[a], Seng Gee Lim, MBBS, MD[a,b],*

KEYWORDS

- Interferon • Nucleoside analogues • HBsAg • qHBsAg • HBV DNA • Treatment
- Stopping therapy • Phase change

KEY POINTS

- Older patients with higher HBV DNA and normal or borderline ALT are at higher risk of cirrhosis or HCC. These patients should be monitored carefully, with consideration for antiviral therapy based on individual risk profile and the presence of other risk factors such as family history and male gender. qHBsAg level may have a role for further risk stratification among HBeAg-negative patients.
- qHBsAg levels can be used to decide when to stop therapy for patients treated with PEG-IFN and nucleos(t)ide analogues.
- Among HBeAg-negative patients, HBsAg level less than 1000 IU/mL and HBV DNA level less than 2000 IU/mL are predictive of a benign disease course, and qHBsAg levels can be used to guide frequency of monitoring.
- On treatment qHBsAg is likely a better predictor of subsequent HBsAg seroclearance compared with baseline HBsAg.

Funded by: NUS.
[a] Division of Gastroenterology and Hepatology, Department of Medicine, National University Hospital, University Medicine Cluster, National University Health System, 1E, Kent Ridge Road, NUHS Tower Block Level 10, Singapore 119228, Singapore; [b] Department of Medicine, Yong Loo Lin School of Medicine, National University of Singapore, Singapore
* Corresponding author. Division of Gastroenterology and Hepatology, Department of Medicine, National University Hospital, University Medicine Cluster, National University Health System, 1E, Kent Ridge Road, NUHS Tower Block Level 10, Singapore 119228, Singapore.
E-mail address: mdclimsg@nus.edu.sg
Twitter: @DrHuangDQ (D.Q.H.)

Clin Liver Dis 25 (2021) 763–784
https://doi.org/10.1016/j.cld.2021.06.005
1089-3261/21/© 2021 Elsevier Inc. All rights reserved.

liver.theclinics.com

INTRODUCTION

Hepatitis B virus (HBV) afflicts more than 250 million individuals worldwide and caused more than 887,000 deaths in 2015 alone.[1] Up to 20% of patients with chronic hepatitis B (CHB) develop cirrhosis, and 15% of these develop hepatocellular carcinoma (HCC).[2] Guidelines provide us with evidence-based criteria to make decisions with regard to prognosis and therapy. There are, however, gray areas where evidence is insufficient or unclear as to prognosis or therapy. Up to now, criteria for prognosis and therapy rely on biomarkers such as alanine aminotransferase (ALT) levels, hepatitis B e antigen (HBeAg) status, and HBV DNA levels, and for fibrosis, noninvasive biomarkers and physical biomarkers.[3] New biomarkers are now available such as quantitative hepatitis B surface antigen (qHBsAg), hepatitis B virus (HBV) RNA, and HBV core-related antigen (HBcrAg)[4] that may provide more information to assist physicians in making clinical decisions.

In this review, we particularly examine the role of qHBsAg in clinical practice.[5,6] HBsAg is the envelope protein of the HBV virion and consists of small, medium, and large proteins translated from pre-S1 mRNA and pre-S2/S mRNA, which are in turn transcribed from covalently closed circular DNA cccDNA.[7] qHBsAg titer is a reflection of the total cccDNA in the liver as well as the transcriptional activity of cccDNA; however, this correlation varies by HBeAg status and disease phase (**Fig. 1**).[8]

Areas of controversy are gray areas in CHB management where there is either insufficient evidence or where opinion is divided and there is no consensus agreement. With the advent of safe easily available oral nucleoside analogue therapy, and the prognostic importance of high HBV DNA levels, the issue of treating patients with high viral load to prevent HCC remains controversial. Another area of controversy is that of antiviral therapy and stopping rules for peginterferon therapy, and for stopping nucleoside analogue therapy. In the latter some patients have achieved HBsAg seroclearance, whereas others have developed HBV flares. Could the use of qHBsAg and HBV DNA provide more precision into the clinical management of such patients? In this review, we focus on the controversial aspects of the management of CHB, with a focus on the role of HBV DNA and qHBsAg.

SHOULD PATIENTS WITH HIGH HEPATITIS B VIRUS DNA LEVELS BUT NORMAL ALANINE AMINOTRANSFERASE LEVELS BE TREATED TO PREVENT HEPATOCELLULAR CARCINOMA?

Several studies have shown that high levels of HBV DNA are associated with increased risk of development of HCC despite normal or relatively normal ALT levels

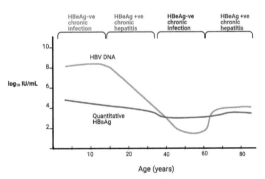

Fig. 1. Variation of qHBsAg and HBV DNA levels with HBeAg status and clinical phase.

(**Table 1**). The World Health Organization (WHO) guidelines recommend that in patients without cirrhosis, treatment should be targeted to patients with persistently abnormal ALT levels and HBV DNA level $\geq$20,000 IU/mL, especially in those older than 30 years, regardless of HBeAg status.[2] The recommended threshold of HBV DNA level $\geq$20,000 IU/mL was derived from a comprehensive systematic review performed by the WHO, which identified 22 observational cohort studies and 1 systematic review that supported this threshold as having increased risk of both HCC and cirrhosis. In the Risk Evaluation of Viral Load Elevation and Associated Liver Disease/Cancer-Hepatitis B Virus (REVEAL-HBV) study, a baseline ALT level of more than 45 U/L was associated with an increased risk of HCC.[9,10] High HBV DNA levels are associated with increased risk of HCC, and antiviral therapy reduces the risk of HCC[11,12]; however, the risk reduction of antiviral therapy was the clearest in those with advanced fibrosis or cirrhosis and less so in those with minimal fibrosis. In the REVEAL-HBV study, the incidence of HCC increased with serum HBV DNA level at study entry in a dose-response relationship of cumulative incidence rate of HCC of 1.3% for HBV DNA level less than 300 copies/mL to 14.9% for an HBV DNA level of 1 million copies/mL or more.[13] This observation led to the development of a 17-point predictive scoring system for HCC (risk estimation for hepatocellular carcinoma in chronic hepatitis B [REACH-B]), which took into account several risk factors such as gender, age, ALT level, HBeAg status, and HBV DNA levels. Despite several cohort and case-control studies (including those with propensity scoring) showing a reduction of HCC in those on antiviral therapy compared with those not on antiviral therapy,[14–18] there has only been a single randomized controlled trial (RCT) that was performed in those with advanced fibrosis or cirrhosis.[19] Consequently, a lack of level 1 evidence makes this unlikely to become a recommendation for therapy, even though long-term antiviral therapy is relatively safe. The utility of qHBsAg as a risk factor was shown in a systematic review, and a meta-analysis of 10 studies reported a pooled odds ratio of 4.99 (95% confidence interval [CI], 3.01–8.29) for HCC when comparing qHBsAg 100 IU/mL or more versus qHBsAg less than 100 IU/mL, and 2.46 (95% CI, 2.15–2.83) when using a threshold of 1000 IU/mL or more versus less than 1000 IU/mL.[20] However, this meta-analysis is limited due to a high level of heterogeneity in the included studies because the investigators included patients with varying HBV phases and degrees of fibrosis and cirrhosis, thereby limiting its application to clinical use. Nonetheless, this meta-analysis provides evidence that there may be a role for qHBsAg to determine HCC risk, but more phase-specific studies are required.

Immune-Tolerant Chronic Hepatitis B

Treatment of patients with high HBV DNA levels to reduce HCC risk has been studied in patients who are in the immune-tolerant phase of CHB, who naturally have high HBV DNA levels. As an example, using the REACH-B risk calculator, a 50-year-old HBeAg-positive male with an ALT level of 20 U/L and HBV DNA level of 100,000 IU/mL would have a 32.0% 10-year risk of HCC. However, current practice guidelines do not routinely recommend antiviral therapy in older immune-tolerant patients, except for EASL, which recommends consideration of antiviral therapy in HBeAg-positive patients aged 30 years and more.[21] A study of immune-tolerant patients (HBeAg-positive, HBV DNA levels > 20,000 IU/mL, ALT levels < 40 IU/L) compared 87 patients in the antiviral treatment group with 397 in the untreated group by balancing baseline characteristics using propensity score matching[22] (see **Table 1**). The investigators found that the antiviral treatment group had a significantly reduced risk for HCC (adjusted hazard ratio [HR], 0.234, P = .046) compared with the control group after, but not before, propensity score matching. This study was limited by the relatively

Table 1
Selected studies evaluating hepatocellular carcinoma risk in patients with high hepatitis B virus DNA level and normal/mildly elevated alanine aminotransferase

Author, Publication Year	Study Period	Study Design	Country	Study Population	HCC Incidence/Risk	Follow-up
Chang et al,[22] 2017	2006–2016	Retrospective observational study	Korea	Comparison of 87 immune-tolerant patients treated with NA vs 397 immune-tolerant patients in the control group	Antiviral treatment group had significantly reduced risk for HCC (HR = 0.234, log-rank $P = .046$) compared with the control group	66.5 mo
Chen et al,[13] 2006	1991–2004	Prospective cohort study	Taiwan	3653 patients with CHB; treatment naive; 164 incident HCC	Cumulative incidence of HCC at the end of follow-up in patients with baseline normal ALT level: 0.98% for patients with baseline HBV DNA <300 copies/mL; 8.6% for patients with baseline HBV DNA 10,000 copies/mL–999,999 copies/mL; 19.5% for patients with baseline HBV DNA>1 million copies/mL	13 y
Tseng,[24] 2012	1985–2000	Prospective cohort study	Taiwan	2688 patients with CHB; 80.5% HBeAg negative; 70.9% ALT level <49; 191 incident HCC	Among HBeAg negative patients with HBV DNA level <2000 IU/mL, the 10-y cumulative incidence of HCC was 0.2% and 2.2% for HBsAg <1000 and ≥1000 IU/mL, respectively. HBsAg was a poor predictor of HCC in HBeAg positive or HBeAg negative/HBV DNA level>2000 IU/mL	14.7 y

Study	Years	Study type	Country	Description	Findings	Follow-up
Kim et al,[23] 2017	2000–2013	Retrospective observational study	Korea	Comparison of 413 untreated immune-tolerant patients with 1497 immune-active patients treated with NA	Significantly higher risk of HCC (adjusted HR 2.54; 95% CI 1.54–4.18) in the untreated immune-tolerant group vs the treated immune-active group	6.3 y
Choi et al,[25] 2019	2000–2013	Retrospective observational study	Korea	Comparison of 900 untreated "replicative phase" patients (normal ALT level, HBV DNA level >2000 IU/mL) with 546 treated immune-active patients	Untreated "replicative phase" group had a higher risk of hepatocellular carcinoma (HCC; HR, 1.76; 95% CI, 1.00–3.10, P = .05) compared with treated immune-active patients	7.8 y
Huang et al,[9] 2021	1997–2016	Retrospective observational study	United States, Taiwan	3366 untreated noncirrhotic CHB (eAg+/-) with high ALT level/low HBV DNA or low HBV DNA/high ALT level	Patients who remained indeterminate had higher 10-y cumulative HCC incidence (4.6% vs 0.5%, P<.0001) and adjusted HR for HCC of 14.1 vs those who remained inactive	12.5 y

Abbreviations: CI, confidence interval; HR, hazard ratio; NA, Nucleos(t)ide analogues.

small numbers in the antiviral treatment group. In addition, although the patients were immune tolerant at baseline, it is possible that these patients experienced a phase change to the immune-active phase during the course of the study, which may have predisposed to the development of complications. Another study of 413 immune-tolerant phase treatment-naive patients (baseline HBV DNA level $\geq$20,000 IU, ALT level in females <19 IU/mL; ALT level in males <30 IU/mL) compared with 1497 treated patients in the immune-active phase (baseline HBV DNA level $\geq$20,000 IU, ALT level $\geq$80 IU/mL)[23] found a significantly higher risk of HCC (adjusted HR [aHR], 2.54; 95% CI, 1.54–4.18) in the untreated immune-tolerant group versus the treated immune-active group. In this analysis, older age, males, and low platelet counts were independent predictors of adverse liver-related outcomes. Although the study team included only patients who remained in the immune-tolerant phase for 1 year before inclusion in the study, the investigators did not account for phase transition to the immune-active phase after the start of the study, therefore it is possible that some patients within the untreated immune-tolerant group had progressed to the immune-active phase before the development of complications. In a Taiwanese study, noncirrhotic patients of varying phases (523 [19.5%] HbeAg positive; 29.1% ALT level $\geq$40 IU/mL) were studied; 64 of the HBeAg-positive patients developed incident HCC.[24] ALT level and HBV DNA both outperformed qHBsAg in the prediction of HCC development within 10 years (area under the receiver operating characteristic curve [ROC] 0.59, 0.48, and 0.35, respectively). However, it must be noted that the patients in the study included both immune-tolerant and immune-active individuals. To date, there are no studies that have used qHBsAg, in addition to ALT and HBV DNA, to further risk stratify immune-tolerant patients, to decide on antiviral therapy. The lack of high-quality large observational studies makes the risk of HCC in truly immune-tolerant patients unclear and the role of qHBsAg uncertain.

Hepatitis B e Antigen-Negative Chronic Hepatitis B with High Viral Load

A study of 5414 HBeAg-negative patients without cirrhosis from Korea identified 900 patients with persistently normal ALT levels but HBV DNA levels greater than 2000 IU/mL (termed *replicative phase*) (see **Table 1**).[25] Compared with treated immune-active patients, the untreated replicative phase patients had almost twice the risk of HCC (HR, 1.76; 95% CI, 1.00–3.10; P = .05). Similarly, a study of 3366 treatment-naive patients with CHB,[9] of which 1303 (38.7%) patients were in the indeterminate phase (with either high HBV DNA level and normal ALT levels, or high ALT and low HBV DNA levels, regardless of HBeAg status) at baseline found that patients who remained in the indeterminate phase throughout follow-up had a 14 times higher risk of HCC versus those who remained in the inactive phase, after adjustment for age, HBeAg status, diabetes, ALT, and HBV DNA. Among patients who were indeterminate, age was the only significant independent predictor for HCC development, with those aged 54 years or greater having the highest risk (aHR, 14.7; 95% CI, 1.84–117.4; P = .01). However, both studies[9,25] did not evaluate the effect of antiviral treatment on HCC risk in the replicative/indeterminate phase; consequently we cannot be certain of the risk reduction benefit (if any) in such patients. In particular, these 2 studies lacked qHBsAg data.

The use of qHBsAg to further risk stratify patients in terms of HCC risk has been examined in a few studies. In the REVEAL HBV cohort, which comprised mostly HBeAg-negative patients with CHB, the cumulative risk of HCC was 1.4%, 4.5%, and 9.2% for those with qHBsAg level less than 100, 100 to 999, and $\geq$1000 IU/mL, respectively.[26] In addition, in another study of inactive CHB carriers, the annual incidence of HCC for patients with normal ALT level was 0.1%, and when qHBsAg levels less than 1000 IU/mL was added to the criteria in the normal ALT group, the HCC risk reduced to 0.03%.[27] In another Taiwanese study, 2688 patients with CHB (80.5% HBeAg negative) without cirrhosis were followed up for 15 years to investigate the association between baseline HBsAg levels and the subsequent risk of HCC. The area under the ROC for predicting HCC development for HBV DNA, ALT, and qHBsAg was 0.70, 0.75, and 0.58 respectively, indicating that qHBsAg level may not be a good tool to predict HCC, when used in patients with HBV in general.[24] However, in a subgroup analysis of patients with HBV DNA less than 2000 IU/mL, the investigators found that qHBsAg level 1000 IU/mL or more was associated with a higher risk of HCC compared with qHBsAg level less than 1000 IU/mL (2.2% vs 0.2%, $P<.001$); multivariable analysis revealed an aHR of 14.4 times higher HCC risk for HBsAg level 1000 IU/mL or more versus less than 1000 IU/mL after adjustment for age, sex, and HBV DNA/HBsAg/ALT dynamics, suggesting that qHBsAg may be useful in selected populations.

At present, there are insufficient data to recommend the routine treatment of patients with high HBV DNA and normal ALT levels to prevent subsequent HCC; however, management should be individualized, with a consideration to treat older patients or those who have multiple risk factors for HCC, such as male gender, age greater than 40 years, HBeAg positivity, and a family history of HCC,[10] particularly because oral antiviral therapy has a good long-term safety record. qHBsAg has a limited role to play in risk stratification of patients with high HBV DNA levels but may be useful in the setting of low HBV DNA levels and may also influence our decision to start antiviral therapy.

In conclusion, studies that examined high viral load in CHB and HCC risk have shown some evidence of increased risk of HCC in such patients. Some observational studies show benefit of antiviral therapy in reducing HCC, but the studies had some methodological concerns that made the conclusions less than convincing. Consequently, only a large well-conducted RCT would provide convincing level 1 evidence that antiviral therapy reduces HCC risk.

SHOULD PATIENTS WITH HIGH HEPATITIS B VIRUS DNA LEVELS BUT NORMAL ALANINE AMINOTRANSFERASE LEVELS BE TREATED TO PREVENT REACTIVATION AND CIRRHOSIS?

Based on the systematic review by WHO, HBV DNA levels greater than a threshold ranging from 4200 to 20,000 IU/mL were significant independent predictors of future active hepatitis, and an HBV DNA level greater than 20,000 IU/mL was predictive of current fibrosis among HBeAg-negative patients in the inactive carrier phase.[2,10] Immune-active patients with high ALT and high HBV DNA levels are at the highest risk of cirrhosis and HCC, and all major society guidelines are in agreement that treatment is indicated.[3,21,28]

However, many patients may have high DNA levels but normal or borderline ALT levels, placing them in an "indeterminate" phase or "gray zone,"[9] and current practice guidelines do not provide clear guidance as to whether these patients with high HBV DNA levels should be treated to prevent reactivation and cirrhosis. In a small study 46 HBeAg-negative patients with CHB with HBV DNA levels between 2000 and 20,000 IU/mL and normal ALT levels (termed low viremic active carriers)[29] **(Table 2)** were followed, and of these 46 patients, 20 (43.5%) became inactive and 1 (2.2%) developed CHB after 57.2 months follow-up. Baseline qHBsAg levels were lower in the inactive phase compared with the low viremic inactive carriers (2.61 $\log_{10}$ IU/mL vs 3.61 $\log_{10}$ IU/mL, $P<.001$). A higher baseline qHBsAg level was associated with developing chronic hepatitis in univariate analysis; however, baseline qHBsAg level was not an

Table 2
Selected studies evaluating reactivation and cirrhosis risk in patients with high hepatitis B virus DNA and normal/mildly elevated alanine aminotransferase

Author, Publication Year	Study Period	Study Design	Country	Study Population and Findings	Follow-up
Oliveri et al,[29] 2017	2000–2001	Prospective cohort study	Italy	153 HBeAg-negative patients with CHB with HBV DNA level $\leq$20,000 IU/mL and normal ALT level. Baseline qHBsAg levels were lower in the inactive phase (HBV level <2000 IU/mL) compared with the low viremic inactive carrier patients (HBV level 2000–20,000 IU/mL) (2.61 $\log_{10}$ IU/mL vs 3.61 $\log_{10}$ IU/mL, P<.001).	4.7 y
Bonacci et al,[54] 2018	1985–2015	Retrospective observational study	Spain	137 inactive and 150 HBeAg-negative CHB "gray zone" patients (either ALT level between 40 and 80 IU/mL and/or HBV DNA level 2000 IU/mL–20,000 IU/mL). Baseline qHBsAg levels were lower in inactive vs "gray zone" patients (338 IU/mL vs 5763 IU/mL, P<.05). 6.3% of "gray zone" patients developed immune-active disease	8.2 y
Lee et al,[26] 2013	1991–2004	Prospective cohort study	Taiwan	3342 patients with CHB; 84.9% HBeAg positive; 94.3% ALT level <45; 327 incident cases of cirrhosis. Cumulative risk for cirrhosis was 4.8%, 8.8%, and 16.2% for participants with serum HBsAg levels <100, 100–999, and $\geq$1000 IU/mL, respectively. qHBsAg was significantly associated with cirrhosis in a dose-response manner (P trend<0.001) among HBeAg-negative individuals with serum HBV DNA levels <10^6 copies/mL, but not those with HBV DNA levels >10^6 copies/mL nor HBeAg-positive individuals	>12 y
Huang et al,[9] 2021	1997–2016	Retrospective observational study	USA, Taiwan	3336 noncirrhotic patients with CHB. Higher 10-y cumulative incidence of cirrhosis among indeterminate patients who remained indeterminate (ALT/HBV DNA not conforming to any of the defined CHB phases by AASLD criteria) vs inactive patients who remained inactive, 8.8% vs 3.5% (P<.0001)	12.5 y

Abbreviations: AASLD, American Association for the Study of Liver Diseases.

independent predictor of developing immune-active disease after adjustment for HBV DNA, HBcrAg, total anti-HBc, and liver stiffness.

In an Italian study, 137 inactive and 150 HBeAg-negative patients with CHB in the "gray zone" (either ALT level between 40 and 80 IU/mL and/or HBV DNA level between 2000 IU/mL and 20,000 IU/mL)[30] were monitored, and baseline quantitative qHBsAg levels were lower in inactive versus "gray zone" patients (338 IU/mL versus 5763 IU/mL, P<.05). After a median follow-up of 8.2 years, 6.3% of "gray zone" patients developed immune-active disease and no patients were found to have developed advanced fibrosis. Owing to the small number of patients, no independent predictors for transiting to the immune-active phase were identified, including qHBsAg levels. A study showed that of 1303 patients in the indeterminate phase (ALT/HBV DNA not conforming to any of the defined CHB phases by American Association for the Study of Liver Diseases [AASLD] criteria), 21.7% of patients transitioned from the indeterminate phase to the inactive phase after a mean follow-up of 12.5 years.[9] Furthermore, the investigators found a higher 10-year cumulative incidence of cirrhosis among indeterminate patients who remained indeterminate versus inactive patients who remained inactive, 8.8% (95% CI, 6.5–11.8) versus 3.5% (95% CI, 2.5–5.0) (P<.0001); however, this study did not report qHBsAg levels.[9] Efficacy and cost-effectiveness data are lacking with regard to antiviral treatment among patients with high HBV and normal ALT levels, and further studies are required before HBV antivirals can be routinely recommended in this subgroup to prevent reactivation and cirrhosis.

A study of 3342 patients with CHB (84.9% HBeAg positive; 94.3% ALT level <45 IU/mL) found that the cumulative risk for cirrhosis was 4.8%, 8.8%, and 16.2% for participants with serum HBsAg levels less than 100, 100 to 999, and $\geq$1000 IU/mL, respectively (P<.001). When stratified by HBeAg status, qHBsAg levels were not associated with cirrhosis among HBeAg-positive patients, but qHBsAg was significantly associated with cirrhosis in a dose-response manner (P trend <.001) among HBeAg-negative individuals with serum HBV DNA levels less than 10^6 copies/mL.

Similar to the findings of HCC risk, studies that examined high viral load in CHB and risk of disease progression have shown some evidence of increased risk of disease progression and phase change. Quantitative HBsAg may be useful in HBeAg-negative patients with HBV DNA less than 10^6 copies/mL to stratify the risk of cirrhosis. However, there were no observational studies examining risk improvement with antiviral therapy. Similarly, only a large well-conducted RCT would provide convincing level 1 evidence that antiviral therapy reduces disease progression in those with high viral load and normal ALT levels. A summary of the studies described earlier is provided in **Table 2**.

CAN QUANTITATIVE HEPATITIS B SURFACE ANTIGEN AND HEPATITIS B VIRUS DNA HELP TO IDENTIFY WHICH PATIENTS WILL REMAIN INACTIVE?

A study of 209 consecutive HBeAg-negative patients with genotype D CHB[31] found that qHBsAg levels were significantly lower in the inactive versus active phase (62.12 vs 3029 IU/mL; P<.001) (**Table 3**). In this study, the combination of baseline HBsAg level less than 1000 IU/mL and HBV DNA level 2000 IU/mL or less provided a 91.1% sensitivity and 95.4% specificity for identifying patients in the inactive phase. In this study, HBsAg and HBV-DNA serum levels correlated weakly ($\rho = 0.638$, P<.001), and HBV DNA level was higher in the active versus inactive phase (389,500 IU/mL vs 49 IU/mL). In a study from the REVEAL-HBV cohort,[32] 1529 HBeAg-negative, genotype B or C patients were assigned as either inactive or active after 18 months of follow-up. The investigators found that a one-time baseline

Table 3
Selected studies evaluating the use of quantitative hepatitis B surface antigen and hepatitis B virus DNA in predicting which patients will remain inactive

Author, Publication Year	Study Period	Study Design	Country	Study Population and Findings	Follow-up
Brunetto et al0,[31] 2010	2000–2006	Prospective cohort study	Italy	209 HBeAg-negative patients, genotype D; qHBsAg levels were significantly lower in the inactive vs active phase (62.12 vs 3029 IU/mL; $P<.001$); the combination of baseline HBsAg level <1000 IU/mL and HBV DNA level ≤2000 IU/mL provided a 91.1% sensitivity and 95.4% specificity for identifying patients in the inactive phase	Median 34.5 mo
Liu et al,[32] 2016	Patients recruited between 1991 and 1992	Retrospective study	Taiwan	1529 HBeAg-negative patients, genotype B or C; one-time baseline measurement of HBsAg level <1000 IU/mL and HBV DNA level <2000 IU/mL was able to predict patients who would remain in the inactive phase, with a sensitivity and specificity of 71% and 85%, respectively.	Up to 18 mo
Pfefferkorn et al,[33] 2017	1998–2015	Retrospective study	Germany	183 treatment-naive patients with CHB and quantified HBV large surface and middle surface proteins across phases; individuals in the inactive carrier phase had significantly lower large surface and middle surface proteins compared with the other phases ($P<.0001$).	Mean 38.5 mo

measurement of HBsAg level less than 1000 IU/mL and HBV DNA level less than 2000 IU/mL was able to predict patients who would remain in the inactive phase, with a sensitivity and specificity of 71% and 85%, respectively. More recently, a study of 183 treatment-naive patients with CHB quantified HBV large surface proteins and HBV middle surface proteins[33] and found lower quantities of both large surface and middle surface proteins in the inactive group compared with the other phases (P<.0001). Further studies are required to validate the role of large and middle surface proteins in the identification of inactive carriers. Taken together, low HBV DNA and qHBsAg levels indicate a favorable and benign course among inactive carriers. The utility of this combined biomarker in identifying inactive patients with low risk of reactivation and HCC development may potentially be used to reduce the frequency of follow-up and could be cost saving.

CAN QUANTITATIVE HEPATITIS B SURFACE ANTIGEN BE USED TO DETERMINE WHEN TO STOP TREATMENT?
Stopping Pegylated Interferon

Among the practice guidelines, European Association for the Study of the Liver (EASL) and Asian Pacific Association for the Study of the Liver (APASL) provide specific recommendations on stopping rules in pegylated interferon (PEG-IFN), but not the AASLD. EASL and APASL recommend that HBeAg-positive patients treated with PEG-IFN should have qHBsAg levels checked at 12 weeks of therapy, and if qHBsAg level is greater than 20,000 IU/mL for genotype B and C, or if there is no decline from baseline for genotype A or D, treatment should be discontinued.[21,28] Among HBeAg-negative patients, both EASL and APASL recommend that those who fail to achieve a decline in qHBsAg level and less than 2 $\log_{10}$ IU/mL reduction in serum HBV DNA levels after 12 weeks of therapy should stop PEG-IFN therapy. By contrast, the AASLD does not recommend specific thresholds for stopping interferon therapy but comment that HBsAg quantification may be useful in guiding the management of such patients.[34]

In a meta-analysis of published studies, conference abstracts and Roche's internal database,[35] including 1423 patients (765 HBeAg positive, 658 HBeAg negative), stopping rules for PEG-IFN therapy based on prespecified biomarker cutoff target performance characteristics were identified. Among HBeAg-negative patients, the investigators only identified sufficient studies in genotype D patients and identified an HBsAg level greater than 20,000 IU/mL or HBV DNA level greater than 6.5 $\log_{10}$ IU/mL at week 12 for genotype D patients as a stopping rule that fulfilled their preset criteria (**Table 4**). However, this study was limited by a lack of sufficient patients to analyze the performance of a decline in HBV DNA or HBsAg levels in HBeAg-negative patients. An RCT of 107 HBeAg-negative patients found that 20 of 20 patients (100%) with a lack of decline of qHBsAg levels and less than 2 log IU/mL reduction in HBV DNA at week 12 subsequently failed PEG-IFN treatment[36] (see **Table 4**). These stopping rules were further validated in a study[37] evaluating 160 HBeAg-negative patients from two independent trials receiving PEG-IFN; the investigators found that the negative predictive value of these stopping rules was 95% for genotypes A to D and 100% for genotype D. A prospective study in Thailand of 98 HBeAg-negative patients[38] (98% genotypes B and C) showed that less than 2 $\log_{10}$ decline in HBV DNA levels and less than 10% $\log_{10}$ decline in HBsAg had negative predictive value (NPV) of 80% and 66% for sustained response.

A meta-analysis[35] identified HBsAg level greater than 20,000 IU/mL, or HBV DNA level greater than 8 $\log_{10}$ IU/mL, at week 12 as a stopping rule for HBeAg-positive

Table 4
Selected studies evaluating the use of quantitative hepatitis B surface antigen in determining when to stop pegylated-interferon treatment

Author, Publication Year	Study Design	Study Population and Findings	Follow-up
Rijckborst et al,[36] 2010	Randomized controlled trial	107 HBeAg-negative patients, mean age 42%, 77% male, mean HBV DNA level 3.8 log IU/mL, 20/20 (100%) with lack of decline of qHBsAg and <2 log IU/mL reduction in HBV DNA level at week 12 did not respond to PEG-IFN	72 wk
Rijckborst et al,[37] 2012	Posthoc analysis of 2 randomized trials	160 HBeAg-negative patients. 21/22 (95.0%) with lack of decline of qHBsAg and <2 log IU/mL reduction in HBV DNA level at week 12 did not respond to PEG IFN	Up to 96 wk
Sonneveld et al,[39] 2013	Posthoc analysis of 3 randomized trials	803 HBeAg-positive patients, 103/103 (100%) with HBV DNA level >20,000 IU/ mL at week 24 did not respond to PEG-IFN	Up to 78 wk
Goulis et al,[55] 2014	Prospective multicenter study	96 HBeAg-negative patients, mean age 42%, 73.3% males, mean HBV DNA level 5.4 log IU/mL, 8/8 (100%) with lack of decline of qHBsAg and <2 log IU/mL reduction in HBV DNA level at week 12 did not respond to PEG IFN	96 wk
Charatcharoenwitthaya et al,[38] 2016	Prospective nationwide cohort study	135 hepatitis HBeAg-positive patients and 98 HBeAg-negative patients, mean age 41.6, 74% male, mean HBV DNA level 6.4 log IU/mL. HBsAg level >20,000 IU/mL at week 12 for HBeAg-positive patients provided a negative predictive value of 96%. 12-week stopping rules of no decline in HBsAg with a <2 log$_{10}$ decline in HBV DNA and a <10% log10 decline in HBsAg among HBeAg-negative patients showed negative predictive values of 80% and 66%, respectively.	At least 24 wk after treatment discontinuation

genotype B and C patients. However, there were insufficient data to analyze stopping rules for genotypes A and D for HBeAg-positive patients. A study analyzed 803 HBeAg-positive patients treated with PEG-IFN and found low response rates at week 12 of therapy in genotypes A or D if there was no decline of HBsAg levels (NPV 97% to 100%), or qHBsAg level was more than 20,000 IU/mL at week 12 for genotypes B and C[39] (see **Table 4**). At week 24 of PEG-IFN therapy, almost all patients with HBsAg levels greater than 20,000 IU/mL failed to achieve a response, irrespective of HBV genotype. In the earlier mentioned Thai study,[38] for HBeAg-positive patients, HBsAg levels greater than 20,000 IU/mL at week 12 provided a good negative predictive value of 96% for sustained response.

By measuring qHBsAg and HBV DNA levels at week 12 of PEG-IFN therapy, physicians can identify nonresponders to treatment and may consider terminating treatment early, hence avoiding unnecessary prolonged treatment and its potential side effects. HBV RNA and HBcrAg have been proposed as potential biomarkers to further tailor therapy with PEG-IFN; however, more data are required before these can be adopted in routine clinical practice.[40,41]

In conclusion, PEG-IFN stopping rules seem to favor genotype D where the evidence seems particularly strong, but there are fewer studies for other genotypes, particularly the Asian genotypes B and C. It is not surprising that EASL guidelines do adopt the stopping rules for PEG-IFN because genotype D is the most prevalent in Europe.

Stopping Nucleos(t)ide Analogues

qHBsAg levels can also help to identify patients who may stop nucleos(t)ide analogues (**Table 5**). In a systemic review,[42] when end of therapy qHBsAg level was less than 100 IU/mL, off-therapy HBV DNA level increased to greater than 200 IU/mL in less than 22% of patients. Among patients with qHBsAg levels less than 200 IU/mL at the end of therapy, less than 7% of patients developed HBV DNA relapse (>2000 IU/mL). In another systematic review,[43] the investigators studied 11 studies with 1716 patients who stopped nucleos(t)ide analogues and found that when qHBsAg level was less than 100 IU/mL, the proportion of off-therapy virological relapse was only 15.4% to 29.4%, compared with 31.4% to 86.8% in patients with qHBsAg levels greater than 100 IU/mL. It was also found that the off-therapy HBsAg loss rates were 21.1% to 58.8% for baseline qHBsAg levels less than 100 IU/mL and 3.3% to 7.4% for qHBsAg level greater than 100 IU/mL at 39 months off therapy. In another study, in patients with end-of-treatment qHBsAg levels 200 IU/mL or less, the 5-year rate of clinical relapse was 27.6%[44] (see **Table 5**). In a large prospective Taiwanese study of 691 HBeAg-negative patients with CHB who stopped nucleos(t)ide analogues,[45] a greater qHBsAg level reduction during therapy of greater than 1 $\log_{10}$, and a lower end-of-treatment qHBsAg level less than 100 IU/mL were significant predictors for off-therapy HBsAg seroclearance (see **Table 5**). This study reported a fairly high virological relapse (HBV DNA level increase of >2000 IU/mL) and clinical relapse rate (HBV DNA level increase of >2000 IU/mL and ALT >2 × upper limit of normal [ULN]) of 79.2% and 60.6%, respectively, for the entire cohort, after a median follow-up of 155 weeks. In this same study, among patients with qHBsAg level reduction during therapy of more than 1 $\log_{10}$, 18 of 142 patients (12.7%) achieved HBsAg seroclearance; and among those with end-of-treatment qHBsAg level less than 100 IU/mL, 24 of 114 patients (21.1%) achieved HBsAg seroclearance.[45] Taken together, a threshold of HBsAg level less than 100 to 200 IU/mL may be used as a threshold to consider safely stopping nucleoside analogues.

Table 5
Selected studies evaluating the use of quantitative hepatitis B surface antigen in determining when to stop nucleos(t)ide analogues

Author, Publication Year	Study Design	Study Population and Findings	Follow-up
Chang et al,[42] 2015	Systematic review	22 studies with a total of 1732 patients on therapy > 6 mo in HBeAg-negative patients with CHB with off-therapy follow-up > 6 mo. Off-therapy HBV DNA level increased > 200 IU/mL in only 9%–22% of patients with end-of-therapy qHBsAg <100 IU/mL, whereas <7% of the patients with end-of-therapy qHBsAg level <200 IU/mL developed HBV DNA relapse to >2000 IU/mL	—
Liu,[43] 2019	Systematic review	11 studies with 1716 patients who stopped nucleos(t)ide analogues. When qHBsAg level was <100 IU/mL, the proportion of off-therapy virological relapse was only 15.4%–29.4%, compared with 31.4%–86.8% in patients with qHBsAg level >100 IU/mL	—
Yao et al,[44] 2017	Prospective cohort study	In 119 patients with CHB who achieved end-of-treatment qHBsAg level ≤200IU/mL; the 5-y rate of clinical relapse was 27.6%	60 mo
Jeng et al,[45] 2018	Prospective multicenter study	In 691 HBeAg-negative patients with CHB who stopped nucleos(t)ide analogues, a greater qHBsAg reduction during therapy of >1 log₁₀, and a lower end-of-treatment qHBsAg level <100 IU/mL predicts off-therapy HBsAg seroconversion. In 142 patients with qHBsAg reduction during therapy of >1, and 114 patients with end-of-treatment qHBsAg level <100 IU/mL, 18 (12.7%) and 24 (21.1%) patients achieved HBsAg seroconversion	155 wk

The issue of stopping long-term nucleos(t)ide analogues therapy in HBeAg-negative CHB still remains controversial despite the accumulating data of the benefits of HBsAg loss. The meta-analysis by Liu was not particularly convincing because the conclusion was not derived through data pooling and no forest plot was generated. Consequently, an RCT to test the benefits and risks of qHBsAg less than 100 IU/mL as the threshold for stopping nucleos(t)ide analogues therapy needs to be performed. A utility of additional biomarkers such as HBV RNA and HBcrAg may provide additional confidence in stopping nucleos(t)ide analogue therapy.

ARE BASELINE FACTORS OR ON-TREATMENT FACTORS BETTER TO PREDICT HEPATITIS B SURFACE ANTIGEN SEROCLEARANCE IN PATIENTS?

HBsAg seroclearance is an uncommon event, with a meta-analysis reporting a pooled annual rate of 1.02%.[46] It was also reported that lower baseline HBV DNA and HBsAg levels were associated with a higher rate of HBsAg seroclearance. A meta-analysis of the efficacy of antiviral therapy in CHB showed that interferon therapy had a small but significant increase in HBsAg loss over nucleos(t)ide analogues (risk difference 3%).[47] However, it is unclear whether baseline versus on-treatment factors are better to predict HBsAg seroclearance in the setting of antiviral therapy. Baseline risk is important in the selection of therapy, whereas on-treatment factors can only be used to decide whether to continue or stop therapy. Hence baseline factors play a more important role.

Predicting Hepatitis B Surface Antigen Loss While on Pegylated Interferon

A posthoc analysis of a randomized trial using peg-interferon ± nucleos(t)ide analogues[48] (114 HBeAg-negative patients) was used to determine the utility of qHBsAg, HBV RNA, and quantitative core-related antigen in predicting HBsAg loss (**Table 6**). In this study, HBsAg loss occurred in 15 of 114 patients (13%). The investigators found that the best predictor of HBsAg seroclearance was qHBsAg at week 8 of treatment (C statistic 0.96 for the univariate model and 0.98 in the multivariate model including treatment arm, age, and sex); in comparison, baseline qHBsAg had a lower C statistic (0.92 in the univariate model and 0.93 in the multivariate model including treatment arm, age, and sex). Incidentally, HBV RNA (C statistic 0.54) and quantitative core-related antigen (C statistic 0.65) were weak predictors of HBsAg loss, both at baseline and on treatment. A study of 335 patients on antiviral therapy[49] (80% PEG-IFN based, 6.9% developed HBsAg loss) found that the change in HBsAg at 6 months and 9 months compared with baseline provided a high C statistic of 0.89 and 0.94, respectively, for HBsAg seroclearance. However, change in core-related antigen was a weak predictor of HBsAg loss, with a C statistic of 0.59 and 0.52, respectively. In another study,[50] 230 patients (12% achieved HBsAg loss) from a randomized study that treated patients with PEG-IFN ± lamivudine found that rates of HBsAg clearance at 1 year were higher in treated patients with a 10% or more $\log_{10}$ decline in HBsAg from baseline versus < $\log_{10}$ decline at week 12 (9.4% vs 1.4%).

Taken together, these findings indicate that on-treatment qHBsAg level kinetics are likely to be better than baseline factors to predict HBsAg seroclearance in patients on PEG-IFN therapy. However, patients already on PEG-IFN who do not belong to the nonresponder group only have a small possibility of HBsAg loss. Although predictors may provide some information on likelihood of this event, this is unlikely to change management. Nonetheless, most patients who complete peg-IFN are likely to be remain quiescent and remain off antiviral therapy.[21]

Table 6
Selected studies evaluating predictors of quantitative hepatitis B surface antigen loss

Author, Publication Year	Study Period	Study Design	Country	Study Population and Findings	Follow-up
Lim et al,[48] 2021	2014–2018	Posthoc analysis of a randomized trial	Singapore	114 HBeAg-negative patients treated with pegylated interferon, 85.1% male; 15/114 (13%) achieved HBsAg loss. AUC for HBsAg loss was 0.96 for HBsAg at week 8 of treatment, 0.92 for HBsAg at baseline	72 wk
Ma et al,[49] 2020	2013–2017	Prospective cohort study	China	335 patients with CHB, mixture of HBeAg +/- (unspecified proportion), 80% treated with pegylated interferon, 20% nucleos(t)ide analogues. ΔHBsAg of 0.64 log10 IU/mL at 6 mo AUC of 0.886. At 12 mo, ΔHBsAg of 1.45 log10 IU/mL at 12 mo had AUC of 0.939. ΔHBcrAg AUC of 0.59 at 6 mo and 0.521 at 12 mo, Δpg RNA had AUC of 0.57 and 0.60	3.6 y
Marcellin et al,[50] 2013	-	Multicenter, randomized trial	Multiple countries	230 HBeAg-negative patients with CHB treated with pegylated interferon ± lamivudine. Among patients with a ≥10% decline in HBsAg from baseline at week 12 and HBV DNA level <2000 IU/mL at 1 y posttreatment, 40% (10/25) achieved HBsAg loss. 44.8% (13/29) of patients with a ≥10% decline in HBsAg from baseline at week 24 and HBV DNA level <2000 IU/mL at 1 y posttreatment achieved HBsAg clearance at 5 y	5 y posttreatment
Peng et al,[52] 2017	-	Prospective cohort study	Taiwan	529 patients (195 HBeAg positive and 334 HBeAg negative) treated with entecavir, 73.2% male. HBsAg levels of <3000 IU/mL at baseline combined with a qHBsAg decline of 75% from baseline was predictive for HBsAg loss (positive and negative predictive values 70% and 100%, respectively)	5 y
Marcellin et al,[53] 2014	2005–2007	Randomized trial	Europe and United States	266 HBeAg positive patients with CHB treated with tenofovir. Multivariable analysis for predictors of HBsAg loss showed that qHBsAg decline of 1 log10 IU/mL at week 24 (HR = 13.7, 95% CI, 5.6–33.7; P<.0001) was an independent predictor, but not baseline HBsAg or HBV DNA	240 wk

Abbreviation: AUC, area under the receiver operating characteristic curve.

Table 7
Summary of advantages and disadvantages in each controversy

Controversy	Advantages	Disadvantages
Treatment of patients with high viral load to prevent HCC	• Strong evidence for increased risk of HCC in individuals with high viral load • Potential to reduce HCC incidence in those currently not eligible for treatment based on guidelines • Oral antiviral therapy safe and well tolerated	• Long-term oral therapy with unclear end points • Low prospect of HBsAg loss • High number needed to treat • Lack of direct evidence demonstrating antiviral therapy reduces HCC in individuals not meeting current treatment thresholds
Treatment of patients with high viral load to prevent cirrhosis	• Some evidence for increased risk of cirrhosis in patients who are in the indeterminate phase • Potential to reduce cirrhosis incidence in those currently not eligible for treatment based on guidelines • Oral antiviral therapy safe and well tolerated	• Long-term oral therapy with unclear end points • Low prospect of HBsAg loss • High number needed to treat • Lack of direct evidence demonstrating a reduced incidence of cirrhosis with antiviral therapy among patients with high viral load but normal ALT level
Use of qHBsAg to determine when to stop treatment in PEG-IFN	• Strong evidence for genotype D validating the use of stopping rules • Reduces exposures to additional doses and potential side effects in the setting of a high risk of futility	• Less data in genotypes B and C
Use of qHBsAg to determine when to stop nucleos(t)ide analogues	• Potentially lower risk of virological relapse when qHBsAg <100–200 IU/mL	• No RCT available • Up to 30% of patients may develop virological relapse after stopping nucleos(t)ide analogues even when HBsAg level <100 IU/mL
Use of HBsAg and HBV DNA to identify patients who will remain inactive	• May identify patients suitable for less-frequent follow-up and enable cost savings	• Marked variation of sensitivity and specificity across studies, more data are required
Baseline HBsAg vs on-treatment HBsAg to predict HBsAg seroclearance	• On-treatment qHBsAg is likely a better predictor of subsequent HBsAg seroclearance compared with baseline HBsAg	• On-treatment qHBsAg is not likely to change clinical management, as PEG-IFN and nucleos(t)ide analogues are likely to be continued to achieve viral suppression even if HBsAg loss is unlikely

Predicting Hepatitis B Surface Antigen Loss While on Nucleo(t)ide Analogues

Among patients treated with nucleos(t)ide analogues, patients who eventually lose HBsAg tend to have a dramatic reduction of qHBsAg to low levels, which may be followed by HBsAg seroconversion.[51] In a prospective study of 529 HBeAg-positive/negative CHB,[52] qHBsAg levels of less than 3000 IU/mL at baseline combined with a qHBsAg decline of 75% or more from baseline provided a predictive algorithm for HBsAg loss (positive predictive value [PPV] and NPV 70% and 100%, respectively; 10 of 215 [4.7%] patients achieved HBsAg loss) during 5 years of treatment with entecavir (see **Table 6**). Among patients with a baseline qHBsAg level less than 3000 IU/mL who did not experience subsequent HBsAg decline of 75%, the PPV for HBsAg seroclearance was only 27%. Similarly, in another study of 266 HBeAg-positive CHB,[53] 23 of 266 (8.6%) patients developed HBsAg loss and a qHBsAg decline of 1 $\log_{10}$ IU/mL or more at week 24 (HR = 13.7; 95% CI, 5.6–33.7; P<.0001) of treatment with tenofovir was found to be an independent predictor of HBsAg loss, whereas baseline qHBsAg and HBV DNA levels were not independently associated with HBsAg loss. Taken together, these data suggest that qHBsAg on treatment is better than baseline qHBsAg for predicting which patients may develop HBsAg seroclearance while on nucleos(tide) analogue therapy. However, the possibility of HBsAg loss is even lower in nucleo(t)ide analogues therapy compared with peg-IFN therapy. In most patients on therapy, long-term therapy seems to be the most likely possibility.

SUMMARY

The utility of qHBsAg in addition to other viral markers is still being explored in CHB management. We have highlighted controversial areas where qHBsAg has been useful in assisting with decision making, with the pros and cons summarized in **Table 7**. The most important issue currently is the utility of qHBsAg in guiding cessation of antiviral therapy in HBeAg-negative CHB; its use as a futility rule in peginterferon therapy is more established in Europe where the findings in genotype D are convincing. For other controversial areas such as therapy for patients with high viral load and normal ALT levels to reduce HCC or liver disease progression RCTs adequately powered to address this subject are required. Finally, there may be a role for qHBsAg to risk stratify HBeAg-negative patients with lower levels of viremia to identify truly inactive CHB carriers; however, more information is required to determine if we can reduce the frequency of follow-up safely.

DISCLOSURE

D.Q. Huang: Advisory board: Eisai; Research support: NMRC Research Training Fellowship, Exxon Mobil-NUS Research Fellowship for Clinicians. G.S. Kew has no disclosures. S.G. Lim: Advisory board: Gilead Sciences, Springbank, Roche, Abbvie, Abbott, Kaleido; Speakers bureau: Gilead Sciences, Abbott, Roche; Research support: Abbott, Merck Sharpe and Dohme, Roche, Gilead Sciences.

REFERENCES

1. World Health Organization. Global hepatitis report 2017. https://apps.who.int/iris/bitstream/handle/10665/255016/9789241565455-eng.pdf;jsessionid=6DB65DA61DB685B218A314037DBE0C09?sequence=1. Accessed 20 May, 2020.

2. World Health Organization. Guidelines for the prevention, care and treatment of persons with chronic hepatitis B infection 2015. https://www.who.int/hepatitis/publications/hepatitis-b-guidelines/en/. Accessed 20 May, 2020.

3. Terrault NA, Lok ASF, McMahon BJ, et al. Update on prevention, diagnosis, and treatment of chronic hepatitis B: AASLD 2018 hepatitis B guidance. *Hepatology* 2018;67(4):1560–99.

4. Coffin CS, Zhou K, Terrault NA. New and old biomarkers for diagnosis and management of chronic hepatitis B virus infection. Gastroenterology 2019;156(2): 355–368 e3.

5. Liao CC, Hsu CW, Gu PW, et al. Comparison of the elecsys HBsAg II assay and the architect assay for quantification of hepatitis B surface antigen in chronic hepatitis B patients. Biomed J 2015;38(3):250–6.

6. Wursthorn K, Jaroszewicz J, Zacher BJ, et al. Correlation between the Elecsys HBsAg II assay and the Architect assay for the quantification of hepatitis B surface antigen (HBsAg) in the serum. J Clin Virol 2011;50(4):292–6.

7. Heermann KH, Goldmann U, Schwartz W, et al. Large surface proteins of hepatitis B virus containing the pre-s sequence. *J Virol* Nov 1984;52(2):396–402.

8. Thompson AJ, Nguyen T, Iser D, et al. Serum hepatitis B surface antigen and hepatitis B e antigen titers: disease phase influences correlation with viral load and intrahepatic hepatitis B virus markers. *Hepatology* 2010;51(6):1933–44.

9. Huang DQ, Li X, Le MH, et al. Natural history and hepatocellular carcinoma risk in untreated chronic hepatitis B patients with indeterminate phase. Clin Gastroenterol Hepatol 2021. https://doi.org/10.1016/j.cgh.2021.01.019.

10. Guideline development for the prevention, care and treatment of persons with chronic hepatitis B Appendix 2: systematic review reports and evidence summaries. Geneva: World Health Organization; 2015.

11. Yang HI, Yuen MF, Chan HL, et al. Risk estimation for hepatocellular carcinoma in chronic hepatitis B (REACH-B): development and validation of a predictive score. Lancet Oncol 2011;12(6):568–74.

12. Jeng WJ, Lok AS. Should treatment indications for chronic hepatitis B be expanded? Clin Gastroenterol Hepatol 2020. https://doi.org/10.1016/j.cgh.2020.04.091.

13. Chen CJ, Yang HI, Su J, et al. Risk of hepatocellular carcinoma across a biological gradient of serum hepatitis B virus DNA level. JAMA 2006;295(1):65–73.

14. Chan SL, Mo FK, Wong VW, et al. Use of antiviral therapy in surveillance: impact on outcome of hepatitis B-related hepatocellular carcinoma. Liver Int 2012;32(2): 271–8.

15. Papatheodoridis GV, Manesis E, Hadziyannis SJ. The long-term outcome of interferon-alpha treated and untreated patients with HBeAg-negative chronic hepatitis B. J Hepatol 2001;34(2):306–13.

16. Thiele M, Gluud LL, Dahl EK, et al. Antiviral therapy for prevention of hepatocellular carcinoma and mortality in chronic hepatitis B: systematic review and meta-analysis. BMJ Open 2013;3(8). https://doi.org/10.1136/bmjopen-2013-003265.

17. Tong MJ, Hsien C, Song JJ, et al. Factors associated with progression to hepatocellular carcinoma and to death from liver complications in patients with HBsAg-positive cirrhosis. Dig Dis Sci 2009;54(6):1337–46.

18. Yuen MF, Seto WK, Chow DH, et al. Long-term lamivudine therapy reduces the risk of long-term complications of chronic hepatitis B infection even in patients without advanced disease. Antivir Ther 2007;12(8):1295–303.

19. Liaw YF, Sung JJ, Chow WC, et al. Lamivudine for patients with chronic hepatitis B and advanced liver disease. N Engl J Med 2004;351(15):1521–31.

20. Thi Vo T, Poovorawan K, Charoen P, et al. Association between hepatitis B surface antigen levels and the risk of hepatocellular carcinoma in patients with chronic hepatitis B infection: systematic review and meta-analysis. Asian Pac J Cancer Prev 2019;20(8):2239–46.
21. EASL 2017 clinical practice guidelines on the management of hepatitis B virus infection. J Hepatol 2017;67(2):370–98.
22. Chang Y, Choe WH, Sinn DH, et al. Nucleos(t)ide analogue treatment for patients with hepatitis B Virus (HBV) e Antigen-Positive Chronic HBV Genotype C infection: a nationwide, multicenter, retrospective study. J Infect Dis 2017;216(11): 1407–14.
23. Kim GA, Lim YS, Han S, et al. High risk of hepatocellular carcinoma and death in patients with immune-tolerant-phase chronic hepatitis B. Gut May 2018;67(5): 945–52.
24. Tseng TC, Liu CJ, Yang HC, et al. High levels of hepatitis B surface antigen increase risk of hepatocellular carcinoma in patients with low HBV load. Gastroenterology 2012;142(5):1140–9.e3 [quiz e13-4].
25. Choi GH, Kim GA, Choi J, et al. High risk of clinical events in untreated HBeAg-negative chronic hepatitis B patients with high viral load and no significant ALT elevation. Aliment Pharmacol Ther 2019;50(2):215–26.
26. Lee MH, Yang HI, Liu J, et al. Prediction models of long-term cirrhosis and hepatocellular carcinoma risk in chronic hepatitis B patients: risk scores integrating host and virus profiles. Hepatology 2013;58(2):546–54.
27. Tseng TC, Liu CJ, Yang HC, et al. Serum hepatitis B surface antigen levels help predict disease progression in patients with low hepatitis B virus loads. Hepatology 2013;57(2):441–50.
28. Sarin SK, Kumar M, Lau GK, et al. Asian-Pacific clinical practice guidelines on the management of hepatitis B: a 2015 update. Hepatol Int 2016;10(1):1–98.
29. Oliveri F, Surace L, Cavallone D, et al. Long-term outcome of inactive and active, low viraemic HBeAg-negative-hepatitis B virus infection: benign course towards HBsAg clearance. Liver Int 2017;37(11):1622–31.
30. Bonacci M, Lens S, Mariño Z, et al. Anti-viral therapy can be delayed or avoided in a significant proportion of HBeAg-negative Caucasian patients in the Grey Zone. Aliment Pharmacol Ther 2018;47(10):1397–408.
31. Brunetto MR, Oliveri F, Colombatto P, et al. Hepatitis B surface antigen serum levels help to distinguish active from inactive hepatitis B virus genotype D carriers. Gastroenterology 2010;139(2):483–90.
32. Liu J, Yang HI, Lee MH, et al. Serum levels of hepatitis B surface antigen and DNA can predict inactive carriers with low risk of disease progression. Hepatology 2016;64(2):381–9.
33. Pfefferkorn M, Böhm S, Schott T, et al. Quantification of large and middle proteins of hepatitis B virus surface antigen (HBsAg) as a novel tool for the identification of inactive HBV carriers. Gut 2018;67(11):2045–53.
34. Terrault NA, Lok ASF, McMahon BJ, et al. Update on prevention, diagnosis, and treatment of chronic hepatitis B: AASLD 2018 hepatitis B guidance. Hepatology 2018;67(4):1560–99.
35. Pavlovic V, Yang L, Chan HL, et al. Peginterferon alfa-2a (40 kD) stopping rules in chronic hepatitis B: a systematic review and meta-analysis of individual participant data. Antivir Ther 2019;24(2):133–40.
36. Rijckborst V, Hansen BE, Cakaloglu Y, et al. Early on-treatment prediction of response to peginterferon alfa-2a for HBeAg-negative chronic hepatitis B using HBsAg and HBV DNA levels. Hepatology 2010;52(2):454–61.

37. Rijckborst V, Hansen BE, Ferenci P, et al. Validation of a stopping rule at week 12 using HBsAg and HBV DNA for HBeAg-negative patients treated with peginterferon alfa-2a. J Hepatol 2012;56(5):1006–11.

38. Charatcharoenwitthaya P, Sukeepaisarnjaroen W, Piratvisuth T, et al. Treatment outcomes and validation of the stopping rule for response to peginterferon in chronic hepatitis B: a Thai nationwide cohort study. J Gastroenterol Hepatol 2016;31(11):1874–81.

39. Sonneveld MJ, Hansen BE, Piratvisuth T, et al. Response-guided peginterferon therapy in hepatitis B e antigen-positive chronic hepatitis B using serum hepatitis B surface antigen levels. Hepatology 2013;58(3):872–80.

40. Caviglia GP, Abate ML, Noviello D, et al. Hepatitis B core-related antigen kinetics in chronic hepatitis B virus genotype D-infected patients treated with nucleos(t)ide analogues or pegylated-interferon-α. Hepatol Res 2017;47(8):747–54.

41. Jansen L, Kootstra NA, van Dort KA, et al. Hepatitis B virus pregenomic RNA is present in virions in plasma and is associated with a response to pegylated interferon alfa-2a and nucleos(t)ide analogues. J Infect Dis 2016;213(2):224–32.

42. Chang ML, Liaw YF, Hadziyannis SJ. Systematic review: cessation of long-term nucleos(t)ide analogue therapy in patients with hepatitis B e antigen-negative chronic hepatitis B. Aliment Pharmacol Ther 2015;42(3):243–57.

43. Liu J, Li T, Zhang L, et al. The role of hepatitis B surface antigen in nucleos(t)ide analogues cessation among asian patients with chronic hepatitis B: a systematic review. Hepatology 2019;70(3):1045–55.

44. Yao CC, Hung CH, Hu TH, et al. Incidence and predictors of HBV relapse after cessation of nucleoside analogues in HBeAg-negative patients with HBsAg </= 200 IU/mL. Sci Rep 2017;7(1):1839.

45. Jeng WJ, Chen YC, Chien RN, et al. Incidence and predictors of hepatitis B surface antigen seroclearance after cessation of nucleos(t)ide analogue therapy in hepatitis B e antigen-negative chronic hepatitis B. Hepatology 2018;68(2):425–34.

46. Yeo YH, Ho HJ, Yang H-I, et al. Factors associated with rates of HBsAg seroclearance in adults with chronic HBV infection: a systematic review and meta-analysis. Gastroenterology 2019;156(3):635–46.e9.

47. Fonseca MA, Ling JZJ, Al-Siyabi O, et al. The efficacy of hepatitis B treatments in achieving HBsAg seroclearance: a systematic review and meta-analysis. J Viral Hepat 2020;27(7):650–62.

48. Lim SG, Phyo WW, Ling JZJ, et al. Comparative biomarkers for HBsAg loss with antiviral therapy shows dominant influence of qHBsAg (qHBsAg). Aliment Pharmacol Ther 2021;53(1):172–82.

49. Ma G, Lou B, Lv F, et al. HBcrAg, pg RNA and HBsAg dynamically supervise the seroconversion of HBsAg with anti-viral therapy: "Loss of HBsAg" maybe not a good end-point of anti-viral therapy. Clin Chim Acta 2020;501:264–9.

50. Marcellin P, Bonino F, Yurdaydin C, et al. Hepatitis B surface antigen levels: association with 5-year response to peginterferon alfa-2a in hepatitis B e-antigen-negative patients. Hepatol Int 2013;7(1):88–97.

51. Cornberg M, Wong VW, Locarnini S, et al. The role of quantitative hepatitis B surface antigen revisited. J Hepatol 2017;66(2):398–411.

52. Peng CY, Lai HC, Su WP, et al. Early hepatitis B surface antigen decline predicts treatment response to entecavir in patients with chronic hepatitis B. Sci Rep 2017;7:42879.

53. Marcellin P, Buti M, Krastev Z, et al. Kinetics of hepatitis B surface antigen loss in patients with HBeAg-positive chronic hepatitis B treated with tenofovir disoproxil fumarate. J Hepatol 2014;61(6):1228–37.

54. Bonacci M, Lens S, Marino Z, et al. Anti-viral therapy can be delayed or avoided in a significant proportion of HBeAg-negative Caucasian patients in the Grey Zone. Aliment Pharmacol Ther 2018;47(10):1397–408.

55. Goulis I, Karatapanis S, Akriviadis E, et al. On-treatment prediction of sustained response to peginterferon alfa-2a for HBeAg-negative chronic hepatitis B patients. Liver Int 2015;35(5):1540–8.

Controversies in the Management of Hepatitis B Hepatocellular Carcinoma

Stuart K. Roberts, MBBS, MD, MPH, FRACP, FAASLD, AGAF[a,b,]*,
Ammar Majeed, MD, PhD, FRACP[a,b], William Kemp, MBBS, PhD, FRACP[a,b]

KEYWORDS

- Hepatitis B • Hepatocellular carcinoma • Risk factors • Screening • Antiviral therapy
- Predictive models

KEY POINTS

- Hepatitis B is the leading cause of liver cancer worldwide.
- HCC incidence is highest in hepatitis B subjects with cirrhosis regardless of age.
- Children with cirrhosis or a first-degree family history of HCC should be included in HCC surveillance programs.
- Antiviral therapy reduces the risk of HCC in HBV-infected subjects and may reduce the risk of HCC recurrence.
- Several risk scores are available to predict the risk of HCC in subjects on antiviral therapy.

INTRODUCTION

Hepatocellular carcinoma (HCC) is the second leading cause of cancer-related death and the seventh most common cancer worldwide.[1,2] Incidence rates are particularly high in East and South-East Asia and sub-Saharan Africa, which collectively account for 85% of all cases, with China alone accounting for half of all cases.[1,2] These high incidence rates parallel the high prevalence of hepatitis B virus (HBV) infection in these regions.[3,4] Indeed, worldwide chronic HBV infection is responsible for more cases of HCC than any other risk factor[5] and together with cirrhosis is responsible for more than half a million deaths each year.[6] Globally, around 50% of HCC cases are attributed to hepatitis B infection, most of which occur in East Asia and sub-Saharan

Author Contributions: contributed to the study design; all authors contributed to the drafting and/or review of the manuscript

[a] The Alfred, 55 Commercial Road, Melbourne 3004, Australia; [b] Monash University, Melbourne, Australia
* Corresponding author. Department of Gastroenterology, The Alfred, 55 Commercial Road, Melbourne 3004, Australia.
E-mail address: s.roberts@alfred.org.au

Clin Liver Dis 25 (2021) 785–803
https://doi.org/10.1016/j.cld.2021.06.006
1089-3261/21/© 2021 Elsevier Inc. All rights reserved.

Africa.[5,7] This is in contrast to developed countries in North America and Western Europe where hepatitis B is responsible for only around 10% to 20% of cases.[5,7]

Several challenges remain in the management of hepatitis B in relation to the development of HCC. This includes a clearer understanding of who is most at risk of HCC, especially among Whites.[8] In addition, the most appropriate HCC screening tools and/or surveillance program in HBV-infected subjects remains a discussion point particularly in the pediatric population, as is the optimal management of HBV and HCC in affected subjects. Moreover, there is ongoing debate about the most appropriate choice of antiviral therapy to reduce the risk of HCC and recurrent HCC in patients with chronic HBV infection and the appropriate patient population that treatment should be targeted at.[6,8,9] Here we discuss these challenges in light of the current best available evidence to better inform clinicians of how to optimally manage HBV-infected subjects with or at risk of HCC.

RISK FACTORS FOR HEPATOCELLULAR CARCINOMA IN HEPATITIS B INFECTION

There are three broad categories of risk factors for HCC development in hepatitis B–infected subjects: (1) host, (2) viral, and (3) environmental/lifestyle. Established host factors associated with increased risk include older age and male sex[6,10]; presence of advanced liver disease[11,12] including cirrhosis[6,10] and chronic hepatitis[6]; coinfections with hepatitis D virus, hepatitis C virus,[13] and HIV[14]; diabetes mellitus[15]; metabolic syndrome[16]; and family history of HCC.[17,18] Also, a recent study suggests an association between PNPLA3 rs738409 polymorphism, a gene linked to fatty acid metabolism, and HCC risk.[19] Key viral factors associated with increased HCC risk predominantly involve markers of viral replication including hepatitis B e antigen (HBeAg) seropositivity,[20] hepatitis B surface antigen (HBsAg) titers, particularly greater than 100 IU/mL,[21,22] and increased viral load (ie, higher HBV DNA levels),[23] and genotype C[24] and presence of basal core/precore viral mutations.[25] Environmental/lifestyle factors associated with HCC development include aflatoxin exposure[26] and heavy ($\geq$60 g/day) alcohol use,[6] whereas coffee intake[27–29] and concomitant statins,[30,31] aspirin,[32,33] and metformin[31,34] seem to reduce HCC risk. Geographic location (ie, Asian vs Western countries)[35,36] and tobacco smoking are not associated with increased risk of HCC in HBV subjects following appropriate adjustment for confounders.[6] Other than cirrhosis, the major risk factors for HCC include older age, male gender, family history of HCC, HBV viral load, HBsAg titers, and HBV genotype C (**Table 1**).

INCIDENT RISK OF HEPATOCELLULAR CARCINOMA IN UNTREATED HEPATITIS B

Early natural history studies reporting HCC incidence in untreated chronic HBV infection yielded inconsistent results with significant variation in study design, geographic region, and risk factors cited as reasons for the disparate outcomes.[35,36] In a recent meta-analysis, Raffetti and colleagues[6] evaluated HCC incidence in untreated subjects with HBV infection according to potential confounders including macrogeographic origin, liver disease status, and risk factors (**Table 2**). Sixty-six studies were included from several regions including North America, Europe, and East Asia. Annual incident HCC rates in asymptomatic carriers with persistent HBsAg positivity across all liver disease stages ranged from 0.07% to 0.42% depending on the region. Inactive carriers with persistently normal alanine aminotransferase (ALT) level, absence of HBeAg, and presence of HBeAb as defined[37] had lower annual incident rates of between 0.03% and 0.17%. In contrast, incident rates were higher in those with more severe liver disease including chronic hepatitis (defined by histology and/or clinical

Table 1
Main risk factors for HCC development in hepatitis B–infected subjects

Risk Factor	Relative Risk	95% Confidence Interval
Host		
Older age (for every 10-y increase in age)[6]	1.7	1.4–2.1
Gender, male vs female[6]	2.7	2.1–3.3
Family history of HCC[17]	2.5	1.6–3.7
Viral		
HBV DNA levels (IU/mL)[22]		
<10	1	
1000–9999	3.8	1.3–18.8
≥10,000	3.3	1.0–17.1
HBsAg titers (IU)[6]		
<100	1	
100–999	3.1	1.6–6.6
≥1000	5.4	3.0–10.8
HBV genotype C vs B[6]	2.5	1.8–3.4

criteria[37]) at 0.12% to 0.49% per year, whereas those with compensated Child-Pugh A cirrhosis had the highest incidence rates of 2% to 3.4% per annum (see **Table 2**). On multivariate analysis a significant increase in incidence rates was noted for age, and for asymptomatic carrier, chronic hepatitis, and cirrhosis status compared with inactive carriers but not for geographic region. In addition, HBV DNA levels greater than 2000 IU/mL and genotype C (vs genotype B) are associated with higher incident rates in Asian studies.

IMPACT OF ANTIVIRAL THERAPY ON INCIDENT RISK OF HEPATOCELLULAR CARCINOMA

Antiviral therapy has several beneficial effects in chronic hepatitis B (CHB) subjects including long-term viral suppression and histologic improvement including reduction in liver fibrosis and reversal of cirrhosis.[38] However, debate continues as to how

Table 2
Incidence rates of HCC in untreated subjects with chronic hepatitis B infection according to geographic region and liver disease status[a]

HCC Incidence	Incidence Rates per 100 Person-Years (95% Confidence Interval)			
	Asymptomatic Carriers	Inactive Carriers	Chronic Hepatitis	Compensated Cirrhosis
Overall	0.31 (0.22–0.41)	0.05 (0.03–0.08)	0.42 (0.27–0.56)	2.97 (2.35–3.59)
North America-Oceania	0.19 (0.07–0.31)	0.17 (0.02–0.62)	0.48 (0.22–0.91)	2.89 (1.23–4.55)
Europe	0.07 (0.05–0.09)	0.03 (0.0–0.10)	0.12 (0.0 0.27)	2.03 (1.3–2.77)
East Asia	0.42 (0.21–0.41)	0.06 (0.02–0.10)	0.49 (0.32–0.66)	3.37 (2.48–4.26)

[a] Adapted from Raffetti et al. *Liver Int.* 2016; 36:1239 to 1251.

effective treatment is at reducing HCC risk particularly with the newer nucleoside analogues (NAs).[10,39] Evidence from several meta-analyses suggests that interferon-α and probably pegylated-interferon-α reduce the incidence of HCC by around 50%, particularly in Asian subjects with cirrhosis, and those with a sustained off-treatment virologic response.[10,40] Recent studies focusing on the recommended first-line NAs, entecavir (ETV) and tenofovir (TDF), seem to show favorable benefit in CHB subjects with a reduction but not elimination of HCC risk, particularly when data from randomized or matched controlled studies are considered. In comparative Asian studies of these agents that included matched untreated control subjects, HCC risk was reduced by 30% overall in patients with cirrhosis and by an overall 80% in patients without cirrhosis (**Fig. 1**).[39] However, thus far no comparative studies evaluating the impact of these agents on HCC risk have been conducted in CHB patients of White origin. Across studies, annual HCC incidence rates ranged from 0.01% to 1.4% in patients without cirrhosis and from 0.9% to 5.4% in subjects with cirrhosis.[39] Of note, achieving an on-treatment virologic response with ETV or TDF was associated with a reduction in HCC risk in Asian but not White studies. Studies comparing current NAs with older agents have found no significant difference in HCC risk reduction.[39,41] Thus, overall the data support a significant reduction in HCC incidence for patients using NAs versus those without.

Recently, there has been considerable interest in the comparative efficacy of TDF versus ETV at reducing HCC risk with at least two large observational studies from Asia reporting a significantly lower risk of HCC in TDF-treated patients compared with those receiving ETV.[42,43] In the largest of these from Korea encompassing a nationwide cohort of more than 24,000 participants, TDF was associated with a significantly lower risk of HCC development compared with ETV-treated patients (0.89 per 100 person-years vs 1.19 per 100 person-years, respectively).[42] Results, however, are not uniform with two other large studies also from Asia finding no significant differences in HCC risk between the two antivirals.[44,45] Moreover the findings of several recent meta-analyses have failed to resolve this issue with at least one major study reporting no difference in HCC risk between the two agents[46] and three others suggesting there may be a lower HCC risk with TDF but with low confidence levels.[47–49] Hence, currently there is no clear evidence to suggest a differential benefit of TDF over ETV at reducing HCC risk and both NAs are therefore appropriate to use at this time.

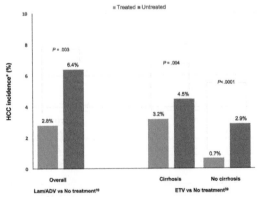

Fig. 1. Incidence of HCC in chronic hepatitis B patients treated with nucleos(t)ide analogues including lamivudine (Lam) with/without adefovir (ADV) and ETV according to cirrhosis status. [a]Refers to overall HCC incidence (Lam/ADV) and annual incidence (ETV).

ROLE OF PREDICTIVE RISK SCORES FOR HEPATOCELLULAR CARCINOMA IN CHRONIC HEPATITIS B

Individual risk factors have limited value in accurately classifying HCC risk, so several scoring systems have been developed to better predict the risk of HBV-related HCC (see **Table 2**).[10] Most of these were developed based on Asian cohorts of untreated CHB patients and typically combine one or more of the known demographic (age, gender), liver disease (ALT, albumin, bilirubin, cirrhosis status, platelets), and viral (HBeAg, HBV DNA) factors associated with increased HCC risk. The most well-known of these are REACH-B,[50] CU-HCC,[51] and GAG-HCC.[52] Over time modifications have been made to these scoring systems to improve their predictive accuracy including addition of liver stiffness measurement and quantitative HBsAg.[39] Importantly, CU-HCC, GAG-HCC, and REACH-B scores remain acceptable in the setting of NA therapy.[53] In a cohort of CHB patients from Hong Kong receiving ETV, the area under curve (AUC) at baseline for CU-HCC, GAG-HCC, and REACH-B for HCC prediction were 0.80, 0.76, and 0.71, respectively, with risk score accuracy improving from Year 2 of treatment onward compared with baseline.[53] However, the applicability and predictably of the previously mentioned HCC risk models are modest in European Whites with CHB treated with ETV or TDF with AUC of 0.63 to 0.75.[54] Consequently, a new model named PAGE-B based on age, platelets, and gender has been developed and validated for White CHB patients and provides a simple and reliable method of predicting 5-year risk of HCC in patients receiving ETV or TDF (**Table 3**).[55]

SHOULD CHILDREN WITH IMMUNE-TOLERANT DISEASE BE SCREENED FOR HEPATOCELLULAR CARCINOMA AND AT WHAT INTERVAL

Although the clinical course of CHB infection during childhood and adolescence is typically benign, up to 4.5% evolve cirrhosis,[56] and 0.01% to 0.03% develop HCC before adulthood.[57] Unfortunately, survival in pediatric HCC remains dismal because most are diagnosed with advanced disease, with 5-year survival rates of 17% to 22%.[58] Observational studies have demonstrated that surveillance is associated with early tumor detection and improved survival.[59] As such, it is important to define pediatric populations with liver disease that have an increased risk of HCC, and who would benefit from appropriate surveillance.

TARGET PEDIATRIC HEPATITIS B VIRUS POPULATION FOR HEPATOCELLULAR CARCINOMA SURVEILLANCE
Children with Cirrhosis with Chronic Hepatitis B Virus

Although liver cirrhosis is the most important risk factor for HCC in adults with hepatitis B,[60] data on the risk of HCC in children with HBV cirrhosis are limited. A 20-year follow-up of White children with HBV showed that cirrhosis, although rare, is an important risk factor for HCC.[61] Several retrospective studies from East Asia have confirmed that most children who present with HBV-associated HCC have underlying cirrhosis.[62,63] Based on these findings, it is appropriate to include the pediatric cirrhotic population in HCC surveillance programs.

Children Without Cirrhosis with Chronic Hepatitis B Virus

In contrast, the issue of HCC surveillance in children without cirrhosis with immunotolerant HBV infection is more contentious because the risk of HCC in this group remains low. Currently, there are insufficient data to identify HBV-infected children without cirrhosis with sufficiently high risk of HCC that would benefit from surveillance. One

Table 3
Risk calculators for HCC development in chronic hepatitis B subjects[a]

Scoring System	Age (y)	Sex	Albumin (g/L)	Bilirubin (μmol/L)	ALT (U/L)	HBeAg	HBV DNA (Copies/mL)	Cirrhosis	Platelets (/mm³)	Risk Scores
GAG-HCC[52]	Per Year 1 (1)	Male: 16 Female: 0	NA	NA	NA	NA	3 × log	Yes: 33 No: 0	NA	Low: <101 High: ≥101
CU-HCC[51]	≤ 50: 0 >50: 3	NA	≤ 35: 20 >35: 0	≤ 18: 0 >18: 1.5	NA	NA	<4 log: 0 4-6 log: 1 >6 log: 4	Yes: 15 No: 0	NA	Low (<5), intermediate (5–20), high (>20)
REACH-B[50]	30–34: 0 35–39: 1 40–44: 2 45–49: 3 50–54: 4 55–59: 5 60–65: 6	Male: 2 Female: 0	NA	NA	<15: 0 15–44: 1 ≥45: 2	+ve: 2 -ve: 0	<4 log: 0 4–5 log: 3 5–6 log: 5 ≥6 log: 4	NA	NA	A 17-point risk scale
PAGE-B[55]	16–29: 0 30–39: 2 40–49: 4 50–59: 6 60–69: 8 ≥70: 10	Male: 6 Female: 0	NA	NA	NA	NA	NA	NA	≥200,000: 0 100,000–199,999: 6 <100,000: 9	A 26-point risk scale (0–25): low (≤ 9), intermediate (10–17), high (≥18)

Abbreviation: NA, not applicable.
[a] Adapted from Varbobotis et al. *Clin Mol Hepatol.* 2016; 22:319 to 326.

potentially important risk factor in this group is a family history of HCC. In a case-control study, the odds ratio of HCC in individuals with viral hepatitis and family history of HCC was 2.4 compared with those with only viral hepatitis and 72.5 compared with those without any risk factor for HCC.[18] Still, although the American Association for the Study of Liver Diseases and European Association for the Study of the Liver recommend HCC screening in adults with chronic HBV and family history of HCC, no similar guidelines exist for children with HBV infection. However, given the evidence linking family history and the risk of HCC in chronic HBV,[17,18] it is reasonable to include children with HBV infection and a first-degree relative with HCC in HCC surveillance programs.

TOOLS USED TO SCREEN FOR HEPATOCELLULAR CARCINOMA IN HEPATITIS B VIRUS SUBJECTS

Worldwide, there is general agreement that HCC surveillance should be offered to all suitable HBsAg-positive subjects with cirrhosis who are willing to undergo treatment and subjects without cirrhosis with CHB infection at increased risk of HCC.[64–66] The latter includes Asian or Black men older than 40 years, Asian women older than 50 years, sub-Saharan Africans older than 20 years, persons with a first-degree relative with a history of HCC, and those with hepatitis D virus infection, all of whom have annual HCC incidence rates greater than the threshold of 0.3% to justify screening. HBsAg seroconversion does not necessarily protect against HCC development in subjects with and without cirrhosis[67] even in those who seroconvert on NA therapy,[68] with males and those older than 50 years most at risk, so these patients should also be offered screening. Established screening tests are abdominal ultrasound (US) with or without serum α-fetoprotein (AFP). Where US is unavailable, high-risk subjects are recommended to be screened with AFP every 6 months.

Nevertheless, because AFP has low sensitivity and specificity for early stage HCC, other HCC-specific tumor markers have been developed as screening tools to improve HCC detection rates in CHB patients. These include Lens culinaris agglutinin-reactive fraction of AFP (AFP-L3), protein induced by vitamin K absence factor II (PIVKA-II), Dickkopf-1 (DKK-1), and circulating IgG antibodies to a variety of target linear peptide antigens associated with HCC.[69] These novel biomarkers alone or in combination have the potential to improve early HCC detection rates in patients with hepatitis B.[69] For example, the combination of PIVKA-II and AFP was reported to have significantly superior performance for HCC detection compared with each biomarker used alone; the weighted AUC for the biomarker combination was 0.859 (95% confidence interval [CI], 0.837–0.882) compared with 0.791 (0.746–0.837) and 0.767 (0.732–0.803) for PIVKA-II and AFP, respectively.[70] Similarly, AFP, AFP-L3, and PIVKA-II in combination was found to have good diagnostic accuracy[71] and improved sensitivity and specificity of early HCC diagnosis[72] such that at least one major Asian society has recommended that these three biomarkers be combined with US for HCC surveillance.[73] Still, further studies are needed at a global level to better understand the clinical utility of these novel biomarkers in the management and surveillance of CHB patients.

SHOULD HISTOLOGIC SEVERITY AFFECT THE FREQUENCY OF HEPATOCELLULAR CARCINOMA SCREENING

Observational studies have demonstrated a strong relationship between the stage of liver disease, degree of inflammation, and the incident risk of HCC in CHB patients as described previously. The incidence of HCC ranges from 0.02 to 0.2 per 100 person-years among inactive HBV carriers, to 0.3 to 0.6 per 100 person-years in those with chronic HBV without cirrhosis, and up to 2.2 to 3.7 per 100 person-years in those with cirrhosis; the corresponding 5-year HCC cumulative incidences were 0.1% to 1%, 1% to 3%, and 10% to 17%, respectively.[6,36]

Hepatic Inflammation and the Risk of Hepatocellular Carcinoma

Ongoing liver inflammation may result in the accumulation of mutations in the host genome, thereby increasing the risk of malignant transformation.[74] Nonmalignant tissue samples from livers affected by HCCs show higher degree of inflammation when compared with samples from livers without tumors.[75] Additionally, longstanding active inflammation increases the risk of fibrosis progression and evolution to cirrhosis, consequently increasing the risk of HCC.[75] The development of cirrhosis, decompensation, and HCC risk were significantly higher in patients whose ALT levels were persistently elevated or who flared-up without normalization than in patients whose ALT flared-up and then normalized or were persistently normal.[76] Overall, these studies highlight the important direct and indirect role of hepatic inflammation in tumorigenesis and HCC development.

The Degree of Fibrosis and Risk of Hepatocellular Carcinoma

The degree of liver fibrosis is strongly associated with the risk of HCC in patients with CHB. The presence of cirrhosis is considered the most important risk factor for the development of HCC, particularly in those with viral hepatitis.[66] In a retrospective study of 330 HCCs resected between 1985 and 1998, 8% of the resected samples showed no fibrosis, 16% demonstrated minimal fibrosis, whereas 76% showed advanced fibrosis or cirrhosis.[77] Similarly, in a prospective Taiwanese study, including 22,070 men of which 3454 were HBsAg positive, the incidence of HCC was 4.7-fold higher in those with cirrhosis compared with individuals without cirrhosis.[78] Several scoring systems for HCC risk prediction in the setting of HBV incorporate the presence of cirrhosis in risk estimation modeling, as noted previously. All major guidelines suggest initiating HCC surveillance for patients with chronic HBV and advanced fibrosis (F3) or cirrhosis using 6-month US with or without AFP.[64–66]

The Presence of Dysplasia

Several histologic abnormalities are prevalent in HBV-related cirrhotic livers containing HCC.[79] "Large cell changes" consists of foci of enlarged cells with nuclear pleomorphism, hyperchromasia, and multinucleation. Chronic HBV patients with large cell changes had a three-fold increased risk of HCC development compared with those without such changes.[80] Conversely, "small cell changes" consist of foci of crowded small hepatocytes with high nuclear/cytoplasmic ratio, increased proliferative activity, and strong morphologic and genetic resemblance to HCC.[81] Such changes are thought to be true precursor lesions of HCC. Aneuploidy (the presence of an abnormal number of chromosomes in a cell) has been observed in the setting of liver cell dysplasia, and is considered an independent risk factor for HCC.[82] Despite these observed associations with the risk of HCC, there are currently no recommendations for obtaining liver biopsies to assess for such changes, and HCC screening guidelines do not take into account the presence of cytologic changes in their recommendations.

FACTORS INFLUENCING THE FREQUENCY OF HEPATOCELLULAR CARCINOMA SURVEILLANCE

The recommendation for surveillance US with or without AFP at 6-month intervals is based on expected tumor growth rate (median doubling time for HCC is 117 days) obtained from observational data[65,83–86] rather than the risk of developing HCC. Hence, the screening interval is not shortened in patients at higher risk for HCC. In a retrospective study of patients with cirrhosis undergoing annual or biannual surveillance, the median survival rate and detection rate of early HCC was higher in patients undergoing 6-month US compared with those undergoing annual surveillance. This was confirmed in a pooled analysis of 19 studies, demonstrating higher sensitivity of US for detecting tumors before clinical presentations when applied at 6-month intervals rather than annually (70% vs 50%).[84] However, in a large randomized multicenter study, patients assigned to a 3-month interval for surveillance US had similar rates of detection of small HCC compared with patients in a 6-month interval group.[87] In summary, there is strong evidence to suggest initiation of biannual HCC surveillance in patients with chronic HBV and advanced fibrosis, and to consider starting screening in the presence of active CHB.

TREATMENT OF HEPATITIS B VIRUS IN PATIENTS WHO DEVELOP HEPATOCELLULAR CARCINOMA NOT ON HEPATITIS B VIRUS THERAPY

Most (70%–90%) patients with HBV-related HCC have preexisting cirrhosis.[88] Even in the absence of HCC, the presence of cirrhosis remains an established indication for the initiation of HBV therapy to preserve liver function, prevent HBV-related flares, and reduce the risk of HCC development.[38,39,89] Consequently, the appropriate use of HBV treatment represents a key primary prevention strategy for reducing the rate of HCC development. However, in patients who have developed HCC and are not on HBV therapy, the introduction of antiviral therapy to reduce recurrence or improve outcomes of HCC therapy is less well established. To that end, existing guidelines provide only weak recommendations made based on moderate-quality evidence.[64]

The primary objectives of commencing HBV therapy in patients with HCC are to prevent HBV reactivation and to reduce the risk of HCC recurrence, both of which represent a major cause of morbidity and mortality following potentially curative treatment.[90] Several large cohort studies have examined the impact of NA usage in improving outcomes for patients undergoing curative HCC resection. These data suggest that CHB patients taking NAs have improved recurrence-free survival (RFS) and overall survival (OS) in comparison with untreated patients. A large cohort study from Taiwan of 4569 HBV-related HCC patients who received curative liver resection found that patients taking NAs had lower rates of HCC recurrence and a significant reduction in all-cause mortality. After adjusting for competing mortality, the treated cohort had a significantly lower HCC recurrence rate and mortality at 6 years than untreated subjects at 45.6% versus 54.6% (P<.001) and 29.0% versus 42.4% (P<.001), respectively (**Fig. 2**).[91] Several meta-analyses evaluating the impact of adjuvant/neoadjuvant HBV therapy on prognosis following HCC curative therapy have been performed with similar findings.[92–95] The most recent analysis of 21 studies with 8742 participants found that NA (predominantly lamivudine/ETV) compared with control subjects, significantly decreased the 1- and 3-year HCC recurrence rates by 21% and 20%, respectively, following resection or ablation. Furthermore, the 1-, 3-, and 5-year OS rates were significantly improved by 5%, 23%, and 27%, respectively.[96] Five-year recurrence rates were not significantly different between the treated and control groups. These findings highlight the potential benefits associated with controlling HBV

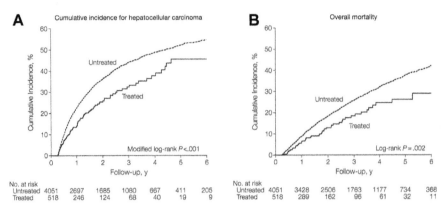

Fig. 2. Impact of nucleoside analogue therapy on cumulative incidences of (*A*) HCC recurrence and (*B*) overall mortality following liver resection. (Reproduced with permission Wu et al. JAMA 2012; 308 (18).)

replication following HCC treatment.[97] One of the few randomized controlled trials in the area found the introduction of adefovir (with add-on lamivudine or ETV monotherapy used for nonresponse or viral resistance) following HCC resection with curative intent significantly improved 5-year RFS (46.1% vs 27.1%; P = .026) and OS (63.1% vs 41.5%; P = .001).[98] The improved RFS and OS of post-resection antiviral therapy is also evident in patients with low preoperative HBV-DNA levels (HBV-DNA <2000 IU/mL)[99] and even among patients who are HBsAg-positive but HBV DNA-negative.[100] A second large study from Hong Kong[101] examining 2198 CHB patients undergoing a variety of HCC therapies reported similar findings of a reduced overall recurrence rate associated with NAs (adjusted subhazard ratio, 0.63; 95% CI, 0.49–0.80). This effect was most significant in patients undergoing resection or local ablation.

CHOICE OF NUCLEOSIDE ANALOGUE THERAPY IN MANAGING HEPATITIS B VIRUS–RELATED HEPATOCELLULAR CARCINOMA

The optimal treatment of HBV following the development of HCC is an NA with a high barrier to resistance, such as ETV and TDF. Whether the type of NA can influence HCC recurrence remains uncertain and future randomized controlled studies would be required to address this issue. Wong and colleagues[101] found that although the reduction in HCC recurrence was evident in lamivudine and ETV cohorts, the magnitude of benefit was greater in patients receiving ETV. In a more recent study Choi and colleagues[102] examined a historical cohort of HCC patients treated with ETV or TDF following curative-intent hepatectomy. Patients in the TDF group had significantly lower rates of HCC recurrence (hazard ratio [HR], 0.82; 95% CI, 0.68–0.98), and death or transplantation (HR, 0.62; 95% CI, 0.44–0.88).[102] Furthermore, TDF was an independent protective factor for early (<2 years; HR, 0.79; P = .03) and late (≥2 years; HR, 0.68; P = .03) postoperative recurrence. These findings are yet to be replicated in other cohorts and no change to current recommendations should be made at this stage.

Reactivation or flare of CHB following HCC resection is association with poor outcomes[103] and the use of NAs following HCC resection can reduce the rates of viral reactivation and also improve survival.[104] Those at highest risk of HBV reactivation seem to be patients undergoing trans-arterial chemoembolization (TACE). A recent meta-analysis found high rates of HBV reactivation in the TACE group compared with control subjects (19.9% vs 7.0%) and that currently available NAs are effective in mitigating the risk of HBV reactivation.[96] Another study from Korea[105] that used propensity score matching in 1084 subjects reported patients receiving prophylactic NAs had significantly better OS than those who did not, with cumulative rates HBV reactivation as high as 44.2% at 3 years observed in the untreated group. Other studies have documented HBV reactivation in 11% of patients who are HBsAg-negative undergoing TACE[106] and highlight the potential for viral reactivation and clinically significant flares of HBV without the use of NAs. Lower but still potentially significant rates of viral reactivation (5.6% vs 14%) have been observed in patients undergoing local ablative therapies versus resection.[107] Viral reactivation is also reported following treatment with tyrosine kinase inhibitors[108] and in patients undergoing radiotherapy.[109] Recent data have highlighted the utility of immunotherapy with immune checkpoint inhibitors in patients with HCC. To date the clinical experience of the use of these agents in patients with hepatitis B remains limited with many studies either excluding patients with hepatitis B or requiring well-controlled HBV on enrollment. Evidence of HBV reactivation in these settings is sporadic and mostly limited to isolated case reports. Two HCC specific trials, Check-Mate-040 trial[110,111] and KEYNOTE-224,[112] included HBV-infected patients on antiviral agents and no HBV-related flares were observed, although 9% HBV participants in the Check-Mate-040 trial had evidence of virologic breakthrough. A recent retrospective study from Taiwan[113] of 62 consecutive patients with HBV who received either pembrolizumab or nivolumab for unresectable HCC found no HBV reactivation in patients receiving NAs and only one of six patients who was not receiving NAs experienced HBV reactivation with a greater than 10-fold increase in HBV DNA level and ALT flare after 9 weeks of treatment.

Given the potential clinical benefits of preventing HBV hepatitis flares, preserving liver function, and avoiding viral reactivation in addition to the potential benefit of reducing the risk of HCC recurrence following curative HCC treatment, it seems prudent to commence NAs in all patients with HBV and HCC. This strategy is not only efficacious, but modeling studies suggest it is also cost-effective.[114] Although acknowledging the need for further studies to establish the role of NAs in prevention or reduction in HCC recurrence,[64] the Asia-Pacific recommend NAs be administered to all patients with detectable HBV viral load at least 1 to 2 weeks before, during, and after chemotherapy, locoregional therapies, resection, or liver transplantation.[115]

TREATMENT OF HEPATITIS B VIRUS IN PATIENTS WHO DEVELOP HEPATOCELLULAR CARCINOMA WHILE ON ANTI–HEPATITIS B VIRUS THERAPY

Optimization of HBV treatment remains a critical component of the broader management of patients with HCC and HBV and should involve timely delivery of individualized strategies to achieve long-term sustained viral suppression and remission of liver disease. This includes the use of appropriate medication with a high barrier to resistance (ie, ETV, TDF, or [tenofovir alafenamide] TAF) at the appropriate time based on patient and viral characteristics, monitoring of therapeutic effect and efficacy, and timely introduction of treatment changes in patients with a suboptimal response to initial therapy.[116] Central to this is a culturally and linguistically appropriate discussion regarding the importance of adherence to treatment as per existing clinical practice guidelines.[89] Optimization of medication adherence has been demonstrated to reduce mortality, the risk of HCC development, and liver disease complications.[117] Despite the controversy surrounding whether NAs with a high barrier to resistance, such as ETV and TDF, are equivalent in achieving HCC recurrence risk reduction,[102] there is no evidence that in the absence of viral replication, switching between NAs represents an acceptable strategy to reduce HCC recurrence or improve liver-related outcomes.

SUMMARY

Hepatitis B is a leading cause of HCC globally with high HCC incidence rates observed among those with high viral load, CHB, and/or cirrhosis. Antiviral therapy with ETV or TDF plays an important role in lowering the risk of HCC across all stages of liver disease, and may lower the risk of HCC recurrence following curative therapy.

CLINICS CARE POINTS

- Surveillance for HCC should be offered to all hepatitis B infected subjects with cirrhosis including children and those at high risk of HCC including those with active disease, advanced fibrosis and those with a family history of HCC.

- Surveillance for HCC in HBV infected subjects should be with twice yearly liver ultrasound with/without alfa-fetoprotein measurement.

- Antiviral therapy should be commenced in all subjects with cirrhosis and in those at high risk for HCC to lower the risk of incident HCC.

- Subjects with chronic hepatitis B who develop HCC should be commenced on anti-viral therapy as it may lower the risk of recurrent HCC after curative therapy.

- Anti-viral therapy in those with hepatitis B should be with a nucleoside analogue with a higher genetic barrier to resistance with either entecavir or tenofovir being acceptable.

DISCLOSURES

Nil to declare relevant to this study.

REFERENCES

1. Bray F, Ferlay J, Soerjomataram I, et al. Global cancer statistics 2018: GLOBO-CAN estimates of incidence and mortality worldwide for 36 cancers in 185 countries. CA Cancer J Clin 2018;68:394–424.
2. Ferlay J, Colombet M, Soerjomataram I, et al. Estimating the global cancer incidence and mortality in 2018: GLOBOCAN sources and methods. Int J Cancer 1941;144:1941–53.
3. Schweitzer A, Horn J, Mikolajczyk RT, et al. Estimations of worldwide prevalence of chronic hepatitis B virus infection: a systematic review of data published between 1965 and 2013. [Review]. Lancet 2015;386:1546–55.
4. Ott JJ, Stevens GA, Groeger J, et al. Global epidemiology of hepatitis B virus infection: new estimates of age-specific HBsAg seroprevalence and endemicity. Vaccine 2012;30:2212–9.
5. Baecker A, Liu X, La Vecchia C, et al. Worldwide incidence of hepatocellular carcinoma cases attributable to major risk factors. [Review]. Eur J Cancer Prev 2018;27:205–12.
6. Raffetti E, Fattovich G, Donato F. Incidence of hepatocellular carcinoma in untreated subjects with chronic hepatitis B: a systematic review and meta-analysis. Liver Int 2016;36:1239–51.
7. Global Burden of Disease Liver Cancer C, Akinyemiju T, Abera S, et al. The burden of primary liver cancer and underlying etiologies from 1990 to 2015 at

the global, regional, and national level: results from the Global Burden of Disease Study 2015. JAMA Oncol 2017;3:1683–91.

8. Arends P, Sonneveld MJ, Zoutendijk R, et al. Entecavir treatment does not eliminate the risk of hepatocellular carcinoma in chronic hepatitis B: limited role for risk scores in caucasians. Gut 2015;64:1289–95.

9. Buti M, Fung S, Gane E, et al. Long-term clinical outcomes in cirrhotic chronic hepatitis B patients treated with tenofovir disoproxil fumarate for up to 5 years. Hepatol Int 2015;9:243–50.

10. Varbobitis I, Papatheodoridis GV. The assessment of hepatocellular carcinoma risk in patients with chronic hepatitis B under antiviral therapy. [Review]. Clin Mol Hepatol 2016;22:319–26.

11. Kim MN, Kim SU, Kim BK, et al. Increased risk of hepatocellular carcinoma in chronic hepatitis B patients with transient elastography-defined subclinical cirrhosis. Hepatology 2015;61:1851–9.

12. Jung KS, Kim SU, Ahn SH, et al. Risk assessment of hepatitis B virus-related hepatocellular carcinoma development using liver stiffness measurement (FibroScan). Hepatology 2011;53:885–94.

13. Cho LY, Yang JJ, Ko KP, et al. Coinfection of hepatitis B and C viruses and risk of hepatocellular carcinoma: systematic review and meta-analysis. [Review]. Int J Cancer 2011;128:176–84.

14. Ioannou GN, Bryson CL, Weiss NS, et al. The prevalence of cirrhosis and hepatocellular carcinoma in patients with human immunodeficiency virus infection. Hepatology 2013;57:249–57.

15. Wang C, Wang X, Gong G, et al. Increased risk of hepatocellular carcinoma in patients with diabetes mellitus: a systematic review and meta-analysis of cohort studies. [Review]. Int J Cancer 2012;130:1639–48.

16. Wong GL, Wong VW, Choi PC, et al. Metabolic syndrome increases the risk of liver cirrhosis in chronic hepatitis B. Gut 2009;58:111–7.

17. Loomba R, Liu J, Yang HI, et al. Synergistic effects of family history of hepatocellular carcinoma and hepatitis B virus infection on risk for incident hepatocellular carcinoma. Clin Gastroenterol Hepatol 2013;11:1636–45.

18. Turati F, Edefonti V, Talamini R, et al. Family history of liver cancer and hepatocellular carcinoma. Hepatology 2012;55:1416–25.

19. Zhang L, Liu C, Xu K, et al. Association between PNPLA3 rs738409 polymorphism and hepatocellular carcinoma risk: an updated meta-analysis. Genes Genomics 2016;38:831–9.

20. Yang HI, Lu SN, Liaw YF, et al. Hepatitis B e antigen and the risk of hepatocellular carcinoma. N Engl J Med 2002;347:168–74.

21. Thi Vo T, Poovorawan K, Charoen P, et al. Association between hepatitis B surface antigen levels and the risk of hepatocellular carcinoma in patients with chronic hepatitis B infection: systematic review and meta-analysis. Asian Pac J Cancer Prev 2019;20:2239–46.

22. Tseng TC, Liu CJ, Yang HC, et al. High levels of hepatitis B surface antigen increase risk of hepatocellular carcinoma in patients with low HBV load. Gastroenterology 2012;142:1140–9.

23. Chen CJ, Yang HI, Su J, et al. Risk of hepatocellular carcinoma across a biological gradient of serum hepatitis B virus DNA level. JAMA 2006;295:65–73.

24. Wong GL, Chan HL, Yiu KK, et al. Meta-analysis: the association of hepatitis B virus genotypes and hepatocellular carcinoma. Aliment Pharmacol Ther 2013; 37:517–26.

25. Wei F, Zheng Q, Li M, et al. The association between hepatitis B mutants and hepatocellular carcinoma. Medicine 2017;96(19):e6835.

26. Hsu IC, Metcalf RA, Sun T, et al. Mutational hotspot in the p53 gene in human hepatocellular carcinomas. Nature 1991;350:427–8.

27. Leung WW, Ho SC, Chan HL, et al. Moderate coffee consumption reduces the risk of hepatocellular carcinoma in hepatitis B chronic carriers: a case-control study. J Epidemiol Community Health 2011;65:556–8.

28. Gelatti U, Covolo L, Franceschini M, et al. Coffee consumption reduces the risk of hepatocellular carcinoma independently of its aetiology: a case-control study. J Hepatol 2005;42:528–34.

29. Bravi F, Bosetti C, Tavani A, et al. Coffee reduces risk for hepatocellular carcinoma: an updated meta-analysis. Clin Gastroenterol Hepatol 2013;11:1413–21.

30. Tsan YT, Lee CH, Wang JD, et al. Statins and the risk of hepatocellular carcinoma in patients with hepatitis B virus infection. J Clin Oncol 2012;30:623–30.

31. Chen CI, Kuan CF, Fang YA, et al. Cancer risk in HBV patients with statin and metformin use: a population-based cohort study. Medicine 2015;94(6):e462.

32. Lee TY, Hsu YC, Tseng HC, et al. Association of daily aspirin therapy with risk of hepatocellular carcinoma in patients with chronic hepatitis B. JAMA Intern Med 2019;179:633–40.

33. Fox RK, Taddei TH, Kaplan DE. Aspirin use and risk of hepatocellular carcinoma in hepatitis B. JAMA Intern Med 2019;179:640–1.

34. Chen HP, Shieh JJ, Chang CC, et al. Metformin decreases hepatocellular carcinoma risk in a dose-dependent manner: population-based and in vitro studies. Gut 2013;62:606–15.

35. Thiele M, Gluud LL, Fialla AD, et al. Large variations in risk of hepatocellular carcinoma and mortality in treatment naive hepatitis B patients: systematic review with meta-analyses. PLoS One 2014;9:e107177.

36. Fattovich G, Bortolotti F, Donato F. Natural history of chronic hepatitis B: special emphasis on disease progression and prognostic factors. [Review] [143 refs]. J Hepatol 2008;48:335–52.

37. Lok AS, McMahon BJ. Chronic hepatitis B. Hepatology 2007;45:507–39.

38. Terrault NA, Bzowej NH, Chang KM, et al. AASLD guidelines for treatment of chronic hepatitis B. Hepatology 2016;63:261–83.

39. Papatheodoridis GV, Chan HL, Hansen BE, et al. Risk of hepatocellular carcinoma in chronic hepatitis B: assessment and modification with current antiviral therapy. [Review]. J Hepatol 2015;62:956–67.

40. Sung JJ, Tsoi KK, Wong VW, et al. Meta-analysis: treatment of hepatitis B infection reduces risk of hepatocellular carcinoma. Aliment Pharmacol Ther 2008;28:1067–77.

41. Singal AK, Salameh H, Kuo YF, et al. Meta-analysis: the impact of oral anti-viral agents on the incidence of hepatocellular carcinoma in chronic hepatitis B. Aliment Pharmacol Ther 2013;38:98–106.

42. Choi J, Kim HJ, Lee J, et al. Risk of hepatocellular carcinoma in patients treated with entecavir vs tenofovir for chronic hepatitis B: a Korean nationwide cohort study. JAMA Oncol 2019;5:30–6.

43. Yip TC, Wong VW, Chan HL, et al. Tenofovir is associated with lower risk of hepatocellular carcinoma than entecavir in patients with chronic HBV infection in China. Gastroenterology 2020;158:215–25.

44. Kim SU, Seo YS, Lee HA, et al. A multicenter study of entecavir vs. tenofovir on prognosis of treatment-naive chronic hepatitis B in South Korea. J Hepatol 2019;71:456–64.

45. Hsu YC, Wong GL, Chen CH, et al. Tenofovir versus entecavir for hepatocellular carcinoma prevention in an International consortium of chronic hepatitis B. Am J Gastroenterol 2020;115:271–80.

46. Tseng CH, Hsu YC, Chen TH, et al. Hepatocellular carcinoma incidence with tenofovir versus entecavir in chronic hepatitis B: a systematic review and meta-analysis. Lancet Gastroenterol Hepatol 2020;5:1039–52.

47. Dave S, Park S, Murad MH, et al. Comparative effectiveness of entecavir versus tenofovir for preventing hepatocellular carcinoma in patients with chronic hepatitis B: a systematic review and meta-analysis. Hepatology 2021;73:68–78.

48. Gu L, Yao Q, Shen Z, et al. Comparison of tenofovir versus entecavir on reducing incidence of hepatocellular carcinoma in chronic hepatitis B patients: a systematic review and meta-analysis. J Gastroenterol Hepatol 2020;35:1467–76.

49. Li M, Lv T, Wu S, et al. Tenofovir versus entecavir in lowering the risk of hepatocellular carcinoma development in patients with chronic hepatitis B: a critical systematic review and meta-analysis. Hepatol Int 2020;14:105–14.

50. Yang HI, Yuen MF, Chan HLY, et al. Risk estimation for hepatocellular carcinoma in chronic hepatitis B (REACH-B): development and validation of a predictive score. Lancet Oncol 2011;12:568–74.

51. Wong VWS, Chan SL, Mo F, et al. Clinical scoring system to predict hepatocellular carcinoma in chronic hepatitis B carriers. J Clin Oncol 2010;28:1660–5.

52. Yuen MF, Tanaka Y, Fong DYT, et al. Independent risk factors and predictive score for the development of hepatocellular carcinoma in chronic hepatitis B. J Hepatol 2009;50:80–8.

53. Wong GL, Chan HL, Chan HY, et al. Accuracy of risk scores for patients with chronic hepatitis B receiving entecavir treatment. Gastroenterology 2013;144:933–44.

54. Papatheodoridis GV, Dalekos GN, Yurdaydin C, et al. Incidence and predictors of hepatocellular carcinoma in caucasian chronic hepatitis B patients receiving entecavir or tenofovir. J Hepatol 2015;62:363–70.

55. Papatheodoridis G, Dalekos G, Sypsa V, et al. PAGE-B predicts the risk of developing hepatocellular carcinoma in caucasians with chronic hepatitis B on 5-year antiviral therapy. J Hepatol 2016;64:800–6.

56. Bortolotti F, Guido M, Bartolacci S, et al. Chronic hepatitis B in children after e antigen seroclearance: final report of a 29-year longitudinal study. Hepatology 2006;43:556–62.

57. Chang MH, Chen TH, Hsu HM, et al. Prevention of hepatocellular carcinoma by universal vaccination against hepatitis B virus: the effect and problems. Clin Cancer Res 2005;11:7953–7.

58. Murawski M, Weeda VB, Maibach R, et al. Hepatocellular carcinoma in children: does modified platinum- and doxorubicin-based chemotherapy increase tumor resectability and change outcome? Lessons learned from the SIOPEL 2 and 3 studies. J Clin Oncol 2016;34:1050–6.

59. Singal AG, Mittal S, Yerokun OA, et al. Hepatocellular carcinoma screening associated with early tumor detection and improved survival among patients with cirrhosis in the US. Am J Med 2017;130:1099–106.e1.

60. Sangiovanni A, Del Ninno E, Fasani P, et al. Increased survival of cirrhotic patients with a hepatocellular carcinoma detected during surveillance. Gastroenterology 2004;126:1005–14.

61. Bortolotti F, Jara P, Crivellaro C, et al. Outcome of chronic hepatitis B in caucasian children during a 20-year observation period. J Hepatol 1998;29:184–90.

62. Zhang XF, Liu XM, Wei T, et al. Clinical characteristics and outcome of hepato-cellular carcinoma in children and adolescents. Pediatr Surg Int 2013;29: 763–70.

63. Hsu HC, Wu MZ, Chang MH, et al. Childhood hepatocellular carcinoma de-velops exclusively in hepatitis B surface antigen carriers in three decades in Taiwan. Report of 51 cases strongly associated with rapid development of liver cirrhosis. J Hepatol 1987;5:260–7.

64. Omata M, Cheng AL, Kokudo N, et al. Asia-Pacific clinical practice guidelines on the management of hepatocellular carcinoma: a 2017 update. Hepatol Int 2017;11:317–70.

65. Marrero JA, Kulik LM, Sirlin CB, et al. Diagnosis, staging, and management of hepatocellular carcinoma: 2018 practice guidance by the American association for the study of liver diseases. Hepatology 2018;68:723–50.

66. European Association for the Study of the Liver. Electronic address eee, Euro-pean association for the study of the L. EASL clinical practice guidelines: man-agement of hepatocellular carcinoma. J Hepatol 2018;69:182–236.

67. Kim JH, Lee YS, Lee HJ, et al. HBsAg seroclearance in chronic hepatitis B: im-plications for hepatocellular carcinoma. J Clin Gastroenterol 2011;45:64–8.

68. Kim GA, Lim YS, An J, et al. HBsAg seroclearance after nucleoside analogue therapy in patients with chronic hepatitis B: clinical outcomes and durability. Gut 2014;63:1325–32.

69. Inoue T, Tanaka Y. Novel biomarkers for the management of chronic hepatitis B. Clin Mol Hepatol 2020;26:261–79.

70. Caviglia GP, Ribaldone DG, Abate ML, et al. Performance of protein induced by vitamin K absence or antagonist-II assessed by chemiluminescence enzyme immunoassay for hepatocellular carcinoma detection: a meta-analysis. Scand J Gastroenterol 2018;53:734–40.

71. Park SJ, Jang JY, Jeong SW, et al. Usefulness of AFP, AFP-L3, and PIVKA-II, and their combinations in diagnosing hepatocellular carcinoma. Medicine 2017;96: e5811.

72. Balaceanu LA. Biomarkers vs imaging in the early detection of hepatocellular carcinoma and prognosis. World J Clin Cases 2019;7:1367–82.

73. Kokudo N, Takemura N, Hasegawa K, et al. Clinical practice guidelines for he-patocellular carcinoma: the Japan Society of Hepatology 2017 (4th JSH-HCC guidelines) 2019 update. Hepatol Res 2019;49:1109–13.

74. Lupberger J, Hildt E. Hepatitis B virus-induced oncogenesis. World J Gastroen-terol 2007;13:74–81.

75. Vaiphei K. Correlative analysis of histological profile of the adjoining liver paren-chyma with liver enzyme levels in hepatocellular carcinoma and their compari-son with chronic liver disease in autopsy cases. Indian J Pathol Microbiol 2007;50:711–7.

76. Park BK, Park YN, Ahn SH, et al. Long-term outcome of chronic hepatitis B based on histological grade and stage. J Gastroenterol Hepatol 2007;22:383–8.

77. Bralet MP, Regimbeau JM, Pineau P, et al. Hepatocellular carcinoma occurring in nonfibrotic liver: epidemiologic and histopathologic analysis of 80 French cases. Hepatology 2000;32:200–4.

78. Beasley RP. Hepatitis B virus. The major etiology of hepatocellular carcinoma. Cancer 1988;61:1942–56.

79. Anthony PP, Vogel CL, Barker LF. Liver cell dysplasia: a premalignant condition. J Clin Pathol 1973;26:217–23.

80. Koo JS, Kim H, Park BK, et al. Predictive value of liver cell dysplasia for development of hepatocellular carcinoma in patients with chronic hepatitis B. J Clin Gastroenterol 2008;42:738–43.

81. Watanabe S, Okita K, Harada T, et al. Morphologic studies of the liver cell dysplasia. Cancer 1983;51:2197–205.

82. Libbrecht L, Craninx M, Nevens F, et al. Predictive value of liver cell dysplasia for development of hepatocellular carcinoma in patients with non-cirrhotic and cirrhotic chronic viral hepatitis. Histopathology 2001;39:66–73.

83. Santi V, Trevisani F, Gramenzi A, et al. Semiannual surveillance is superior to annual surveillance for the detection of early hepatocellular carcinoma and patient survival. J Hepatol 2010;53:291–7.

84. Singal A, Volk ML, Waljee A, et al. Meta-analysis: surveillance with ultrasound for early-stage hepatocellular carcinoma in patients with cirrhosis. Aliment Pharmacol Ther 2009;30:37–47.

85. Trevisani F, De Notariis S, Rapaccini G, et al. Semiannual and annual surveillance of cirrhotic patients for hepatocellular carcinoma: effects on cancer stage and patient survival (Italian experience). Am J Gastroenterol 2002;97:734–44.

86. Sheu JC, Sung JL, Chen DS, et al. Growth rate of asymptomatic hepatocellular carcinoma and its clinical implications. Gastroenterology 1985;89:259–66.

87. Trinchet JC, Chaffaut C, Bourcier V, et al. Ultrasonographic surveillance of hepatocellular carcinoma in cirrhosis: a randomized trial comparing 3- and 6-month periodicities. Hepatology 2011;54:1987–97.

88. El-Serag HB. Epidemiology of viral hepatitis and hepatocellular carcinoma. Gastroenterology 2012;142:1264–1273 e1.

89. European Association for the Study of the Liver. Electronic address eee, European Association for the Study of the Liver. EASL 2017 clinical practice guidelines on the management of hepatitis B virus infection. J Hepatol 2017;67: 370–98.

90. Jaeck D, Bachellier P, Oussoultzoglou E, et al. Surgical resection of hepatocellular carcinoma. Post-operative outcome and long-term results in Europe: an overview. Liver Transpl 2004;10:S58–63.

91. Wu CY, Chen YJ, Ho HJ, et al. Association between nucleoside analogues and risk of hepatitis B virus-related hepatocellular carcinoma recurrence following liver resection. JAMA 2012;308:1906–14.

92. Wong JS, Wong GL, Tsoi KK, et al. Meta-analysis: the efficacy of anti-viral therapy in prevention of recurrence after curative treatment of chronic hepatitis B-related hepatocellular carcinoma. Aliment Pharmacol Ther 2011;33:1104–12.

93. Sun P, Dong X, Cheng X, et al. Nucleot(s)ide analogues for hepatitis B virus-related hepatocellular carcinoma after curative treatment: a systematic review and meta-analysis. PLoS One 2014;9:e102761.

94. Xia BW, Zhang YC, Wang J, et al. Efficacy of antiviral therapy with nucleotide/nucleoside analogs after curative treatment for patients with hepatitis B virus-related hepatocellular carcinoma: a systematic review and meta-analysis. Clin Res Hepatol Gastroenterol 2015;39:458–68.

95. Liu GM, Huang XY, Shen SL, et al. Adjuvant antiviral therapy for hepatitis B virus-related hepatocellular carcinoma after curative treatment: a systematic review and meta-analysis. Hepatol Res 2016;46:100–10.

96. Zhang G, Yu X, Liu P, et al. Efficacy of nucleoside analogs for chronic hepatitis B virus-related hepatocellular carcinoma after curative treatment: a meta-analysis. Dig Dis Sci 2018;63:3207–19.

97. Hung IF, Wong DK, Poon RT, et al. Risk factors and post-resection independent predictive score for the recurrence of hepatitis B-related hepatocellular carcinoma. PLoS One 2016;11:e0148493.

98. Huang G, Lau WY, Wang ZG, et al. Antiviral therapy improves postoperative survival in patients with hepatocellular carcinoma: a randomized controlled trial. Ann Surg 2015;261:56–66.

99. Huang G, Li PP, Lau WY, et al. Antiviral therapy reduces hepatocellular carcinoma recurrence in patients with low HBV-DNA levels: a randomized controlled trial. Ann Surg 2018;268:943–54.

100. Li C, Li ZC, Ma L, et al. Perioperative antiviral therapy improves the prognosis of HBV DNA-negative patients with HBV-related hepatocellular carcinoma. Expert Rev Gastroenterol Hepatol 2020;14:749–56.

101. Wong GL, Tse YK, Chan HL, et al. Oral nucleos(t)ide analogues reduce recurrence and death in chronic hepatitis B-related hepatocellular carcinoma. Aliment Pharmacol Ther 2016;43:802–13.

102. Choi J, Jo C, Lim YS. Tenofovir versus entecavir on recurrence of hepatitis B virus-related hepatocellular carcinoma after surgical resection. Hepatology 2021;73:661–73.

103. Thia TJ, Lui HF, Ooi LL, et al. A study into the risk of exacerbation of chronic hepatitis B after liver resection for hepatocellular carcinoma. J Gastrointest Surg 2007;11:612–8.

104. Huang S, Xia Y, Lei Z, et al. Antiviral therapy inhibits viral reactivation and improves survival after repeat hepatectomy for hepatitis B virus-related recurrent hepatocellular carcinoma. J Am Coll Surg 2017;224:283–93.e4.

105. Jang JW, Yoo SH, Nam HC, et al. Association of prophylactic anti-hepatitis B virus therapy with improved long-term survival in patients with hepatocellular carcinoma undergoing transarterial therapy. Clin Infect Dis 2020;71:546–55.

106. Jang JW, Kim YW, Lee SW, et al. Reactivation of hepatitis B virus in HBsAg-negative patients with hepatocellular carcinoma. PLoS One 2015;10:e0122041.

107. Dan JQ, Zhang YJ, Huang JT, et al. Hepatitis B virus reactivation after radiofrequency ablation or hepatic resection for HBV-related small hepatocellular carcinoma: a retrospective study. Eur J Surg Oncol 2013;39:865–72.

108. Shiba S, Kondo S, Ueno H, et al. Hepatitis B virus reactivation during treatment with multi-tyrosine kinase inhibitor for hepatocellular carcinoma. Case Rep Oncol 2012;5:515–9.

109. Jun BG, Kim YD, Kim SG, et al. Hepatitis B virus reactivation after radiotherapy for hepatocellular carcinoma and efficacy of antiviral treatment: a multicenter study. PLoS One 2018;13:e0201316.

110. El-Khoueiry AB, Sangro B, Yau T, et al. Nivolumab in patients with advanced hepatocellular carcinoma (CheckMate 040): an open-label, non-comparative, phase 1/2 dose escalation and expansion trial. Lancet 2017;389:2492–502.

111. Yau T, Kang YK, Kim TY, et al. Efficacy and safety of nivolumab plus ipilimumab in patients with advanced hepatocellular carcinoma previously treated with sorafenib: the CheckMate 040 randomized clinical trial. JAMA Oncology 2020;6(11):e204564.

112. Zhu AX, Finn RS, Edeline J, et al. Pembrolizumab in patients with advanced hepatocellular carcinoma previously treated with sorafenib (KEYNOTE-224): a non-randomised, open-label phase 2 trial. Lancet Oncol 2018;19:940–52.

113. Lee PC, Chao Y, Chen MH, et al. Risk of HBV reactivation in patients with immune checkpoint inhibitor-treated unresectable hepatocellular carcinoma. J Immunother Cancer 2020;8(2):e001072.

114. Xie L, Yin J, Xia R, et al. Cost-effectiveness of antiviral treatment after resection in hepatitis B virus-related hepatocellular carcinoma patients with compensated cirrhosis. Hepatology 2018;68:1476–86.

115. Sarin SK, Kumar M, Lau GK, et al. Asian-Pacific clinical practice guidelines on the management of hepatitis B: a 2015 update. Hepatol Int 2016;10:1–98.

116. Chen EQ, Tang H. Optimization therapy for the treatment of chronic hepatitis B. World J Gastroenterol 2014;20:5730–6.

117. Shin JW, Jung SW, Lee SB, et al. Medication nonadherence increases hepatocellular carcinoma, cirrhotic complications, and mortality in chronic hepatitis B patients treated with entecavir. Am J Gastroenterol 2018;113:998–1008.

Controversies in Treating Chronic Hepatitis B Virus Infection

Discordant Serologic Results

Arif Sarowar, BSc, Grishma Hirode, MSc,
Harry L.A. Janssen, PhD, MD, Jordan J. Feld, MPH, MD*

KEYWORDS

- Hepatitis B • Discordant serologies • Chronic infection • Occult hepatitis

KEY POINTS

- Discordant serologic findings can lead to misinterpretation and doubt in treating chronic hepatitis B virus (HBV) infection.
- Defective antigen/antibody recognition can disrupt normal serologic levels in HBV.
- Optimized testing assays, additional tests, and screening strategies can prevent misdiagnosis of those with discordant serologies.

INTRODUCTION

The natural history of chronic hepatitis B virus (HBV) infection is dynamic, with multiple phases of infection that vary in duration, severity, and outcome. Current guidelines recommend a combination of serologic, virologic, and biochemical markers in order to understand the phase in the natural history of chronic HBV infection for proper treatment management.[1–4] Assessment of liver fibrosis also is recommended, which may guide therapeutic decision making to prevent progression to cirrhosis and hepatocellular carcinoma (HCC).[2]

The hallmark of active HBV infection is the presence of hepatitis B surface antigen (HBsAg). At the onset of infection, most individuals have circulating hepatitis B e antigen (HBeAg), which is associated with high levels of viral replication and increased infectivity. Those who acquire infection early in life typically go through a prolonged period of HBeAg-positive infection with high levels of HBV DNA but no active liver injury, often referred to as the immune tolerant phase of infection. After many years or even decades of this profile, a transition to active hepatitis occurs with elevations in liver enzymes and associated active inflammation, which may lead to progressive

Toronto Centre for Liver Disease, University Health Network, 200 Elizabeth Street, Toronto, Ontario M5G 2C4, Canada
* Corresponding author.
E-mail address: jordan.feld@uhn.ca

Clin Liver Dis 25 (2021) 805–816
https://doi.org/10.1016/j.cld.2021.06.007
1089-3261/21/© 2021 Elsevier Inc. All rights reserved.

liver fibrosis. During this immune active phase of disease, HBV DNA levels typically fall as alanine aminotransferase (ALT) rises, and eventually clearance of HBeAg occurs. Although loss of HBeAg usually results in the development of HBeAg antibodies, there may be periods of overlap where both HBeAg and anti-HBe are present or where both are absent. HBeAg seroconversion may be the end of active hepatitis and signify the beginning of the immune control phase of disease, characterized by low or undetectable levels of HBV DNA and normal liver enzymes. Alternatively, flares of hepatitis may occur after HBeAg clearance with increases in HBV DNA levels and associated ALT elevations. HBeAg-negative chronic hepatitis B may cause progressive liver injury and fibrosis if left untreated. With prolonged inactive disease, either spontaneously or with suppressive antiviral therapy, HBsAg clearance eventually may occur with or without the development of HBsAg antibodies (anti-HBs), indicating the end of active HBV infection. Those who have cleared HBsAg usually still harbor antibodies to hepatitis B core antigen (anti-HBc), which typically persist lifelong. Reactivation of HBV can occur even after HBsAg loss due to the persistence of replication-competent covalently closed circular DNA (cccDNA) in infected hepatocytes; however, loss of immune control after HBsAg loss occurs only with fairly profound immunosuppression.

The phase of disease is determined by the serologic profile along with the liver enzymes and HBV DNA levels. There are exceptions, however, to the usual serologic patterns observed during different stages of HBV infection (**Fig. 1**). Uncommon serologic profiles may be deceptive and potentially lead to suboptimal management decisions. Discordant serologic results may occur via different mechanisms; recognition and understanding are key to help guide clinical decision making. Although the cause of some discordant results remains controversial, this article aims to discuss possible explanations for these scenarios and recommend strategies to guide clinical management (**Table 1**).

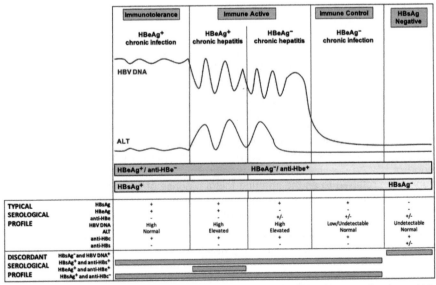

Fig. 1. Typical and atypical serologic profiles during chronic HBV infection. The natural history of chronic HBV infection is shown, highlighting the antigens and antibodies as well as the HBV DNA and ALT levels found in each phase of infection. Phases of infection affected by different discordant serologies are also shown.

Table 1
Key characteristics of discordant serologic profiles observed during hepatitis B virus infection

Discordant Profile	Prevalence	Key Mechanisms	Clinical Relevance
HBsAg⁻ and HBV DNA⁺	0.1%–3% of HBsAg⁻/anti-HBc⁺ individuals[5–13]	• Occult hepatitis • S gene mutations • Low assay sensitivity	• Antiviral therapy not recommended except to prevent HBV reactivation with potent immunosuppression
HBsAg⁺ and anti-HBs⁺	2.8%–5.8% of HBsAg-positive individuals[14–17]	• Immune escape S gene mutations • Heterologous HBsAg serotypes • HBV superinfection	• Dual positivity does not affect disease course or management. • Monitored and treated as per standard for chronic HBV infection
HBeAg+ and anti-HBe⁺	Common but transient	• PC/basic core promoter mutations • Transitional phase to HBeAg negative state • Low assay sensitivity	• Management determined by disease phase, levels of viral replication, and liver histology
HBsAg⁺ and anti-HBc⁻	0.1% of HBsAg-positive individuals[18]	• Immunodeficiency of B-cell/T-cell response • Vertical transmission (transient) • Core gene deletions	• May be indicative of immunodeficiency, but unlikely to affect disease course or alter management

IDENTIFYING CHRONIC HEPATITIS B VIRUS WHEN SEROLOGIC RESULTS ARE DISCORDANT

Hepatitis B Surface Antigen Negative with Hepatitis B Virus DNA Positive

Most patients who clear HBsAg have undetectable HBV DNA as well. Some patients have persistent low-level HBV DNA replication, however, despite the absence of detectable HBsAg. This pattern often is referred to as occult hepatitis B infection (OBI), in which persistent low levels of HBV DNA are present despite absence of viral protein expression.[19] Most individuals with OBI are positive for anti-HBc and less commonly for anti-HBs; however, there also are instances where the presence of HBV DNA is found entirely in isolation with no other markers of past or current HBV infection.[19] The clinical significance of OBI is controversial. Some studies have reported an increased risk of inflammation, progressive fibrosis and even an increased incidence of cirrhosis and HCC.[20,21] Those with OBI also may be at higher risk of HBV reactivation due to immunosuppressive therapy, in particular, B-cell depleting agents or hematopoietic stem cell transplantion.[22,23] Potent immunosuppression may result in reappearance of HBsAg, followed by high HBV DNA levels and resultant severe or even fatal flares of hepatitis.[23]

The prevalence of OBI varies widely between populations but also may be difficult to interpret due to differences in assay sensitivity and sampling frequency. Globally, HBV DNA is detected in 0.1% to 3% of HBsAg-negative/anti-HBc–positive blood donors, with higher prevalence found in Middle Eastern and Asian populations (1.09%–3%) compared with North American (0.1%–1.05%) and European (0%–1.59%) populations.[5–13] Higher rates of OBI have been reported in those with other risk factors, such as HCC, cirrhosis, and human immunodeficiency virus/HBV coinfections.[24–26] Importantly, studies of patients with unexplained cirrhosis and/or HCC have reported higher rates of OBI, raising concern that low-level HBV replication and/or HBV integration may be driving negative outcomes.[24,26–30]

An important consideration in the diagnosis of OBI is the sensitivity of the HBsAg assay used. Current commercial HBsAg assays use a lower limit of detection (LOD) of 0.05 IU/mL. However, 1% to as high as 48% of samples reported as negative on a standard 0.05-IU/mL LOD assay yield a positive result with assays with 0.0005-IU/mL LOD.[31–33] Whether these very low levels of HBsAg are clinically relevant is unknown, because the beneficial natural history seen after HBsAg clearance is based on standard 0.05-IU/mL LOD assays. It would be interesting to look back at old epidemiologic studies to determine if very low levels of HBsAg (<0.05 IU/mL) were associated with negative clinical outcomes compared with those who were negative even by these more sensitive assays. Understanding the clinical relevance of very low levels of HBsAg will be important in the future to help define true functional HBV cure (HBsAg loss), the current therapeutic target for new agents.

In addition to assay sensitivity, mutations in the HBV S genes also may contribute to false OBI occurence where altered HBsAg is undetected by commercially approved assays.[34] Mutations P142L, D144A, and D144E have been found to produce false-negative HBsAg tests as well as other mutations occurring in the "a" determinant region in the HBV S gene.[35,36] Some "a" determinant mutants not only are difficult to detect but also lack ability to be neutralized by antibodies generated by the HBV vaccine.[37] Such mutations are concerning due to the ineffectiveness of routine screening both for detecting active infection and for those at risk for reactivation.[38] Concern that increasing prevalence of vaccine escape mutants could thwart global vaccination efforts has been raised. Studies from Taiwan, the first country to introduce universal HBV vaccination, found increasing prevalence of "a" determinant mutants in children, rising from 7.8% to 23.1% 15 years after implementation of universal HBV vaccination.[39] Although the relative prevalence increased, the absolute number of people with mutants in the total population of children decreased due to a reduction in the overall number of HBsAg-positive individuals, highlighting the importance of universal vaccination and limiting concerns of mutant prevalence.[39,40] Nevertheless, better assays and understanding of the physiochemical changes that affect S gene antigenicity in the presence of such mutations would be helpful. Currently, the use of more standardized, improved assays with higher sensitivity and detection of mutant variants may prevent misdiagnosis, avoiding discordant findings.

Current clinical guidelines do not recommend antiviral therapy or liver cancer surveillance for individuals with OBI, because, despite the questionable associations with outcomes, the absolute risks of HCC and liver-related mortality are low.[19,27] The additional relevance of OBI for the risk of HBV reactivation should be considered, however, when undergoing immunosuppressive therapies.[41] For those scheduled to receive immunosuppression, in particular B-cell depleting agents or other potent regimens, HBV DNA should be measured in those who test HBsAg-negative/anti-HBc–positive with a plan to either monitor carefully or initiate antiviral therapy if HBV DNA is detectable.[42] Whether HBV DNA measurement is required in those receiving less potent immunosuppression is less clear. In the rare circumstance of active HBV-related hepatitis with high HBV DNA and/or HBeAg positivity with undetectable HBsAg, HBsAg mutants should be considered, which can be detected with specialized assays. Further studies on OBI are warranted, particularly with more sensitive HBsAg assays to better understand whether a subset of patients with this profile merit closer follow-up and/or antiviral therapy.

HBsAg Positive and Anti-HBs Positive

In most circumstances, the presence of anti-HBs indicates the end of active HBV infection, because antibodies typically develop after clearance of HBsAg and are associated with a lower risk of HBV reactivation. Although it might be imagined that the appearance of anti-HBs in people who are HBsAg-positive indicates impending HBsAg loss, this usually is not the case. Active HBV infection and replication may persist despite high levels of anti-HBs.[14]

The prevalence of dual HBsAg and anti-HBs positivity has been found in large cohorts to range from 2.8% to 5.8%.[14–17] One large study observed anti-HBs positivity in 2.9% of the HBsAg-positive populations, with 85% of these patients continuing this serologic pattern after 1 year of follow-up.[15] Rather than indicating impending clearance, the presence of anti-HBs actually has been reported to be associated with an increase in liver-related outcomes, with 1 study finding a 3.08-fold higher risk of HCC ($P = .014$), but the investigators also observed higher HBsAg seroclearance (hazard ratio 1.43; $P = .046$) with no significant differences in mortality compared with patients positive for only HBsAg during 5.4 years of follow-up.[17] Another study reported increased presence of active chronic hepatitis and advanced fibrosis, with significantly higher HBV DNA levels compared with lone HBsAg-positive patients.[14]

The molecular mechanisms for dual positivity are not entirely understood. Several studies have attributed this discordant finding to immune escape mutations that could allow viral replication and infection to escape the neutralizing effect of anti-HBs. One recent study with detailed viral sequencing in 131 HBsAg-positive/anti-HBs-positive patients, identified significantly higher numbers of substitutions within the "a" determinant region in the HBsAg gene, compared with a control group of lone HBsAg-positive patients, suggesting immune pressure by the anti-HBs antibodies was responsible for these changes.[16] Mutations/deletions in the pre-S/S gene have been observed to induce production of altered surface proteins, which are not recognized by anti-HBs antibodies.[43,44] These same pre-S/S gene mutations have been suggested to play an important role in the development of HCC.[10] Presence of heterologous serotype-specific anti-HBs also has been postulated to explain concurrent HBsAg/anti-HBs levels, in which heterologous specific anti-HBs antibodies do not target the circulating HBsAg proteins.[45] Unlike anti-HBs induced by vaccination with high affinity to all HBsAg serotypes, anti-HBs antibodies in those with HBsAg positivity have been shown to have low affinity for heterologous HBsAg serotypes.[46] Further evidence for the immune escape hypothesis was found when switching from a *y* to *d* epitope via a single point mutation, allowing the virus to replicate in the presence of anti-HBs.[47]

One postulated explanation for mismatched anti-HBs and HBsAg is reinfection or superinfection with the inability of preexisting antibodies to neutralize a newly encountered strain of the virus.[48] Such patients may have persistent active viral replication following superinfection, following the usual course of infection due to limited or no protective ability of existing anti-HBs antibodies. HBV mutants and superinfection have been found to be stable and, although rare, can be transmitted horizontally to other people.[48]

Studies have shown that false positivity for detection of anti-HBs assays is not likely a reason for the dual-positive phenomenon, because most commercially available assays cannot detect low levels of antibodies, even postvaccination.[49]

Although the clinical significance of HBsAg/anti-HBs positivity is not entirely clear, most data support managing these patients as if they did not have anti-HBs and were lone HBsAg-positive. Although some studies have found dual positivity associated with more active disease and advanced fibrosis,[14] a recent report from the large Hepatitis B Research Network (HBRN) found that concurrent HBsAg/anti-HBsAg positivity did not affect the natural history or risk of clinical outcomes. The HBRN investigators found that anti-HBs levels were persistently low in HBsAg/anti-HBsAg–positive patients, with anti-HBs disappearing in approximately 50% after 4 years mean follow-up.[50] Based on these and other data, guidelines recommend that patients with concurrent HBsAg and anti-HBs should be monitored and treated as if the anti-HBs were not present.[2,3]

HBeAg Positive and Anti-HBe Positive

The presence of HBeAg indicates active HBV replication and high levels of infectivity. In the natural course of chronic HBV infection, loss of circulating HBeAg usually is followed by emergence of HBe antibodies (anti-HBe), often with a transition to a less active phase of disease. Concurrent HBeAg and anti-HBe positivity is not observed infrequently in chronic HBV infection.[51]

During the HBeAg-positive phases of chronic HBV infection, HBeAg is made in huge quantities and anti-HBe is not detectable because HBeAg is in great excess with only free Ag or antibody being measurable. HBeAg loss occurs most commonly because of the development of the precore (PC) and/or basal core promotor (BCP) mutations.[52] The PC mutation (G1896A) results in the insertion of a premature stop codon, preventing the translation of the PC protein, a precursor to HBeAg, whereas the BCP mutation (A1762T/G1764A) reduces expression of the PC protein at the transcriptional level.[53] As the prevalence of PC/BCP mutants in the viral quasispecies increases, the amount of circulating HBeAg decreases.[54] Eventually, levels of HBeAg fall below the level of circulating anti-HBe. When HBeAg and anti-HBe are produced at similar levels, both or neither may be detectable in serum. When HBeAg loss occurs without the appearance of PC/BCP mutations, it is thought to suggest reduced cccDNA transcription, leading to reduced HBeAg levels with the same result in terms of balance with anti-HBe.[55]

Clearance of HBeAg and even HBeAg seroconversion may not be a stable state, with many patients experiencing a period as flip-floppers; chronic hepatitis B patients in whom HBeAg and anti-HBe flip-flop back and forth.[56] The flip-flopper phenotype may persist for a prolonged period but usually eventually leads to stable HBeAg loss, with or without appearance of anti-HBe. The clinical significance of flip-flopping, dual positivity, or dual negativity is not clear, but most data suggest that such patients are in transition to HBeAg-negative disease, either to an immune control or HBeAg-negative chronic HBV phenotype.

Assay sensitivity also may play a part in the classification of HBeAg and anti-HBe status.[51,57,58] Similar to the occurrence of concurrent HBsAg and anti-HBs detection, decreased affinity between HBeAg and anti-HBe is hypothesized to be another possible explanation for concurrent HBeAg and anti-HBe positivity.[51]

For HBeAg and anti-HBe–positive patients, management is based on levels of viral replication and degree of liver inflammation and fibrosis.[2,3,59] With serial evaluation of HBeAg and anti-HBe, many patients ultimately clear HBeAg with or without persistence of anti-HBe.

HBsAg Positive and Anti-HBc Negative

Most HBsAg-positive patients also test positive for antibodies towards core antigen (anti-HBc). During acute infection, HBsAg is the first viral marker to appear, which rarely may be detected before IgM anti-HBc have developed. Such findings are not common in chronic HBV infection. During the natural history of HBV, chronic HBV infection is associated with persistence of HBsAg in the blood and presence of anti-HBc.[60] Although spontaneous clearance of HBsAg can occur, anti-HBc typically continue to be detectable in blood long term, if not lifelong.[60] Loss or lack of anti-HBc in the presence of HBsAg occurs only in rare clinical scenarios.

The lack of anti-HBc in patients with chronic HBV infection is due most commonly to significant immunodeficiency impairing antibody production. B-cell or plasma disorders like common variable immunodeficiency or malignancies like chronic lymphocytic leukemia and multiple myeloma may lead to global and/or selective antibody deficiencies if B-cell clones responsible for specific antibody production are lost.[61] Similarly, B-cell–depleting therapies, like rituximab or other anti-CD20 agents, may lead to loss of specific antibody production.[62] In patients with known HBV infection, emergence of one of these immunodeficiency scenarios may lead to loss of anti-HBc. The finding of HBsAg-positivity without anti-HBc should prompt testing for immunodeficiency. In those who previously cleared HBsAg, with anti-HBc as the only marker of past HBV exposure, loss of anti-HBc due to immunodeficiency may lead to a risk of HBV reactivation that would be hard to prevent with standard HBsAg and anti-HBc testing prior to chemotherapy.[63,64] Accordingly, past HBV infection should be considered in patients with hematologic malignancies with risk factors for HBV (eg, born in an endemic country), even if they test negative for all HBV markers, leading to prompt HBV testing with any evidence of hepatitis.

In addition to B-cell deficiencies, T-cell defects also may affect anti-HBc production. Increases in antigen-specific activation of CD4$^+$ T lymphocytes have been found to correspond to increases in anti-HBc titer.[65] T-cell exhaustion, where lymphocytes become functionally inactive following antigen exposure, also can affect production of anti-HBc.[66] Mutations can affect T-cell recognition of HBc epitopes in several ways, including anergy induction of the HBc-specific CD4$^+$ T-cell responses, which may lead to reduced or rarely absent anti-HBc.[67]

Another possible explanation for lack of anti-HBc is the formation of HBcAg/anti-HBc immune complexes. Immune complexes of anti-HBc with excess HBc antigen in the bloodstream can result in undetectable levels with commercially available tests.[68,69] Such anti-HBc complexes can be detected after immune complex dissociative treatments, such as polyethylene glycol precipitation with ion chaotropic treatment; however, this is not used routinely commercially.[70]

This atypical profile also has been seen transiently following vertical transmission of HBV from HBeAg-positive carrier mothers that can result in initial absence of anti-HBc in immune incompetent infants.[71] HBeAg can traverse the placenta form mother to fetus, leading to tolerance in the infant to HBeAg, which is antigenically very similar to HBcAg, leading to initial failure to produce antibodies to HBcAg. With maturation of the infant immune system during early infancy, however, the typical profile (HBsAg-positive/anti-HBc-positive) usually emerges.[18]

Agent-related factors also have been used to explain anti-HBc nonproduction in hosts.[72] Nucleotide sequence deletions in the core gene have been shown to affect antigen recognition by immune cells.[73] Presence of immunodominant epitopes are important for HBcAg recognition, which can contribute to lack of effective immune responses for clearance.[73] Additionally, previous studies have found the interdimer interface of core protein affecting several stages of genome replication and secretion, such as capsid assembly, pregenomic RNA packaging, and reverse transcription.[74] The presence of amino acid substitutions in the core protein can lead to lower production or secretion of HBcAg and HBeAg, which may result in anti-HBc negativity in some cases.[75]

The absence of anti-HBc with HBsAg positivity is rare, with blood donor studies reporting such occurrence in 0.1% of HBsAg-positive donors.[18] Although this atypical finding can indicate defective immune responses, not much is known on its effect on the natural history of HBV.[76] Identification of this profile should prompt a search for immunodeficiency but, if absent, is unlikely to affect the clinical course of disease or management.

SUMMARY

In conclusion, although discordant HBV serologic results are relatively uncommon, they can lead to confusion and suboptimal clinical management if identified improperly. Understanding when discordant serology may occur, key mechanisms involved, and how it has an impact on the natural history of disease can have important implications for disease monitoring and therapeutic decision making. The mechanisms causing discordant serologies continue to be studied; however, most explanations recognize variations in assay sensitivity and the role of mutations that hinder normal antigen/antibody production or recognition. Continued study of areas of uncertainty and development of tools to avoid discordant results may help in the future. For now, to avoid misdiagnosis, use of other tools, including HBV DNA and ALT, in particular, can be performed to accurately classify the phase of chronic HBV infection.

CLINICS CARE POINTS

- Those with HBsAg loss should be further monitored with other serological testing to prevent misdiagnosis of HBV infection
- Managing patient's serological findings should be determined by disease phase, viral activity and liver histology.
- Patient medical history (was thinking mutations/history of chemotherapy) should be considered to understand atypical serological findings.

FINANCIAL DISCLOSURES

H.L.A. Janssen: Consulting, grant, and research support for AbbVie, Arbutus, ARENA, Enyo, Gilead Sciences, Bristol Myers Squibb, GlaxoSmithKline, Janssen Medimmune, Merck, Roche, Vir Biotechnology Inc., and Viroclinics. J.J. Feld: Consulting and/or research support from Abbvie, Antios, Arbutus, Enanta, Eiger, Gilead, GlaxoSmithKline, Janssen, and Roche. The other authors report nothing to disclose.

REFERENCES

1. Liaw Y-F, Sung JJY, Chow WC, et al. Lamivudine for patients with chronic hepatitis B and advanced liver disease. N Engl J Med 2004;351(15):1521–31.
2. Terrault NA, Lok ASF, McMahon BJ, et al. Update on prevention, diagnosis, and treatment of chronic hepatitis B: AASLD 2018 hepatitis B guidance. Hepatology 2018;67(4):1560–99.
3. Lampertico P, Agarwal K, Berg T, et al. EASL 2017 clinical practice guidelines on the management of hepatitis B virus infection. J Hepatol 2017;67(2):370–98.
4. Sarin SK, Kumar M, Lau GK, et al. Asian-Pacific clinical practice guidelines on the management of hepatitis B: a 2015 update. Hepatol Int 2016;10(1):1–98.

5. Hourfar MK, Jork C, Schottstedt V, et al. Experience of German Red Cross blood donor services with nucleic acid testing: results of screening more than 30 million blood donations for human immunodeficiency virus-1, hepatitis C virus, and hepatitis B virus. Transfusion 2008;48(8):1558–66.

6. O'Brien SF, Fearon MA, Yi QL, et al. Hepatitis B virus DNA-positive, hepatitis B surface antigen-negative blood donations intercepted by anti-hepatitis B core antigen testing: the Canadian Blood Services experience. Transfusion 2007;47(10): 1809–15.

7. Kleinman SH, Kuhns MC, Todd DS, et al. Frequency of HBV DNA detection in US blood donors testing positive for the presence of anti-HBc: implications for transfusion transmission and donor screening. Transfusion 2003;43(6):696–704.

8. Brojer E, Grabarczyk P, Liszewski G, et al. Characterization of HBV DNA +/ HBsAg - blood donors in Poland identified by triplex NAT. Hepatology 2006; 44(6):1666–74.

9. Fang Y, Shang QL, Liu JY, et al. Prevalence of occult hepatitis B virus infection among hepatopathy patients and healthy people in China. J Infect 2009;58(5): 383–8.

10. Lin CL, Liu CH, Chen W, et al. Association of pre-S deletion mutant of hepatitis B virus with risk of hepatocellular carcinoma. J Gastroenterol Hepatol 2007;22(7): 1098–103.

11. Linauts S, Saldanha J, Strong DM. PRISM hepatitis B surface antigen detection of hepatits B virus minipool nucleic acid testing yield samples. Transfusion 2008; 48(7):1376–82.

12. Chevrier MC, St-Louis M, Perreault J, et al. Detection and characterization of hepatitis B virus of anti-hepatitis B core antigen-reactive blood donors in Quebec with an in-house nucleic acid testing assay. Transfusion 2007;47(10):1794–802.

13. Papatheodoridis G, Vlachogiannakos I, Cholongitas E, et al. Discontinuation of oral antivirals in chronic hepatitis B: a systematic review. Hepatology 2016; 63(5):1481–92.

14. Colson P, Borentain P, Motte A, et al. Clinical and virological significance of the co-existence of HBsAg and anti-HBs antibodies in hepatitis B chronic carriers. Virology 2007;367(1):30–40.

15. Pu Z, Li D, Wang A, et al. Epidemiological characteristics of the carriers with coexistence of HBsAg and anti-HBs based on a community cohort study. J Viral Hepat 2016;23(4):286–93.

16. Hou W, Huo Z, Du Y, et al. Characteristics of amino acid substitutions within the "a" determinant region of hepatitis B virus in chronically infected patients with co-existing HBsAg and anti-HBs. Clin Res Hepatol Gastroenterol 2020;44(6):923–31.

17. Kwak MS, Chung GE, Yang JI, et al. Long-term outcomes of HBsAg/anti-HBs double-positive versus HBsAg single-positive patients with chronic hepatitis B. Sci Rep 2019;9(1):1–7.

18. Laperche S, Guitton C, Smilovici W, et al. Blood donors infected with the hepatitis B virus but persistently lacking antibodies to the hepatitis B core antigen. Vox Sang 2001;80(2):90–4.

19. Raimondo G, Locarnini S, Pollicino T, et al. Update of the statements on biology and clinical impact of occult hepatitis B virus infection. J Hepatol 2019;71(2): 397–408.

20. Raimondo G, Pollicino T, Romanò L, et al. A 2010 update on occult hepatitis B infection l'hépatite B occulte. Pathol Biol 2010;58:254–7.

21. Covolo L, Pollicino T, Raimondo G, et al. Occult hepatitis B virus and the risk for chronic liver disease: a meta-analysis. Dig Liver Dis 2013;45(3):238–44.

22. Seto WK, Chan TSY, Hwang YY, et al. Hepatitis B reactivation in occult viral carriers undergoing hematopoietic stem cell transplantation: a prospective study. Hepatology 2017;65(5):1451–61.

23. Loomba R, Liang TJ. Hepatitis B reactivation associated with immune suppressive and biological modifier therapies: current concepts, management strategies, and future directions. Gastroenterology 2017;152(6):1297–309.

24. Re V, Frank I, Gross R, et al. Prevalence, risk factors, and outcomes for occult hepatitis B virus infection among HIV-infected patients. J Acquir Immune Defic Syndr 2007;44(3):315–20.

25. Cacciola I, Pollicino T, Squadrito G, et al. Occult hepatitis B virus infection in patients with chronic hepatitis C liver disease. N Engl J Med 1999;341(1):22–6.

26. Chan HL-Y, Tsang SW-C, Leung NW-Y, et al. Occult HBV infection in cryptogenic liver cirrhosis in an area with high prevalence of HBV infection. Am J Gastroenterol 2002;97(5):1211–5.

27. Hassan ZK, Hafez MM, Mansor TM, et al. Occult HBV infection among Egyptian hepatocellular carcinoma patients. Virol J 2011;8.

28. Ghisetti V, Marzano A, Zamboni F, et al. Occult Hepatitis B virus infection in HBsAg negative patients undergoing liver transplantation: clinical significance. Liver Transplant 2004;10(3):356–62.

29. Kao JH, Chen PJ, Lai MY, et al. Occult hepatitis B virus infection and clinical outcomes of patients with chronic hepatitis C. J Clin Microbiol 2002;40(11):4068–71.

30. Shi Y, Wu YH, Wu W, et al. Association between occult hepatitis B infection and the risk of hepatocellular carcinoma: a meta-analysis. Liver Int 2012;32(2):231–40.

31. Yang R, Song G, Guan W, et al. The Lumipulse G HBsAg-Quant assay for screening and quantification of the hepatitis B surface antigen. J Virol Methods 2016;228:39–47.

32. Seto WK, Tanaka Y, Wong DKH, et al. Evidence of serologic activity in chronic hepatitis B after surface antigen (HBsAg) seroclearance documented by conventional HBsAg assay. Hepatol Int 2013;7(1):98–105.

33. Ozeki I, Nakajima T, Suii H, et al. Analysis of hepatitis B surface antigen (HBsAg) using high-sensitivity HBsAg assays in hepatitis B virus carriers in whom HBsAg seroclearance was confirmed by conventional assays. Hepatol Res 2018;48(3):E263–74.

34. Raimondo G, Allain JP, Brunetto MR, et al. Statements from the Taormina expert meeting on occult hepatitis B virus infection. J Hepatol 2008;49(4):652–7.

35. Kim KH, Lee KH, Chang HY, et al. Evolution of hepatitis B virus sequence from a liver transplant recipient with rapid breakthrough despite hepatitis B immune globulin prophylaxis and lamivudine therapy. J Med Virol 2003;71(3):367–75.

36. Lazarevic I. Clinical implications of hepatitis B virus mutations: recent advances. World J Gastroenterol 2014;20(24):7653–64.

37. Zuckerman AJ. Effect of hepatitis B virus mutants on efficacy of vaccination. Lancet 2000;355(9213):1382–4.

38. Purdy M. Hepatitis B virus S gene escape mutants. Asian J Transfus Sci 2007;1(2):62.

39. Chang M-H. Review breakthrough HBV infection in vaccinated children in Taiwan: surveillance for HBV mutants. Antivir Ther 2010;15:463–9.

40. Ni YH, Huang LM, Chang MH, et al. Two decades of universal hepatitis B vaccination in Taiwan: impact and implication for future strategies. Gastroenterology 2007;132(4):1287–93.

41. Lok ASF, McMahon BJ. Chronic hepatitis B: update 2009. Hepatology 2009;50(3): 661–2.

42. Hwang JP, Feld JJ, Hammond SP, et al. Hepatitis B virus screening and management for patients with cancer prior to therapy: ASCO provisional clinical opinion update. J Clin Oncol 2020;38(31):3698–715.

43. Mun HS, Lee SA, Jee Y, et al. The prevalence of hepatitis B virus preS deletions occurring naturally in Korean patients infected chronically with genotype C. J Med Virol 2008;80(7):1189–94.

44. Chen BF, Liu CJ, Jow GM, et al. High prevalence and mapping of pre-S deletion in hepatitis B virus carriers with progressive liver diseases. Gastroenterology 2006;130(4):1153–68.

45. Pondé RAA. The underlying mechanisms for the "simultaneous HBsAg and anti-HBs serological profile". Eur J Clin Microbiol Infect Dis 2011;30(11):1325–40.

46. Author H, Gerlich WH. Editorial commentary: the enigma of concurrent hepatitis B surface antigen (HBsAg) and antibodies to HBsAg. Clin Infect Dis 2007;44(9): 1170–2.

47. Margeridon SV, Lachaux A, Trepo C, et al. A quasi-monoclonal anti-HBs response can lead to immune escape of 'wild-type' hepatitis B virus. J Gen Virol 2005.

48. Krastev ZA. The "return" of hepatitis B. World J Gastroenterol 2006;12(44): 7081–6.

49. Heijtink RA, Schneeberger PM, Postma B, et al. Anti-HBs levels after hepatitis B immunisation depend on test reagents: routinely determined 10 and 100 IU/l seroprotection levels unreliable. Vaccine 2002;20(23–24):2899–905.

50. Lee WM, King WC, Schwarz KB, et al. Prevalence and clinical features of patients with concurrent HBsAg and anti-HBs: evaluation of the hepatitis B research network cohort. J Viral Hepat 2020;27(9):922–31.

51. Wang J, Zhou B, Lai Q, et al. Clinical and virological characteristics of chronic hepatitis B with concurrent hepatitis B e antigen and antibody detection. J Viral Hepat 2011;18(9):646–52. .

52. Papatheodoridis GV, Hadziyannis SJ. Diagnosis and management of pre-core mutant chronic hepatitis B. J Viral Hepat 2001;8:311–21.

53. Xiao L, Zhou B, Gao H, et al. Hepatitis B virus genotype B with G1896A and A1762T/G1764A mutations is associated with hepatitis B related acute-on-chronic liver failure. J Med Virol 2011;83(9):1544–50.

54. Qin Y, Zhang J, Mao R, et al. Prevalence of basal core promoter and precore mutations in Chinese chronic hepatitis B patients and correlation with serum HBeAg titers. J Med Virol 2009;81(5):807–14.

55. Malmström S, Larsson SB, Hannoun C, et al. Hepatitis B viral DNA decline at loss of HBeAg is mainly explained by reduced cccdna load - down-regulated transcription of PgRNA has limited impact. PLoS One 2012;7(7).

56. Davis GL, Hoofnagle JH, Waggoner JG. Spontaneous reactivation of chronic hepatitis B virus infection. Gastroenterology 1984;86(2):230–5.

57. Robbins D, Wright T, Coleman C, et al. Serological detection of HBeAg and anti-HBe using automated microparticle enzyme immunoassays. J Virol Methods 1992;38(3):267–81.

58. Dow BC, Macvarish I, Barr A, et al. Significance of tests for HBeAg and anti-HBe in HBsAg positive blood donors. J Clin Pathol 1980;33(11):1106–9.

59. Hatzakis A, Magiorkinis E, Haida C. HBV virological assessment. J Hepatol 2006; 44(Suppl. 1):71–6.

60. Chevaliez S, Pawlotsky JM. Diagnosis and management of chronic viral hepatitis: antigens, antibodies and viral genomes. Best Pract Res Clin Gastroenterol 2008; 22(6):1031–48.

61. Ahn S, Cunningham-Rundles C. Role of B cells in common variable immune deficiency. Expert Rev Clin Immunol 2009;5(5):557–64.

62. Caligiuri P, Cerruti R, Icardi G, et al. Overview of hepatitis B virus mutations and their implications in the management of infection. World J Gastroenterol 2016; 22(1):145–54.

63. Avettand-Fenoel V, Thabut D, Katlama C, et al. Immune suppression as the etiology of failure to detect anti-HBc antibodies in patients with chronic hepatitis B virus infection. J Clin Microbiol 2006;44(6):2250–3.

64. Yeo W, Chan TC, Leung NWY, et al. Hepatitis B virus reactivation in lymphoma patients with prior resolved hepatitis B undergoing anticancer therapy with or without rituximab. J Clin Oncol 2009;27(4):605–11.

65. Jung M-C, Diepolder HM, Spengler U, et al. Activation of a Heterogeneous Hepatitis B (HB) Core and e Antigen-Specific CD4+ T-cell population during seroconversion to Anti-HBe and Anti-HBs in hepatitis B virus infection. J Virol 1995;69: 3358–68.

66. Schwartz RH. T cell anergy. Annu Rev Immunol 2003;21:305–34.

67. Diepolder HM, Jung M-C, Wierenga E, et al. Anergic TH1 clones specific for hepatitis B virus (HBV) core peptides are inhibitory to other HBV core-specific CD4+ T cells in vitro. J Virol 1996;70:7540–8.

68. Lazizi Y, Dubreuil P. Excess HBcAg in HBc antibody-negative chronic hepatitis B virus carriers. Hepatology 1993;17(6):966–70.

69. Maruyama T, McLachlan A, Lino S, et al. The serology of chronic hepatitis B infection revisited. J Clin Invest 1993;91(6):2586–95.

70. Bredehorst R, Von Wulffen H, Granato C. Quantitation of hepatitis B virus (HBV) core antigen in serum in the presence of antibodies to HBV core antigen: comparison with assays of serum HBV DNA, DNA polymerase, and HBV e antigen. J Clin Microbiol 1985;21(4):593–8.

71. Hsu H-Y, Chang M-H, Hsieh K-H, et al. Cellular immune response to HBcAg in mother-to-infant transmission of hepatitis B virus. Hepatology 1992;15(5):770–6.

72. Pondé RAA. Atypical serological profiles in hepatitis B virus infection. Eur J Clin Microbiol Infect Dis 2013;32(4):461–76.

73. Fiordalisi G, Primi D, Tanzi E, et al. Hepatitis B virus C gene heterogeneity in a familial cluster of anti-HBc negative chronic carriers. J Med Virol 1994;42(2):109–14.

74. Tan Z, Pionek K, Unchwaniwala N, et al. The interface between hepatitis B virus capsid proteins affects self-assembly, pregenomic RNA packaging, and reverse transcription. J Virol 2015;89(6):3275–84.

75. Chen J, Liu B, Tang X, et al. Role of core protein mutations in the development of occult HBV infection. J Hepatol 2021.

76. Melegari M, Jung MC, Schneider R, et al. Conserved core protein sequences in hepatitis B virus infected patients without anti-HBc. J Hepatol 1991;13(2):187–91.

Chronic Hepatitis B Virus in Patients with Chronic Hepatitis C Virus

Nelson E. Airewele, MD[a,b,*], Mitchell L. Shiffman, MD[a,b]

KEYWORDS

- Chronic hepatitis B virus • Chronic hepatitis C virus • HBV-HCV coinfection
- HCV treatment • HBV treatment

KEY POINTS

- Because of overlapping risk factors current or previous infection with hepatitis B virus (HBV) is common in patients with chronic hepatitis C virus (HCV).
- HCV and HBV interact within the host and, in most cases, HCV dominates and suppresses HBV.
- Eradication of HCV with direct-acting antiviral (DAA) therapy removes these suppressive effects, allows HBV replication to increase, and may cause HBV reactivation with flare in liver enzymes.
- All patients with chronic HCV should be checked for hepatitis B surface antigen (HBsAg), anti–hepatitis B (HB) core, and anti–HB surface before initiating treatment with a DAA.
- All patients with detectable HBsAg are at increased risk of flare during or following HCV treatment and should be treated with an HBV antiviral agent before or at the time HCV treatment is initiated. Patients with isolated anti–HB core may have occult HBV and should be monitored closely during and after HCV treatment.

EPIDEMIOLOGY OF HEPATITIS B VIRUS, HEPATITIS C VIRUS, AND COINFECTION

Hepatitis B virus (HBV) and hepatitis C virus (HCV) infections represent the most common cause of chronic liver disease in many countries. Worldwide, an estimated 350 million persons have chronic HBV.[1] Areas of the world with the highest prevalence for HBV include many Asian countries, sub-Saharan Africa, Eastern Europe, and Central and South America. Approximately half the population of these countries have serologic markers of current or previous HBV infection.[2] The United States, Canada, and many countries in the European Union (EU) are considered to have a low prevalence of HBV. In these countries, less than 2% of the population has serologic markers

[a] Liver Institute of Richmond, Bon Secours Mercy Health, Richmond, VA, USA; [b] Liver Institute of Hampton Roads, Bon Secours Mercy Health, Newport News, VA, USA
* Corresponding author. Liver Institute of Richmond, 5855 Bremo Road, Suite 509, Richmond, VA 23226, USA.
E-mail address: Nelson_airewele@bshsi.org

Clin Liver Dis 25 (2021) 817–829
https://doi.org/10.1016/j.cld.2021.06.008
1089-3261/21/© 2021 Elsevier Inc. All rights reserved.

liver.theclinics.com

of exposure to HBV.[3,4] In the United States, chronic HBV is estimated to be present in 1.25 million to 2.2 million persons, or about 0.5% of the population. However, half of these infections are in persons who have immigrated to the United States from areas of the world with high prevalence.[2,3] As discussed elsewhere in this issue, increased migration of persons from countries where HBV is common to the United States, Canada, and many countries of the EU is expected to increase the prevalence of HBV in these countries (See Tout and colleagues's article "The Changing Demographics of Hepatitis B Virus Infection," in this issue).

As opposed to HBV, the prevalence of chronic HCV is distributed relatively evenly throughout the world.[1] The peak prevalence of HCV occurred in 1990, just before the identification of this virus and the development of the first serologic test.[5,6] Before this, the primary mode of transmitting HCV was through the transfusion of blood products. By 1990, an estimated 123 million persons worldwide had acquired HCV, or about 1% to 4% of the population in most countries. The primary exception was Egypt, where 25% of the population was infected with HCV because of health care–associated transmission in the 1960s.[7] In the United States, approximately 5 million persons had serologic evidence of infection, and 4 million were estimated to have chronic HCV.[8]

Since 1990, when HCV was essentially eliminated from the blood supply, the most common route by which persons became infected with this virus was through the intravenous and intranasal use of illicit drugs.[9] The highest incidence of HCV infection is now in young adults between the ages of 20 and 39 years. Globally, 28% of persons who inject drugs are less than 25 years of age. In the United States, the number of newly reported cases within this age group has tripled between 2010 and 2015.[10,11] This second wave of HCV has changed the demographics of HCV from a disease of baby boomers with mean age in the 50s to a relatively flat prevalence between the ages of 20 and 60 years. HCV is only rarely acquired via sexual interaction between long-standing heterosexual couples.[12]

The incidence of acute HBV has declined dramatically in many countries since the 1990s through vaccination practices of specific high-risk populations.[13] Risk factors for acquiring HBV are also discussed (See Dekker and colleagues's article "Treatment and Prevention of Acute Hepatitis B Virus," in this issue). The global push for vaccination has increased nonvaccinated teenagers and young adults to the pinnacle of acute HBV infection.[10,13] Persons in this age group acquire HBV through sexual interactions and/or by using illicit drugs. Because the primary risk factor for acquiring both HBV and HCV are similar, it is not surprising that patients can become coinfected with both viruses.

The prevalence of HBV-HCV coinfection throughout the world has been difficult to assess because those studies that have investigated this have used different markers to screen for these viruses.[14–18] For example, some studies defined HBV infection by the presence of HBV surface antigen (HBsAg), whereas others used antibodies to HBV core protein (anti–HB core). No studies have used HBV DNA testing to confirm whether patients had active or inactive HBV. Similarly, HCV infection has been defined by the presence of antibodies to HCV (anti-HCV) or by HCV RNA. The best estimates indicate that 9% to 30% of persons with markers of previous exposure to HBV also have markers for HCV, and about 40% to 60% of persons with chronic HCV have serologic markers of prior exposure to HBV. However, because about 15% to 20% of patients with anti-HCV achieve spontaneous resolution shortly after exposure and most persons exposed to HBV as adults resolve this virus, the prevalence of patients who harbor both viruses seems to be only 1% to 6%. In areas of the world where HBV is endemic, such as many Asian countries, the prevalence of HBV and HCV coinfection is greater than in places where HBV is less common.[19]

HBV and HCV coinfection is associated with a more severe clinical course than in patients with either HBV or HCV. Coinfected patients seem to have a higher rate of fibrosis progression to cirrhosis than patients with chronic HBV, and a higher risk of developing hepatic decompensation and hepatocellular carcinoma than patients with either chronic HBV or HCV alone.[20–24] The largest study in a non-Asian population compared 95 patients who were coinfected and positive for HBsAg and HCV RNA with 375 patients with only HBV and 380 patients with only HCV infection. Patients with HCV or HBV monoinfection were matched 1:4:4 by age, sex, and presumed duration of infection to a coinfected patient.[25] Stage 3 fibrosis or cirrhosis was present in 58% of patients with HBV and HCV coinfection compared with 58% of patients with HCV infection but only 32% of patients with HBV infection. The lower rate of cirrhosis in the HBV group was likely caused by the inclusion of patients with inactive HBV, who were also HBsAg positive, and a higher rate of HBV treatment in the HBV monoinfected group versus the coinfected group. Hepatic decompensation was more common in patients with coinfection, 11%, compared with 2% and 4% for patients with HBV and HCV monoinfection respectively. This finding was likely caused by reactivation of inactive HBV in patients with cirrhosis contributing to hepatic decompensation, and multivariate analysis confirmed an association between HBV and hepatic decompensation.

INTERACTION OF HEPATITIS VIRUSES

Both HCV and HBV require host proteins for translation, replication, and other critical steps in their viral life cycles. As a result, when a patient is coinfected, both viruses must share or compete for these host proteins. Host immunologic and viral factors affect how these viruses compete and explains why 1 virus may dominate the other. Four serologic profiles can be observed in patients with coinfection: HCV dominant, HBV dominant, codominant, and neither replicative.[26,27] The serologic and virologic pattern for each of these is summarized in **Table 1**. The neither-replicative pattern simply reflects patients who resolved HBV following acute infection and achieved spontaneous seroconversion of HCV. It is not known whether simultaneous infection with both HBV and HCV alters the ability of the host to resolve either or both infections.

Hepatitis C Virus Dominant

This serologic pattern is the most common and is observed in 47% of patients with HCV-HBV coinfection.[26,27] In these patients, HCV actively suppresses HBV

Table 1
Patterns of hepatitis B virus/hepatitis C virus coinfection

	HCV Dominant	HBV Dominant	Codominant	Neither Replicative
Frequency (%)	47	14	18	21
Anti-HCV	Positive	Positive	Positive	Positive
HCV RNA	High	Low or undetectable	Moderate	Undetectable
HBsAg	Positive or negative	Positive	Positive	Negative
Anti–HB Core	Positive	Positive	Positive	Positive
Anti–HB Surface	Positive or negative	Negative	Negative	Positive or negative
HBV DNA	Low or undetectable	Positive	Moderate	Undetectable

The HCV-dominant group also includes those patients with occult HBV. These patients are positive for only anti–HB core and have no detectable HBsAg and HBV DNA. This finding may account for up to 20% of patients in the HCV-dominant group.

replication. HCV RNA levels in serum are high and HBV DNA is either low or undetectable. Serologic markers of HBV infection are typically positive, including HBsAg and anti–HB core.

There are several mechanisms that allow HCV to dominate HBV. Probably the most important is that HCV core protein directly suppresses HBV enhancer activity and downregulates HBV transcription.[28,29] In vitro cell culture studies have shown that the intracellular activity of HBV polymerase and production of HB core antigen are reduced when HCV is added to cell culture medium.[29] Gamma interferon and IP-10 (interferon gamma-inducible protein), known suppressors of HBV, have been shown to be increased in patients in whom HCV dominates HBV.[30] In humanized mouse models coinfected with HBV and HCV, HBV DNA synthesis increases when interferon production is inhibited, and following treatment of HCV with a direct-acting antiviral agent (DAA).[31] Suppression of HBV replication seems to be more pronounced with HCV genotype 1.[26,27] The suppressive effects of HCV following acute infection in patients who already have chronic HBV may be so profound that seroconversion of HBV occurs. In these patients, loss of hepatitis B e antigen (HBeAg) and HBsAg and appearance of antibodies to HBe protein and anti–HB surface have been observed.[32]

In some patients, HCV can shut down HBV replication to such a degree that HBsAg and HBV DNA are below the level of detection of standard assays or are not produced at all. These patients are referred to as having occult HBV infection, and this is estimated to occur in about 9% of patients with HBV-HCV coinfection or 20% of patients in the HCV-dominant group.[26,27,33] The presence of occult HBV explains why some patients with isolated anti–HB core may develop reactivation of HBV and a biochemical flare when HCV is eradicated during and following treatment with DAA therapy.[33] However, this seems to be a very uncommon event. In 1 large retrospective study, reactivation of occult HBV was observed to occur in less than 1% of patients with HCV treated with DAA therapy.[34] In another study of 40 patients with chronic HCV and occult HBV, HBV DNA was assessed before, during, and after DAA therapy.[35] In this study, 25% of patients had detectable HBV DNA before treatment with mean viral load of 42 IU/mL. Three months after treating HCV with DAA therapy, the percentage of patients with detectable HBV DNA increased to 57% but mean HBV DNA increased to only 85 IU/mL. Serum liver transaminase levels remained normal and HBsAg remained undetectable in all patients.

Hepatitis B Virus Dominant

This serologic pattern is the least common seen in patients with HBV-HCV coinfection and is observed in only 14% of patients.[26,28] These patients typically have active HBV, are HBeAg positive, and have high serum levels of HBV DNA and low levels or undetectable HCV RNA. This pattern is more likely seen in patients with chronic HCV who then develop acute HBV.[22,26] The high replication rate of HBV observed in these patients suppresses HCV replication, reduces the production of HCV core protein, and downregulates other host immunologic effects that typically lead to HCV dominance. The lower prevalence of the HBV-dominant pattern is likely caused by the lower prevalence of E antigen–positive HBV in the population where the host immune system is already tolerant of HBV and cannot achieve spontaneous seroconversion.

In some patients in whom HBV dominates, anti-HCV is positive but HCV RNA is undetectable. Although some studies have detected fragments of HCV RNA in the liver tissue of patients who are anti-HCV positive and HCV RNA is undetectable in serum, there is no good evidence to suggest that occult HCV that could reemerge and cause liver injury exists.[36] Instead, patients who are anti-HCV positive with undetectable HCV RNA have either been previously cured of HCV with antiviral therapy or have had spontaneous resolution of HCV. The latter is known to occur in 20% to 25% of persons following acute HCV infection.[37]

TREATMENT OF HEPATITIS B VIRUS AND HEPATITIS C VIRUS

The treatment of chronic HBV with either peginterferon (PEGINF) or a DAA is the focus of several articles in this issue. PEGINF administered once weekly for 48 weeks to patients with E antigen–positive chronic active HBV achieves seroconversion to inactive HBV in about 33% of patients. However, PEGINF seems to be most effective in patients with HBV genotype A where seroconversion exceeds 50%. Oral DAA therapy for HBV is highly effective and suppresses HBV DNA to undetectable levels in about 90% of patients regardless of E-antigen status. Up to 33% of patients with E antigen–positive active HBV seem to achieve seroconversion over 5 years.

Standard interferon and then PEGINF were the first therapies used for treatment of chronic HCV. Sustained virologic response (SVR) with PEGINF and ribavirin (RBV) is achieved in 33% to 50% of patients with genotype 1, 80% with genotype 2, and 70% for genotype 3.[38,39] The duration of therapy is 48 weeks but can be reduced to 24 weeks in patients with a rapid virologic response.[40] Long-term follow-up studies have shown that patients with HCV who achieved SVR have a recurrence rate of only 0.5% over 8 years of follow-up and it is unclear whether this low rate of recurrence reflects reinfection or true relapse.[41,42] Curing HCV leads to resolution of many of the extrahepatic effects of chronic HCV and improves quality of life.[43] PEGINF and RBV are no longer used for treatment of chronic HCV in most in the world because of the side effects of this regimen and the lower SVR rates compared with DAA therapy across all genotypes.

The first highly effective PEGINF-free regimens used to treat HCV emerged in 2013 with the availability of the polymerase inhibitor sofosbuvir.[44] Over the next several years, the combination of ledipasvir-sofosbuvir, sofosbuvir-velpatasvir, sofosbuvir-velpatasvir-voxilaprevir, and glecaprevir-pibrentasvir became available.[45–48] Each of these DAA combinations achieves an SVR in about 90% to 98% of patients, including those with cirrhosis, with few to no side effects in most patients. Because of this high rate of SVR with a limited duration of therapy, all patients with chronic HCV who are HCV RNA positive in serum should be treated.

In the past 6 years, since DAA combination therapy has become readily available, the burden of HCV in many countries throughout the world has significantly declined. The latest data suggest that chronic HCV is now present in less than 1% of the population in the United States and many European countries.[49] The World Health Organization has set a goal to eradicate all HCV globally by the year 2030.[50]

TREATMENT OF PATIENTS WITH HEPATITIS B VIRUS–HEPATITIS C VIRUS COINFECTION

Reactivation and/or flare of HBV in patients with HCV coinfection did not occur during the 15 years HCV was treated with PEGINF, because PEGINF suppresses replication of both HCV and HBV and, historically,[51] had been the primary treatment of each of these viral infections.[38,52] In addition, because achieving SVR was not common in patients with HCV treated with PEGINF, except in patients with HCV genotypes 2 or 3,[38,39] the pattern of HBV or HCV dominance was not likely altered and this blunted any reactivation and/or flare of HBV following PEGINF therapy.

The nucleoside analogues currently used for treatment of HBV have no effect on HCV, and the DAAs used for HCV have no effect on HBV. The current DAAs for HCV are highly effective. Treatment leads to rapid eradication of intracellular HCV, removes the suppressive effect of HCV on HBV, and allows unopposed replication of HBV, which can then precipitate HBV reactivation and/or flare. The initial report by the US Food and Drug Administration of this scenario described 28 patients who developed a flare in liver enzymes during or following HCV treatment and were subsequently found to have active HBV.[53] Three patients in this report developed acute liver failure during the flare; 2 of whom died and 1 received a liver transplant. Most of the patients in this report had incomplete serologic studies for HBV before initiating HCV treatment and the risk of flare could not be calculated. Since then, several reports describing risk factors for HBV reactivation and/or flare have appeared. The topic was recently reviewed in *Clinics in Liver Disease* and elsewhere.[54,55]

Recognizing patients at risk of developing HBV reactivation and/or flare mandates that all patients with HCV be tested for HBV before initiating treatment of HCV. The various serologic and virologic tests available to assess HBV are discussed in Philippe J. Zamor and Ashley M. Lane's article "Interpretation of HBV serologies," in this issue. Initial testing must include all common HBV serologies, including HBsAg, anti–HB core, and anti–HB surface. Patients who are HBsAg positive should then be tested for HBeAg, anti-HBe and HBV DNA as outlined in **Fig. 1**. Similarly, patients who have serologic evidence of current infection or previous exposure to HBV should be tested for anti-HCV.

The 3 major liver societies, American Association for the Study of Liver Disease (AASLD), European Association for the Study of the Liver (EASL), and Asian Pacific Association for the Study of the Liver (APASL) differ only slightly in their recommendations for treating patients with HBV-HCV coinfection.[56–58] The primary difference is how patients with inactive HBV are handled. This question is discussed here. **Table 2** summarizes the various serologic and virologic patterns of HBV that could be observed in patients with coinfection and defines the treatments that the authors think are optimal for each situation. These recommendations are based on the clinical guidelines of AASLD, EASL, and APASL, our review of the existing literature, and our institute's experience treating patients with coinfection where we have observed and managed several patients with flares in HBV.

Immune-Tolerant Hepatitis B Virus

None of the 3 society guidelines address how to approach this type of patient if the patient is coinfected with HCV.[56–58] These patients are HBsAg positive, HBeAg

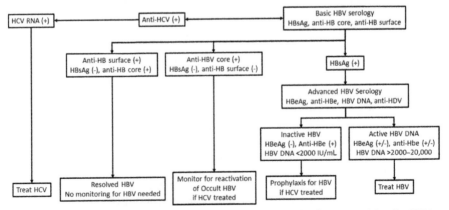

Fig. 1. Serologic testing to be performed in patients who initially test positive for HBV or HCV.

Table 2
Hepatitis B virus serology and treatment recommendations in patients with hepatitis B virus–hepatitis C virus coinfection during hepatitis C virus treatment

HBV Description	Immune Tolerant	Active E Antigen Positive	Active E Antigen Negative	Inactive	Isolated Anti–HB Core	Resolved
HBsAg	+	+	+	+	—	—
Anti–HB core	+	+	+	+	+	+
Anti–HB surface	—	—	—	—	—	+
HBeAg	+	+	—	—	—	—
Anti-HBe	—	—	+	+/−	+	+
HBV DNA (IU/mL)	>2 million	>20,000	>2000	< 2000	UD	UD
Treat for HBV during HCV treatment	Prophylaxis[a]	Yes[b]	Yes	Prophylaxis	Monitor[c]	No
Cirrhosis	Yes	Yes	Yes	Yes	No	No

Abbreviation: UD, undetectable.

[a] Prophylaxis for HBV requires that treatment of HBV with a nucleoside analogue be initiated simultaneously with HCV DAA treatment. HBV treatment can be stopped 6 months after treatment of HCV was completed. Patients should then be monitored periodically for evidence of reactivation and biochemical flare.

[b] "Yes" indicates that patients have indications for treatment of HBV regardless of HCV. Treatment of HBV should be initiated before or simultaneously with HCV treatment. HBV treatment should be continued long term after HCV treatment has stopped.

[c] "Monitor" indicates that patients with isolated anti–HB core should be monitored at periodic intervals during and after HCV treatment. Patients who develop reactivation of HBV by becoming HBsAg positive and develop increasing HBV DNA to greater than 2000 IU/mL should be started on antiviral therapy.

positive, have very high levels of HBV DNA, and typically are HBV dominant. Because these patients already have high levels of HBV DNA, the authors think they are at high risk for biochemical flare when HCV is eradicated with DAA therapy. These patients should therefore receive prophylaxis to prevent HBV flare with an oral DAA during HCV treatment and for 3 to 6 months after HCV DAA therapy has been completed. Once the HBV DAA is stopped, these patients should continue to be monitored at periodic intervals, every 3 to 6 months, to see whether they convert to active HBV and require additional treatment or return to the immune-tolerant state.

Active Hepatitis B Virus and E Antigen Positive

These patients are HBsAg positive, HBeAg positive, and have increased levels of HBV DNA greater than 20,000 IU/mL. They may have an HBV, HCV, or codominant pattern depending on the serum levels of HBV DNA and HCV RNA. These patients meet all criteria for HBV treatment regardless of the HCV infection. HBV treatment with an oral DAA should be initiated before or simultaneously with HCV treatment, and both HBV DNA and HCV RNA should be monitored. Once HCV treatment has been completed, HBV treatment should be continued long term until seroconversion to inactive HBV has occurred.

An alternative approach would be to treat HBV and HCV simultaneously with PEGINF and RBV. This approach would be particularly effective in a patient with HBV genotype A and HCV genotypes 2 or 3 coinfection where the chance for HBV seroconversion is greater than 50% and the likelihood of achieving an SVR for HCV would be about 80% and 70% respectively. Following the initiation of PEGINF and RBV, HCV RNA should be assessed at week 4 to determine whether a rapid virologic response was achieved and RBV can be stopped after 12 weeks or should be continued for 24 weeks.[40] Methods to assess HBV response to PEGINF are discussed elsewhere in this issue. In patients who are responding to treatment, PEGINF should be continued for up to 48 weeks.

Active E Antigen–Negative Hepatitis B Virus

These patients are HBsAg positive, HBeAg negative, anti-HBe positive or negative, and have increased HBV DNA levels greater than 2000 IU/mL. They may have an HBV, HCV, or codominant pattern depending on the serum levels of HBV DNA and HCV RNA. These patients meet all criteria for treatment of the HBV regardless of the HCV infection. HBV treatment with an oral DAA should be initiated before or simultaneously with HCV treatment and both HBV DNA and HCV RNA should be monitored. Once HCV treatment has been completed, HBV treatment should continue long term because seroconversion to inactive HBV cannot occur.

Inactive E Antigen–Negative Hepatitis B Virus

The 3 society guidelines differ in how to approach these patients if they are coinfected with HCV.[56–58] These patients are HBsAg positive, HBeAg negative, anti-HBe positive or negative, and have serum HBV DNA levels less than 2000 IU/mL. In some cases, HBV DNA is undetectable. These patients are HCV dominant. In the absence of HCV treatment, there is no indication for treating a patient with inactive HBV. However, these patients are at increased risk for biochemical and virologic flare when immune suppressed during cancer chemotherapy and when treated with high-dose immune suppression, especially monoclonal biologics that target the immune response.[59] All 3 societies recommend that these patients receive prophylaxis with an HBV DAA while they are receiving cancer chemotherapy or immune-modulating agents.[56–58] The authors think these patients are also at risk for flare and should be treated for HBV when HCV is treated with a DAA.[60] HBV and HCV treatment with nucleoside analogues and DAAs, respectively, should be started simultaneously and HBV treatment should be continued for 3 to 6 months after completing HCV treatment. Once HBV treatment is stopped, HBV DNA and serum liver transaminase levels should be monitored at periodic intervals for an additional 3 to 6 months to assess for HBV flare. If a flare in liver transaminases and HBV DNA does occur, the patient should be placed back on an HBV nucleoside analogue lifelong.

Occult Hepatitis B Virus

The 3 society guidelines agree on how to approach this type of patient if the patient is coinfected with HCV.[56–58] Patients with occult HBV have HCV dominance that is so strong, and replication of HBV that is so slow, that HBsAg and HBV DNA are less than the level of detection with standard assays or are not present at all. These patients are anti–HB core positive but negative for HBsAg and anti–HB surface and are serologically indistinguishable from patients who have long ago resolved HBV and in whom anti–HB surface has decreased to less than the level of detection with standard assays. However, it is not possible to determine which patients with this serologic pattern have occult HBV or resolved HBV. However, previous studies have shown that occult HBV is uncommon and reactivation of HBV in patients with isolated anti–HB core occurs only rarely.[60,61] It is therefore recommended that patients who are isolated anti–HB core positive be monitored more frequently when treated for HCV with a DAA but not treated with an HBV nucleoside analogue. These patients should be tested for HBsAg midway thought treatment; about 4 to 6 weeks after starting an HCV DAA; at the end of HCV treatment; and at 1, 3, and 6 months after HCV treatment has been completed. If HBsAg remains negative, no further monitoring is necessary. In contrast, if HBsAg becomes positive, HBV DNA should be measured and monitored at intervals of 1 to 3 months. If HBV DNA increases to the level where treatment is indicated, an HBV nucleoside analogue should be initiated or the patient should be treated with PEGINF, if appropriate. In contrast, if HBV DNA level remains low, the patient should continue to be monitored at intervals typically used for patients with inactive HBV.

Resolved Hepatitis B Virus

These patients are HBsAg negative, anti–HB core positive, and anti–HB surface positive. There is no indication for HBV treatment. HCV should be treated with a DAA and there is no need to monitor HBV during treatment. If liver transaminase levels do not normalize or flare either during or after HCV therapy, additional testing to evaluate for other causes of increased liver transaminases should be performed, including HBV serologies and HBV DNA. The risk of developing recurrence of HBV with flare in liver transaminases in a patient with resolved infection is extremely small.

Patients with Cirrhosis

Patients with HBsAg and cirrhosis are at increased risk for developing hepatocellular carcinoma and hepatic decompensation. It is recommended that these patients be placed on lifelong antiviral treatment of HBV regardless of serum HBV DNA level and even if HBV is inactive.[56–58] The same is true if there is coinfection with HCV. Patients with isolated anti–HB core do not require HBV treatment even if they have cirrhosis. However, a patient with occult HBV and cirrhosis who has reappearance of HBsAg during or following HCV treatment should be placed on an oral HBV nucleoside analogue long term.

SUMMARY

HBV and HCV coinfection is uncommon but not rare owing to both viruses sharing similar routes of transmission. All patients with chronic HCV must therefore be evaluated for chronic HBV or previous exposure before initiating HCV therapy with a DAA. Patients who are HBsAg positive are at increased risk of developing reactivation and/or flare of HBV and develop severe liver injury. All patients with HBsAg should therefore be treated for HBV when HCV is treated with a DAA. Patients with occult HBV should be monitored more frequently during HCV therapy with a DAA but do not require treatment of HBV unless they develop reactivation with recurrence of HBsAg and flare.

ACKNOWLEDGMENTS

The authors thank our team of advanced practice clinicians, Phil Alexander NP, Sarah Hubbard PA, Karla Pray NP, Ashley Foster NP, and April Ashworth NP, for their knowledge, compassion, and dedication in the management and treatment of our patients with chronic HBV.

DISCLOSURE

Dr N.E. Airewele receives research grant funding from Gilead. Dr M.L. Shiffman is a consultant and advisor to Gilead and AbbVie; receives honorarium as a speaker for Gilead and AbbVie; and receives research grant funding from Gilead.

REFERENCES

1. Te HS, Jensen DM. Epidemiology of hepatitis B and C viruses: a global overview. Clin Liver Dis 2010;14:1–21.
2. Lavanchy D. Hepatitis B virus epidemiology, disease burden, treatment, and current and emerging prevention and control measures. J Viral Hepat 2004;11: 97–107.
3. Kowdley KV, Wang CC, Welch S, et al. Prevalence of chronic hepatitis B among foreign-born persons living in the United States by country of origin. Hepatology 2012;56:422–33.
4. Lin CL, Kao JH. The clinical implications of hepatitis B virus genotype: recent advances. J Gastroenterol Hepatol 2011;26(Suppl 1):123–30.
5. Alter MJ. The epidemiology of acute and chronic hepatitis C. Clin Liver Dis 1997; 1:559–68.
6. Armstrong FL, Alter MJ, McQuillan GM, et al. The past incidence of hepatitis C virus infection: implications for the future burden of chronic liver disease in the United States. Hepatology 2000;31:777–82.
7. Frank C, Mohamed MK, Strickland GT, et al. The role of parenteral antischistosomal therapy in the spread of hepatitis C virus in Egypt. Lancet 2000;355:887–91.
8. Armstrong GL, Wasley A, Simard EP, et al. The prevalence of hepatitis C virus infection in the United States, 1999 through 2002. Ann Intern Med 2006;144: 705–14.
9. Shiffman ML. The next wave of hepatitis C virus: the epidemic of intravenous drug use. Liver Int 2018;38(Suppl 1):34–9.
10. Degenhardt L, Peacock A, Colledge S, et al. Global prevalence of injecting drug use and sociodemographic characteristics and prevalence of HIV, HBV, and HCV in people who inject drugs: a multistage systematic review. Lancet Glob Health 2017;5:e1192–207.
11. Doerrbecker J, Behrendt P, Mateu-Gelabert P, et al. Transmission of hepatitis C virus among people who inject drugs: viral stability and association with drug preparation equipment. J Infect Dis 2013;207:281–7.
12. Terrault NA, Dodge JL, Murphy EL, et al. Sexual transmission of hepatitis C virus among monogamous heterosexual couples: the HCV partners study. Hepatology 2013;57:881–9.
13. Shiffman ML. Management of acute hepatitis B. Clin Liver Dis 2010;14:75–91.
14. Basnayake SK, Easterbrook PJ. Wide variation in estimates of global prevalence and burden of chronic hepatitis B and C infection cited in publish literature. J Viral Hepat 2016;23:545–59.
15. Cheruvu S, Marks K, Talal AH. Understanding the pathogenesis and management of hepatitis B/HIV and hepatitis B/Hepatitis C virus coinfection. Clin Liver Dis 2007;11:917–43.
16. Tyson GI, Kramer JR, Duan Z, et al. Prevalence and predictors of hepatitis B coinfection in a United States cohort of hepatitis C infected patients. Hepatology 2013;58:538–45.
17. Bini EJ, Permalswami PV. Hepatitis B virus infection among America patients with chronic hepatitis C virus infection: prevalence, racial ethnic differences, and viral interaction. Hepatology 2013;51:759–66.
18. Liaw YF. Role of Hepatitis C virus in dual and triple hepatitis virus infection. Hepatology 1995;22:1101–8.

19. Zhang Q, Qi W, Wang X, et al. Epidemiology of hepatitis B and hepatitis C infections and benefits of programs for hepatitis prevention in Northeastern China: a cross-sectional study. Clin Infect Dis 2016;62:305–12.
20. Crockett SD, Keeffe EB. Natural history and treatment of hepatitis B and hepatitis C virus co-infection. Ann Clin Microbiol Antimicrob 2005;4:13.
21. Konstantinou D, Deutsch M. The spectrum of HBV/HCV coinfection: epidemiology, clinical characteristics, viral interactions and management. Ann Gastroenterol 2015;28:221–8.
22. Zampino R, Pisaturo MA, Cirillo G. Hepatocellular Carcinoma in chronic HBV-HCV co-infection is correlated to fibrosis and disease duration. Ann Hepatol 2015;14:75–82.
23. Crespo J, Lozano JL, de la Cruz F, et al. Prevalence and significance of hepatitis C viremia in chronic active hepatitis B. Am J Gastroenterol 1994;89:1147–51.
24. Shi J, Zhu L, Liu S, et al. A meta-analysis of case-control studies on the combined effect of hepatitis B and C virus infections in causing hepatocellular carcinoma in China. Br J Cancer 2005;92:607–12.
25. Pol S, Haour G, Fontaine H, et al. The negative impact of HBV/HCV coinfection on cirrhosis and its consequences. Aliment Pharmacol Ther 2017;46:1054–60.
26. Mavilia MG, Wu GY. HBV-HCV Coinfection: viral interactions, management and viral reactivation. J Clin Transl Hepatol 2018;6:296–3015.
27. Raimondo G, Brunetto MR, Pontisso P, et al. Longitudinal evaluation reveals a complex spectrum of virological profiles in hepatitis B virus/hepatitis C virus-coinfected patients. Hepatology 2006;43:100–7.
28. Chen SY, Kao CF, Chen CM, et al. Mechanisms for inhibition of hepatitis B virus gene expression and replication by hepatitis C virus core protein. J Biol Chem 2003;278:591–607.
29. Schuttler CG, Fiedler N. Suppression of hepatitis B virus enhancer 1 and 2 by hepatitis C virus core protein. J Hepatol 2002;37:855–62.
30. Wiegand SB, Jaroszewicz J, Potthoff A, et al. Dominance of hepatitis C virus (HCV) is associated with lower quantitative hepatitis B surface antigen and higher serum interferon g-induced protein 10 levels in HBV/HCV-coinfected patients. Clin Microbiol Infect 2015;21. 710.e1-9.
31. Eyre NS, Phillips RJ, Bowden S, et al. Hepatitis B virus and hepatitis C virus interaction in Huh-7 cells. J Hepatol 2009;51:446–57.
32. Sheen IS, Liaw YF, Chu CM, et al. Role of hepatitis C virus infection in spontaneous hepatitis B surface antigen clearance during chronic hepatitis B virus infection. J Infect Dis 1992;165:831–4.
33. Cardoso C, Alves AL, Augusto F, et al. Occult hepatitis B infection in Portuguese patients with chronic hepatitis C liver disease: prevalence and clinical significance. Eur J Gastroenterol Hepatol 2013;25:142–6.
34. Jaroszewicz J, Pawłowska M, Simon K, et al. Low risk of HBV reactivation in a large European cohort of HCV/HBV coinfected patients treated with DAA. Expert Rev Anti Infect Ther 2020;18:1045–54.
35. Musolino C, Cacciola I, Tripodi G, et al. Behaviour of occult HBV infection in HCV-infected patients under treatment with direct-acting antivirals. Antivir Ther 2019;24:187–92.
36. Haydon GH, Jarvis LM, Blair CS, et al. Clinical significance of intrahepatic hepatitis C virus levels in patients with chronic HCV infection. Gut 1998;42:570–5.
37. Westbrook RH, Dusheiko G. Natural history of hepatitis C. J Hepatol 2014;61:S58–68.

38. McHutchison JG, Lawitz EJ, Shiffman ML, et al. Peginterferon alfa-2b or alfa-2a with ribavirin for treatment of hepatitis C infection. N Engl J Med 2009;361: 580–93.

39. Shiffman ML, Suter F, Bacon BR, et al. Peginterferon alfa-2a and ribavirin for 16 or 24 weeks in HCV genotype 2 or 3. N Engl J Med 2007;357:124–34.

40. Fried MW, Hadziyannis SJ, Shiffman ML, et al. Rapid virological response is the most important predictor of sustained virological response across genotypes in patients with chronic hepatitis C virus infection. J Hepatol 2011;55:69–75.

41. Swain MG, Lai MY, Shiffman ML, et al. A sustained virologic response is durable in patients with chronic hepatitis C treated with peginterferon alfa-2a and ribavirin. Gastroenterology 2010;139:1593–601.

42. Manns MP, Pockros PJ, Norkrans G, et al. Long-term clearance of hepatitis C virus following interferon α-2b or peginterferon α-2b, alone or in combination with ribavirin. J Viral Hepat 2013;20:524–9.

43. Shiffman ML, Benhamou Y. Cure of HCV related liver disease. Liver Int 2015; 35(Suppl 1):71–7.

44. Shiffman ML, James AM, Long AG, et al. Treatment of chronic HCV with sofosbuvir and simeprevir in patients with cirrhosis and contraindications to interferon and/or ribavirin. Am J Gastroenterol 2015;110:1179–85.

45. Afdhal N, Zeuzem S, Kwo P, et al. Ledipasvir and sofosbuvir for untreated HCV genotype 1 infection. N Engl J Med 2014;370:1889–98.

46. Feld JJ, Jacobson IM, Hézode C, et al. Sofosbuvir and velpatasvir for HCV genotype 1, 2, 4, 5, and 6 infection. N Engl J Med 2015;373:2599–607.

47. Bourlière M, Gordon SC, Flamm SL, et al. Sofosbuvir, velpatasvir, and voxilaprevir for previously treated HCV infection. N Engl J Med 2017;376:2134–46.

48. Forns X, Lee SS, Valdes J, et al. Glecaprevir plus pibrentasvir for chronic hepatitis C virus genotype 1, 2, 4, 5, or 6 infection in adults with compensated cirrhosis (EXPEDITION-1): a single-arm, open-label, multicentre phase 3 trial. Lancet Infect Dis 2017;17:1062–8.

49. Polaris Observatory HCV Collaborators. Global prevalence and genotype and distribution of hepatitis C virus infection in 2015: a modeling study. Lancet Gastroenterol Hepatol 2017;2:161–76.

50. Pedrana A, Munari S, Stoové M, et al. The phases of hepatitis C elimination: achieving WHO elimination targets. Lancet Gastroenterol Hepatol 2021;6:6–8.

51. Samuel CE. Antiviral actions of interferons. Clin Microbiol Rev 2001;14:778–809.

52. Liaw YF, Jia JD, Chan HL, et al. Shorter durations and lower doses of peginterferon alfa-2a are associated with inferior hepatitis B e antigen seroconversion rates in hepatitis B virus genotypes B or C. Hepatology 2011;54:1591–9.

53. Bersoff-Matcha SJ, Cao K, Jason M, et al. Hepatitis B virus reactivation associated with direct-acting antiviral therapy for chronic hepatitis C virus: a review of cases reported to the U.S. food and drug administration adverse event reporting system. Ann Intern Med 2017;166:792–8.

54. Abdelaal R, Yanny B, El Kabany M. HBV/HCV coinfection in the era of HCV-DAAs. Clin Liver Dis 2019;23:463–72.

55. Shiffman ML, Gunn NT. Management and treatment of chronic HBV and HCV coinfection and the impact of antiviral therapy. Curr Hepatol Rep 2017;16:169–77.

56. Terrault N, Lok ASF, McMahon BJ, et al. Update on prevention, diagnosis and treatment of chronic hepatitis B: AASLD 2018 hepatitis B guidance. Hepatology 2018;67:1560–99.

57. EASL 2017 clinical practice guidelines on the management of hepatitis B virus infection. J Hepatol 2017;67:370–98.

58. Kanda T, Lau GKK, Wei L, et al. APASL HCV guidelines of virus-eradicated patients by DAA on how to monitor HCC occurrence and HBV reactivation. Hepatol Int 2019;13:649–61.

59. Shouval D, Shibolet O. Immunosuppression and HBV reactivation. Semin Liver Dis 2013;33:167–77.

60. Belperio PS, Shahoumian TA, Mole LA, et al. Evaluation of hepatitis B reactivation among 62,920 veterans treated with oral hepatitis C antivirals. Hepatology 2017; 66:27–36.

61. Tamori A, Abiru S, Enomoto H, et al. Low incidence of hepatitis B virus reactivation and subsequent hepatitis in patients with chronic hepatitis C receiving direct acting antiviral therapy. J Viral Hepat 2018;25:608–11.

New Treatments for Chronic Hepatitis B Virus/Hepatitis D Virus Infection

Lisa Sandmann, MD[a], Heiner Wedemeyer, MD[a,b],*

KEYWORDS

- Hepatitis delta • Antiviral treatment • Interferon • Bulevirtide • Nucleic acid polymers • Interferon lambda • siRNA

KEY POINTS

- HBV/HDV coinfection is associated with a faster progression of liver disease leading to liver cirrhosis and an increased risk for the development of hepatocellular carcinoma.
- Pegylated interferon-alpha or the recently approved entry inhibitor bulevirtide (if available) are recommended treatment options for patients with compensated liver disease.
- Novel antiviral compounds that interfere with the viral life cycle are currently tested in clinical and preclinical trials.

INTRODUCTION

Hepatitis D virus (HDV) infection causes the most severe form of chronic viral hepatitis.[1] HDV infection occurs only as a coinfection in patients who are hepatitis B surface antigen (HBsAg) positive. Recently, it has been suggested that HDV may also be transmitted with other envelopes than HBsAg. In vitro, envelopes derived from the vesicular stomatitis virus or the hepatitis C virus E1/E2 proteins allowed viral packaging, egress, and entry in cells expressing the relevant receptors.[2] However, so far there is no clinical evidence that other viruses may be responsible for frequent HDV transmissions in the absence of hepatitis B virus (HBV) infection. Because HDV is a defective virus that does not encode for own viral enzymes, viral replication depends on host proteins. The two HDV proteins, small and large hepatitis delta antigen (HDAg), fulfill important functions in regulating replication, viral assembly, and coating with HBV envelope proteins, which are essential for cell egress and reinfection of hepatocytes.[3]

[a] Department of Gastroenterology, Hepatology and Endocrinology, Hannover Medical School, Carl-Neuberg-Str. 1, Hannover 30625, Germany; [b] German Center for Infection Research (DZIF), Partner Side Hannover/Braunschweig
* Corresponding author. Department of Gastroenterology, Hepatology and Endocrinology, Hannover Medical School, Carl-Neuberg-Str. 1, Hannover 30625, Germany.
E-mail address: Wedemeyer.Heiner@mh-hannover.de

Clin Liver Dis 25 (2021) 831–839
https://doi.org/10.1016/j.cld.2021.06.011
1089-3261/21/© 2021 Elsevier Inc. All rights reserved.

EPIDEMIOLOGY AND NATURAL HISTORY OF HEPATITIS D VIRUS INFECTION

HDV infection shows a very heterogeneous pattern worldwide. At least 8 different HDV genotypes have been described.[4] These genotypes show distinct geographic distributions: although the HDV genotype 1 is the most frequent and dominant virus in Northern America, Europe, and Central Asia, HDV genotype 2 can be found particularly in Eastern Asia. The HDV genotype 3 is endemic in the Amazonas, and genotypes 5 to 8 have been mainly described in Africa. The HDV genotype 1 also shows genetic diversity in Europe, which allows classification into genotype 1 subtypes.[5] HDV genotype 1 subtypes may show distinct features in natural history as well as response to type 1 interferon therapy. The importance of HDV genotypes in general for both the risk of progression to liver cirrhosis and hepatocellular carcinoma as well as response to interferon-alpha–based antiviral therapies is becoming more and more evident. For example, HDV genotype 5 compared with genotype 1 has been shown to take a much milder course and has also been associated with higher response rates to interferon therapy.[6] In recent years, there has been some discussion about the overall frequency of HDV infection worldwide. Many studies show a significant selection bias as either referral center cohorts have been investigated for HDV infection or only patients with advanced liver disease have been included. In these populations, a much higher frequency of HDV infections has been observed. In contrast, population-based studies show a very low frequency of HDV infection. Recent meta-analyses suggested that between 10 and 20 million individuals may carry HDV.[7] Other systematic reviews suggested much higher frequencies of up to 70 million HDV carriers worldwide.[8–10] What is quite clear is that HDV infection is associated with a significantly increased risk for rapid disease progression.[7,11] Particular risk factors for more advanced disease progression have been suggested. These include HIV coinfection, male gender, and Eastern Mediterranean origin.[7,12,13] Simple clinical markers may classify the individual risk for disease progression. The baseline event-anticipation score includes markers of portal hypertension (platelet levels), liver synthesis function (albumin) as well as epidemiologic features such as age, gender, and region of origin. It is important to note that every HDV-infected patient may rapidly progress to liver cirrhosis; this has recently been highlighted by a large study from Sweden, which included approximately 80% of all HDV-infected patients in Sweden. Here, patients who had not yet developed liver cirrhosis displayed a rather mild course of disease with a follow-up of up to 18 years. On the other hand, patients with already developed liver cirrhosis showed a very aggressive course of disease with almost 50% of patients developing liver-related clinical complications within 5 years of additional follow-up.[12] This has also been confirmed by a large study of patients recruited in France.[14] Further studies to characterize the individual course of HDV infection are needed; this is in particular important because interferon-alpha has been thus far the only recommended treatment option. To understand which patients may benefit from novel antiviral therapies, a clear individual risk determination would be needed to select the optimal treatment regimen for each individual. In this context, another particular feature of HDV needs to be considered: in HDV infection features of autoimmune hepatitis can frequently be found in liver histology. The importance of autoimmune liver disease in HDV infection is that during interferon treatment the underlying autoimmune hepatitis may be unmasked and severe flares of hepatitis have been described during interferon-based therapies.[15]

In addition to an advanced risk to develop liver cirrhosis HDV has also been associated with a significantly increased risk to develop hepatocellular carcinoma.[16] This effect has been in particular observed in Asian cohorts and in more recent studies published after 2020.

VIROLOGY OF HEPATITIS B VIRUS/HEPATITIS D VIRUS COINFECTION AND SEROLOGIC AND VIROLOGIC TESTING FOR HEPATITIS D VIRUS

The HDV is a defective RNA virus with a genome only encoding the hepatitis D protein. Therefore, viral replication depends on host proteins, and the presence of the HBV envelope protein HBsAg is essential for the virion's egress from and entry into hepatocytes. After attachment to heparan sulfate proteoglycans and binding of the pre-S1 region of L-HBsAg to hNTCP (human sodium taurocholate co-transporting polypeptide), viral particles enter the cytoplasm via endocytosis, and the ribonucleoprotein (RNP) is released and translocates into the nucleus. In the nucleus, HDV replication is carried out by host RNA polymerases. The HDV open reading frame encodes 2 forms of hepatitis delta proteins, the small (S-) and large (L-) HDAg. These proteins fulfill important functions in regulating genome replication, RNP assembly, and its coating with HBsAg. They undergo excessive posttranslational modifications including farnesylation of the L-HDAg, which is essential for RNP's coating with HBsAg and virion assembly.[3] An overview of the viral replication cycle is depicted in **Fig. 1**.

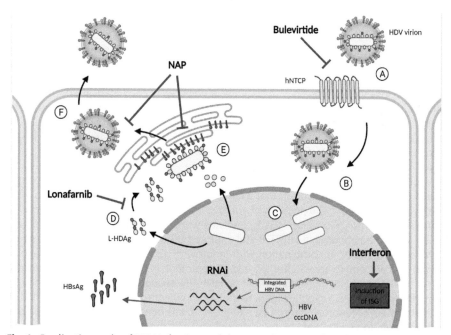

Fig. 1. Replication cycle of HDV infection and therapeutic approaches. (A) HDV virion's binding to hNTCP, the HBV/HDV specific receptor. The viral ribonucleoprotein (RNP) is released in the cytoplasm. (B) Translocation to the nucleus. (C) HDAg mRNA transcription and replication of HDV RNA. (D) Farnesylation of L-HDAg by a cellular farnesyltransferase. (E) Formation of the RNP and interaction with HBsAg at the endoplasmic reticulum to induce envelopment. (F) Secretion of HDV virions. cccDNA, covalently closed circular DNA; HBsAg, hepatitis B surface antigen; HDV, hepatitis D virus; hNTCP, human sodium taurocholate co-transporting polypeptide; ISG, interferon stimulated genes; L-HDAg, large hepatitis D antigen; NAP, nucleic acid polymers; RNAi, RNA interference compounds. The figure was created with BioRender.com.

Because of the progressive clinical course of HDV infection, national and international guidelines stress the importance of HDV testing in HBsAg positive patients.[17,18] The recommended screening test is anti-HDV, which, if positive, should be followed by testing of HDV RNA to identify active HDV infection. Importantly, HDV RNA levels can fluctuate over time and differences in the extraction method of the test may lead to variation in the assay's lower detection limit.[19] In addition, even if HDV is often the predominant virus in HBV/HDV coinfection, fluctuating viral activity of HBV can be seen during the natural course of the chronic coinfection. Nucleoside or nucleotide analogues (NAs) do not influence HDV replication and are therefore not recommended in patients with suppressed or low HBV DNA levels (<2000 IU/mL) except in patients with liver cirrhosis.[17] Theoretically, long-term suppression of HBV infection by NA treatment may lead to reduction of HBsAg, which should have beneficial effects on HDV infection.[18]

INTERFERON-BASED TREATMENT OF CHRONIC HEPATITIS D VIRUS INFECTION

Interferon has been used to treat HDV infection since the early 1980s after the discovery of HDV by Mario Rizzetto.[20] In early days, response to treatment was difficult to determine because HDV RNA polymerase chain reaction assays were not standardized and had a very low sensitivity. The first study investigating different doses of interferon-alpha showed significant response rates with undetectable HDV RNA in 1994.[21] However, when these patients were retested 10 years later, several patients initially classified as HDV RNA responders proved to show residual levels of HDV RNA. Still, patients with a relative reduction of HDV RNA in the absence of complete undetectable HDV RNA showed an improved clinical long-term outcome if treated with high doses of interferon.[22] Additional studies with pegylated interferon-alpha either alone or in combination with lamivudine or ribavirin have been published.[23,24] At that time the largest randomized controlled trial to treat HDV infection was the Hepatitis Delta International Intervention Trial (HIDIT-I).[15] In that trial, 48 weeks of treatment with pegylated interferon-alpha either alone or in combination with adefovir dipivoxil was compared with a monotherapy with adefovir dipivoxil. About 25% to 30% of patients were HDV RNA-undetectable at the end of treatment in both arms including pegylated interferon-alpha, whereas this was not achieved in patients with adefovir monotherapy. The addition of adefovir had no effect on virological responses regarding HDV RNA. However, HBsAg declines were more pronounced in the combination arm. The subsequent HIDIT II trial explored 96 weeks of pegylated interferon-alpha either alone or in combination with tenofovir.[25] Extending treatment durations did not prevent viral relapses after the end of treatment. In addition, the coadministration of tenofovir had no significant effect on HDV RNA suppression rates, even though numerically there was a slightly higher response in patients receiving tenofovir. Thus, a potential effect of tenofovir cannot be excluded. In this context it is interesting to note that tenofovir administration has been associated with induction of interferon-lambda in HBV-infected patients.[26,27] Still, most of the patients with HDV infection cannot be treated with interferon-alpha, as the compound is contraindicated in patients with decompensated cirrhosis. In particular, patients with platelet levels lower that 90,000 per μl should not be treated with pegylated interferon-alpha, as the risk for decompensation and severe complications is high. However, it is important to note that successful interferon treatment has been associated with improved clinical long-term outcomes. This has been shown already in cohorts from Italy,[28] France,[14] England,[6] Sweden,[12] Germany,[29] and Turkey.[30] It has to be noted that this improvement in clinical long-term outcomes did not require a complete suppression of HDV

RNA even though a negative HDV RNA status is clearly associated with improved long-term outcome.[31] Another important notion is that long-term follow-up of all HDV-infected patients is required. In contrast to hepatitis C virus infection postinterferon undetectability of the virus does not mean cure of the infection. Late relapses have already been observed in the 5-year follow-up of the HIDIT I trial.[32] But later relapses after even 7 or 8 years of initial responses were described in the 10-year follow-up of the HIDIT I trial.[31]

Another issue to be considered in the treatment of interferon is that low levels of on-treatment viremia have recently been associated with a high risk for posttreatment relapse.[33] Patients, who were negative at the end of the HIDIT I trial with a less sensitive in-house HDV RNA assay but positive in a recently introduced highly sensitive commercial assay (RoboGene), were at risk for posttreatment relapse of about 60% to 70%, whereas in contrast only 20% of patients who tested negative in both assays relapsed after the end of treatment. Thus, in any antiviral treatment of HDV infection sensitive assays should be used to detect residual viremia, which may give important information to personalize treatment duration.

NOVEL TREATMENTS AGAINST HEPATITIS D VIRUS INFECTION

The primary goal of treatment of HDV and HBV coinfection should be HBsAg clearance. With the clearance of HBsAg HDV RNA should also decline; this has been shown very nicely in the context of liver transplantation for HBV/HDV coinfection. Here the decline of HBsAg induced by administration of hepatitis B immunoglobulins during the first days after transplantation paralleled with HDV RNA declines. Therefore, all novel antiviral therapies aiming to induce HBsAg clearance should also be explored in HDV infection. Trials are already ongoing exploring small interfering RNAs targeting HBsAg in HDV infection (Clinical Trials.gov, NCT04535544). Until these approaches will be available, alternative treatments for HDV infection are urgently needed. Because interferon-alpha shows efficacy against HDV infection, it was straightforward to also explore the potential efficacy of interferon-lambda against HDV. Interferon-lambda shows antiviral efficacy both in vitro as well as in humanized mouse models against HDV.[34] Subsequently, interferon-lambda has also been explored in pivotal clinical trials that were presented during recent liver meetings.[35,36] In these trials, an antiviral effect has clearly been demonstrated. However, the safety of interferon-lambda in patients with advanced cirrhosis still needs to be determined. The potential advantage of interferon-lambda is that less systemic side effects would be expected. Further trials are ongoing.

Another antiviral approach would be the so-called prenylation inhibitor lonafarnib. Prenylation is a key step in the hepatitis D viral life cycle and is important for virus packaging. The role of prenylation for HDV has already been described more than 25 years ago by Jeffrey Glenn,[37] and the proof-of-concept in a mouse model has been determined in 2005.[38] Recently, lonafarnib has been explored at different doses in different cohorts of HDV infection.[39] The drug can be boosted with ritonavir, which allows lower doses and reduces side effects. Still, there is a significant gastrointestinal toxicity leading to substantial weight loss described in the first trials. Importantly, HDV RNA declines were observed in most of the patients. Some patients even showed a remarkable off-treatment control of HDV infection associated with improved liver histology and disappearance of advanced fibrosis. The drug is currently investigated in phase III studies. Here, monotherapy with lonafarnib is explored as well as combination with pegylated interferon-alpha 2a.

Nucleic acid polymers (NAP) were also explored in HDV infection. They have a variety of proposed mechanisms of action including blocking of secretion of viral particles as well as interfering with virion packaging. For chronic HDV infection, NAPs have been studied in 12 patients treated in Moldavia.[40] In this study, the patients received once weekly intravenous NAP injections for 15 weeks followed by 15 weeks of combination therapy for pegylated interferon-alpha and NAPs. Thereafter, treatment was completed with additional 33 weeks of pegylated interferon-alpha monotherapy, leading to a total interferon treatment duration of 48 weeks. During NAP monotherapy significant declines in HBsAg and HDV RNA were observed in most of the patients. After switching to interferon significant ALT flares were observed in several patients. When nucleic acid polymers were stopped, few patients experienced viral breakthrough during ongoing interferon treatment or developed postinterferon relapses. The long-term follow-up of this cohort has been recently published.[41] It became evident that those patients who cleared HBsAg also remained HDV RNA-negative, and even patients with severe hepatitis flares did not experience hepatic decompensations. Further trials are currently planned or already ongoing to explore the ideal formulation of these nucleic acid polymers. In addition, further developments of this class of compounds are currently also studied in clinical phase I trials for HBV monoinfection. S-antigen transport-inhibiting oligonucleotides polymers (STOPS), which interfere with intracellular HBsAg trafficking, have successfully been tested in preclinical animal models. Because of the subcutaneous application mode, STOPS represent interesting compounds targeting HBsAg, and a clinical phase I study is currently ongoing for HBV monoinfected patients.

The final approach that is explored in HDV infection includes the HBV/HDV entry inhibitor bulevirtide. The drug targets the bile acid transporter hNTCP. Thus, by mode of action, an increase in bile acids should be observed during treatment, which exactly has been observed in all clinical trials. In these trials, bulevirtide has been used as subcutaneous injection of 2 to 10 mg daily either alone or in combination with tenofovir or pegylated interferon-alpha. Treatment with bulevirtide induces a linear on-treatment decline of HDV RNA. However, it is currently unknown how many patients may achieve posttreatment virological control. In phase II trials the drug has been given for 24 to 48 weeks either alone or in combination with tenofovir or pegylated interferon-alpha. A >2 log HDV RNA decline was observed in 46% to 77% and 13% to 60% at 24 or 48 weeks of treatment, respectively. Of note, this antiviral response was associated with a marked improvement in liver enzymes as well as improvement in liver elastographies.[42–44] A phase III trial is currently exploring 2 mg versus 10 mg of treatment for 2 or 3 years. Recently, the compound has received conditional approval by the European Medical Agency and can be prescribed for patients with compensated liver disease in Europe.

The currently evolving landscape of antiviral treatments against HDV is promising. However, treatments for patients with decompensated cirrhosis are lacking. At this stage, liver transplantation remains the only treatment option for patients with decompensated HDV infection. Here, it is important to note that posttransplantation maintenance of anti-hepatitis B surface antibody levels is required, as HBV antigen may persist in the liver after transplantation for several years.[45]

CLINICS CARE POINTS

- HBV/HDV coinfection is the most severe form of chronic viral hepatitis and is associated with an accelerated course of liver disease.

- Every HBV positive patient should be tested for HDV coinfection.
- The primary goal of treatment of HBV/HDV coinfection should be HBsAg clearance.
- For patients with compensated liver disease antiviral treatment with pegylated interferon-alpha or the recently approved entry inhibitor bulevirtide is recommended (if available).
- Novel antiviral compounds that interfere with the viral life cycle are currently tested in clinical and preclinical trials (eg, interferon lambda, the prenylation inhibitor lonafarnib, nucleic acid polymers [NAP] or S-antigen transport-inhibiting oligonucleotide polymers [STOPS]).
- Antiviral treatment opitions for patients with decompensated liver disease are lacking and liver transplantation remains the only treatment option.

REFERENCES

1. Rizzetto M, Hamid S, Negro F. The changing context of hepatitis D. J Hepatol 2021. https://doi.org/10.1016/j.jhep.2021.01.014.
2. Perez-Vargas J, Amirache F, Boson B, et al. Enveloped viruses distinct from HBV induce dissemination of hepatitis D virus in vivo. Nat Commun 2019;10(1):2098.
3. Sureau C, Negro F. The hepatitis delta virus: replication and pathogenesis. J Hepatol 2016;64(1 Suppl):S102–16.
4. Le Gal F, Brichler S, Drugan T, et al. Genetic diversity and worldwide distribution of the deltavirus genus: a study of 2,152 clinical strains. Hepatology 2017;66(6):1826–41.
5. Karimzadeh H, Usman Z, Frishman D, et al. Genetic diversity of hepatitis D virus genotype-1 in Europe allows classification into subtypes. J Viral Hepat 2019; 26(7):900–10.
6. Spaan M, Carey I, Bruce M, et al. Hepatitis delta genotype 5 is associated with favourable disease outcome and better response to treatment compared to genotype 1. J Hepatol 2020;72(6):1097–104.
7. Stockdale AJ, Kreuels B, Henrion MYR, et al. The global prevalence of hepatitis D virus infection: systematic review and meta-analysis. J Hepatol 2020;73(3):523–32.
8. Wedemeyer H. The burden of hepatitis D - defogging the epidemiological horizon. J Hepatol 2020;73(3):493–5.
9. Chen H-Y, Shen D-T, Ji D-Z, et al. Prevalence and burden of hepatitis D virus infection in the global population: a systematic review and meta-analysis. Gut 2019;68(3):512–21.
10. Miao Z, Zhang S, Ou X, et al. Estimating the global prevalence, disease progression, and clinical outcome of hepatitis delta virus infection. J Infect Dis 2020; 221(10):1677–87.
11. Béguelin C, Moradpour D, Sahli R, et al. Hepatitis delta-associated mortality in HIV/HBV-coinfected patients. J Hepatol 2017;66(2):297–303.
12. Kamal H, Westman G, Falconer K, et al. Long-term study of hepatitis delta virus infection at secondary care centers: the impact of viremia on liver-related outcomes. Hepatology 2020. https://doi.org/10.1002/hep.31214.
13. Calle Serrano B, Großhennig A, Homs M, et al. Development and evaluation of a baseline-event-anticipation score for hepatitis delta. J Viral Hepat 2014;21(11): e154–63.
14. Roulot D, Brichler S, Layese R, et al. Origin, HDV genotype and persistent viremia determine outcome and treatment response in patients with chronic hepatitis delta. J Hepatol 2020;73(5):1046–62.

15. Wedemeyer H, Yurdaydìn C, Dalekos GN, et al. Peginterferon plus adefovir versus either drug alone for hepatitis delta. N Engl J Med 2011;364(4):322–31.
16. Alfaiate D, Clément S, Gomes D, et al. Chronic hepatitis D and hepatocellular carcinoma: a systematic review and meta-analysis of observational studies. J Hepatol 2020;73(3):533–9.
17. EASL 2017 Clinical Practice Guidelines on the management of hepatitis B virus infection. J Hepatol 2017;67(2):370–98.
18. Terrault NA, Lok ASF, McMahon BJ, et al. Update on prevention, diagnosis, and treatment of chronic hepatitis B: AASLD 2018 hepatitis B guidance. Hepatology 2018;67(4):1560–99.
19. Bremer B, Anastasiou OE, Ciesek S, et al. Automated nucleic acid isolation methods for HDV viral load quantification can lead to viral load underestimation. Antivir Ther 2019;24(2):117–23.
20. Rizzetto M, Bonino F, Crivelli O, et al. Complement fixing hepatitis B core antigen immune complexes in the liver of patients with HBs antigen positive chronic disease. Gut 1976;17(11):837–43.
21. Farci P, Mandas A, Coiana A, et al. Treatment of chronic hepatitis D with interferon alfa-2a. N Engl J Med 1994;330(2):88–94.
22. Farci P, Roskams T, Chessa L, et al. Long-term benefit of interferon alpha therapy of chronic hepatitis D: regression of advanced hepatic fibrosis. Gastroenterology 2004;126(7):1740–9.
23. Niro GA, Ciancio A, Gaeta GB, et al. Pegylated interferon alpha-2b as monotherapy or in combination with ribavirin in chronic hepatitis delta. Hepatology 2006; 44(3):713–20.
24. Wolters LM, van Nunen AB, Honkoop P, et al. Lamivudine-high dose interferon combination therapy for chronic hepatitis B patients co-infected with the hepatitis D virus. J Viral Hepat 2000;7(6):428–34.
25. Wedemeyer H, Yurdaydin C, Hardtke S, et al. Peginterferon alfa-2a plus tenofovir disoproxil fumarate for hepatitis D (HIDIT-II): a randomised, placebo controlled, phase 2 trial. Lancet Infect Dis 2019;19(3):275–86.
26. Murata K, Asano M, Matsumoto A, et al. Induction of IFN-λ3 as an additional effect of nucleotide, not nucleoside, analogues: a new potential target for HBV infection. Gut 2018;67(2):362–71.
27. Murata K, Tsukuda S, Suizu F, et al. Immunomodulatory mechanism of acyclic nucleoside phosphates in treatment of hepatitis B virus infection. Hepatology 2020;71(5):1533–45.
28. Romeo R, Del Ninno E, Rumi M, et al. A 28-year study of the course of hepatitis Delta infection: a risk factor for cirrhosis and hepatocellular carcinoma. Gastroenterology 2009;136(5):1629–38.
29. Wranke A, Serrano BC, Heidrich B, et al. Antiviral treatment and liver-related complications in hepatitis delta. Hepatology 2017;65(2):414–25.
30. Yurdaydin C, Keskin O, Kalkan Ç, et al. Interferon treatment duration in patients with chronic delta hepatitis and its effect on the natural course of the disease. J Infect Dis 2018;217(8):1184–92.
31. Wranke A, Hardtke S, Heidrich B, et al. Ten-year follow-up of a randomized controlled clinical trial in chronic hepatitis delta. J Viral Hepat 2020;27(12): 1359–68.
32. Heidrich B, Yurdaydın C, Kabaçam G, et al. Late HDV RNA relapse after peginterferon alpha-based therapy of chronic hepatitis delta. Hepatology 2014;60(1): 87–97.

33. Bremer B, Anastasiou OE, Hardtke S, et al. Residual low HDV viraemia is associated HDV RNA relapse after PEG-IFNa-based antiviral treatment of hepatitis delta: results from the HIDIT-II study. Liver Int 2021;41(2):295–9.

34. Giersch K, Homs M, Volz T, et al. Both interferon alpha and lambda can reduce all intrahepatic HDV infection markers in HBV/HDV infected humanized mice. Sci Rep 2017;7(1):3757.

35. Etzion O, Hamid SS, Lurie Y, et al. PS-052-End of study results from LIMT HDV study: 36% durable virologic response at 24 weeks post-treatment with pegylated interferon lambda monotherapy in patients with chronic hepatitis delta virus infection. J Hepatol 2019;70(1):e32.

36. Koh C, Da BL, Surana P, et al. A phase 2 study of lonafarnib, ritonavir and peginterferon lambda for 24 weeks: interim end-of-treatment results from the LIFT HDV study. AASLD 2020. Late breaking abstract L08.

37. Glenn JS, Watson JA, Havel CM, et al. Identification of a prenylation site in delta virus large antigen. Science 1992;256(5061):1331–3.

38. Bordier BB, Ohkanda J, Liu P, et al. In vivo antiviral efficacy of prenylation inhibitors against hepatitis delta virus. J Clin Invest 2003;112(3):407–14.

39. Yurdaydin C, Kalkan C, Karakaya F, et al. Subanalysis of the LOWR HDV-2 study reveals high response rates to Lonafarnib in patients with low viral loads. J Hepatol 2018;68:S89.

40. Bazinet M, Pântea V, Cebotarescu V, et al. Safety and efficacy of REP 2139 and pegylated interferon alfa-2a for treatment-naive patients with chronic hepatitis B virus and hepatitis D virus co-infection (REP 301 and REP 301-LTF): a nonrandomised, open-label, phase 2 trial. Lancet Gastroenterol Hepatol 2017; 2(12):877–89.

41. Bazinet M, Pântea V, Placinta G, et al. Safety and efficacy of 48 Weeks REP 2139 or REP 2165, tenofovir disoproxil, and pegylated interferon alfa-2a in patients with chronic HBV infection Naïve to Nucleos(t)ide therapy. Gastroenterology 2020; 158(8):2180–94.

42. Wedemeyer H, Bogomolov P, Blank A, et al. Final results of a multicenter, open-label phase 2b clinical trial to assess safety and efficacy of Myrcludex B in combination with Tenofovir in patients with chronic HBV/HDV co-infection. J Hepatol 2018;68:S3.

43. Wedemeyer H, Schöneweis K, Bogomolov PO, et al. GS-13-Final results of a multicenter, open-label phase 2 clinical trial (MYR203) to assess safety and efficacy of myrcludex B in cwith PEG-interferon Alpha 2a in patients with chronic HBV/HDV co-infection. J Hepatol 2019;70(1):e81.

44. Wedemeyer H, Schöneweis K, Bogomolov PO, et al. 48 weeks of high dose (10 mg) bulevirtide as monotherapy or with peginterferon alfa-2a in patients with chronic HBV/HDV co-infection. J Hepatol 2020;73:S52–3.

45. Mederacke I, Filmann N, Yurdaydin C, et al. Rapid early HDV RNA decline in the peripheral blood but prolonged intrahepatic hepatitis delta antigen persistence after liver transplantation. J Hepatol 2012;56(1):115–22.

Use of Hepatitis B Virus–Positive Organs in Organ Transplantation

Saro Khemichian, MD, Jeffrey Kahn, MD,
Norah A. Terrault, MD, MPH*

KEYWORDS

- Donor-transmitted hepatitis • Reactivation • Hepatitis B surface antigen
- Antibody to hepatitis B core • Hepatitis B immunoglobulin

KEY POINTS

- Use of HBV positive organs in transplantation has gained broader application due to availability of highly effective antivirals and use of hepatitis B immunoglobulin.
- Testing of organ donors is of utmost importance to mitigate the risk to the recipient with a recent change in guidelines recommending testing in living donors within 28 days of donation and in deceased donors within 96 hours.
- Risk of donor transmitted HBV can vary based on organs and donor and recipient serologies with the highest risk seen in hepatitis B surface antigen positive donors and HBV naïve liver transplant recipients.
- While there have been some data regarding stopping of antiviral prophylaxis for HBV after liver transplantation currently this is not recommended.
- HBV vaccination remains one of the key steps in minimizing risk of donor-transmitted HBV infection. All HBV naïve transplant candidates are recommended to undergo vaccination, with re-vaccination in those that the anti-HBs titers have waned.

HISTORICAL PERSPECTIVE

Transplantation of organs from hepatitis B virus (HBV)–exposed donors dates back to the 1980s.[1] The significant morbidity and mortality of people with end-stage renal, liver, heart, and lung diseases in need of transplantation provided justification for consideration of donor-transmitted HBV infection as a manageable risk. Over the decades, this practice has expanded, supported by positive outcomes, particularly with the availability of safe and effective therapies.

The need to consider the use of HBV-positive donors is particularly important in countries with a high prevalence of hepatitis B. For example, in a study of liver

Division of Gastrointestinal and Liver Diseases, Keck School of Medicine at University of Southern California, 1520 San Pablo Street, Suite 1000, Los Angeles, CA 90033, USA
* Corresponding author.
E-mail address: terrault@usc.edu

transplant (LT) recipients from Asia, 43% of donors had evidence of current or prior HBV infection.[2] In the United States, urban transplant centers reported rates of HBV infection (current/prior) as high as 15%.[3] HBV vaccination programs, introduced in the 1980s, have helped to decrease the prevalence of HBV infection among donors. A study from Spain supports this finding, with the prevalence of anti-hepatitis B core (HBc) being 27% in donors more than 60 years of age, but only 3.6% in those aged 1 to 20 years of age.[4] However, with many countries experiencing immigration from countries with high prevalence of HBV, the prevalence of HBV-positive donors might be expected to increase.[5]

Early studies highlighted differences in the risk of HBV transmission from donor to recipient by serologic status. Hepatitis B surface antigen (HBsAg)-positive donors are at a high risk of transmission, whereas anti-HBc–positive/HBsAg–negative donors are lower. The type of organ transplant influenced risk also, with LT recipients at the highest risk compared with other solid organ transplants. This finding is not surprising, given that HBV resides in the form of covalently closed circular DNA (cccDNA) within the nucleus of hepatocytes and persists even among persons who have cleared HBsAg and HBV DNA from the blood.

The availability of prophylactic therapies such as hepatitis B immunoglobulin (HBIG) as well as safe and highly effective antivirals for HBV has allowed a broader application of HBV positive organs in transplantation. Hepatitis B immune globulin became an established component of prophylaxis in LT recipients with chronic hepatitis B in the early 1990s and its use extended to other solid organs as prophylaxis against infection from HBV-positive donors. Lamivudine, the first nucleoside analogue for HBV, was approved in the mid-1990s and paved the way to use of monotherapy and combination prophylaxis approaches. These days, entecavir and tenofovir (disoproxil or alafenamide) are the preferred drugs for preventing HBV infection in the context of organ transplantation, owing their higher barrier to viral resistance than first-generation drugs, such as lamivudine.

HEPATITIS B TESTING OF ORGAN DONORS

The likelihood of encountering HBsAg-positive or anti-HBc–positive/HBsAg–negative donors is related to the regional HBV epidemiology. In 2010, there were an estimated 248 million HBsAg-positive individuals worldwide and approximately 2 billion people with past or current infection,[6,7] with the highest overall seroprevalence of current infection being in the World Health Organization African region (8.9%) and the lowest, in the region of the Americas (0.81%)[6]; prevalence in the United States is 0.27%.[6] Rates of HBV exposure, as measured by the presence of anti-HBc, are higher. In the 2011 to 2016 National Health and Nutrition Examination Survey of the US population, 4.7% were HBV exposed, with higher rates in non-Hispanic Blacks (11%), Asians (23%) and Hispanics (6%) compared with non-Hispanic Whites (2.4%) and higher among foreign-born (12.3%) versus US-born persons (3.0%).[8] Another National Health and Nutrition Examination Survey from 2001 to 2016 found anti-HBc positivity among persons who inject drugs was 19.7% compared with 4.6% in the general population,[9] a proportion likely to be impacted by the ongoing opioid epidemic.

Testing donors for HBV status is crucial in mitigating risk to the recipient and guiding measures to prevent HBV transmission and reactivation if the HBV-positive organ is transplanted. After exposure, HBV infection is generally detectable by serology (HBsAg/anti-HBc) at 38 to 50 days after exposure with HBV DNA detected early, typically 20 to 26 days.[10] The early period of infection before the detection of HBV DNA in blood is the eclipse period, with HBV still potentially transmissible, particularly to LT recipients.

The Public Health Services guidelines, published in 2013, require that all solid organ donors be tested for the presence of HBsAg, anti-HBc, and HBV DNA (by nucleic acid testing [NAT]), and these tests should occur within 96 hours of organ procurement. For living donation, testing should be as close to the transplant as possible, but within 28 days. The Organ Procurement and Transplant Network policies had not been fully aligned with Public Health Services guidelines regarding testing for HBV exposure until this year. The Organ Procurement and Transplant Network previously required that a donor considered at risk for HBV transmission be based on potential exposure within 12 months of organ donation, but recent data show that the risk of undetected HBV infection is less than 1/1,000,000 after 35 days, prompting a policy change to 1 month.[11] Previously, the required donor testing had been HBsAg and anti-HBc, but not HBV NAT, unless the donor met Public Health Services guidelines for being at increased risk. However, as of March 1, 2021, living donors should be tested within 28 days of organ donation, and deceased donors, within 96 hours, for HBV DNA by NAT in addition to serologic tests for HBsAg and anti-HBc.[12] A study of 9643 deceased donors who were HBV seronegative revealed that only 1 donor (0.02%) was NAT positive for HBV and that 7.8% of HBV seropositive donors were negative by NAT,[13] providing reassurance that an HBV NAT-negative donor is at very low risk for disease transmission, especially for no-liver organ transplant recipients.

Anti-HBc testing of blood donors began in the 1980s, initially as a surrogate for what was later identified as hepatitis C, because of similarities in the risk profiles of infected individuals. The presence of anti-HBc in the absence of HBsAg generally represents a convalescent state of HBV infection, but donors are at risk for disease transmission. HBV NAT testing may help to determine HBV transmission risk, especially for non-LT recipients. HBV replication is low in these donors,[14,15] resulting in undetectable or low levels of HBV DNA in the serum, yet with virus residing in the liver in the form of cccDNA or integrated virus, with the ability for reactivate in the face of immunosuppression.[16] Studies of anti-HBc–positive/HBsAg–negative organ and tissue donors report rates of HBV DNA positivity of 1.25% to 13.00%.[17–19] Evaluating donors for the presence anti-HBs increases the likelihood that the anti-HBc result is a true positive, especially in a donor who was unlikely to have been vaccinated. Identifying a true-positive versus false-positive anti-HBc has potentially important implications, because organs with no risk of HBV transmission may be discarded, and, conversely, long-term antivirals after transplantation may be used unnecessarily.[20]

NATURAL HISTORY AND OUTCOMES WITH USE OF ANTI–HEPATITIS B CORE ANTIGEN–POSITIVE, HEPATITIS B SURFACE ANTIGEN–NEGATIVE DONORS

The risks for LT recipients of anti-HBc positive donors differs from that of non-liver solid organ transplant recipients (**Table 1**). The post-transplant manifestations of transmitted infection range from asymptomatic seroconversion, mild hepatitis (alanine aminotransferase elevation accompanying the HBV DNA detection), to more severe forms of hepatitis, including fibrosing cholestatic HBV and acute liver failure.

Liver Transplant Recipients

Case series from the mid-1980s to the early 1990s highlighted the dismal outcomes of HBsAg-negative recipients who received livers from anti-HBc–positive/HBsAg–negative donors without prophylaxis, with 25% to 94% of HBsAg-negative recipients of livers from anti-HBc–positive donors developing HBsAg.[21–24] The significant risk

Table 1
Level of risk of donor-transmitted infection in the absence of HBV prophylaxis

Donor Serology	Solid Organ Recipient Type	Recipient Serology	Risk
HBsAg+	Liver	Any	High
	Nonliver	HBV naive	Moderate to high?
		Anti-HBs positive	Low
Anti-HBc positive, HBsAg negative	Liver	HBV naive	High
		Anti-HBc positive only	Intermediate
		Anti-HBs positive	Low
	Non-Liver	HBV naive	Low
		Anti-HBc positive only	Low
		Anti-HBs positive	Very low

identified in these early studies provides strong rationale for prophylaxis in all LT recipients of HBV-positive donors.

Prophylaxis protocols using either HBIG, antivirals such as lamivudine, or a combination of HBIG plus antiviral therapy have been used with the goal of decreasing donor-transmitted HBV. In a systematic review of 39 studies with 903 recipients of anti-HBc–positive donors, among recipients who were HBsAg-negative and received no prophylaxis, HBsAg developed in 48% who were anti-HBc–/anti-HBs–negative and 15% in those anti-HBc–/anti-HBs–positive, with prophylaxis decreasing these rates to 12% and 3%, respectively, and lamivudine superior to HBIG alone and the same as HBIG and lamivudine combined.[25] The authors' proposed algorithm was for no prophylaxis for anti-HBc–/HBs–positive recipients and lamivudine for all others.[25] Another systematic review published in 2009 found the risk of HBsAg development to be 2.7% versus 3.6% with lamivudine alone versus lamivudine plus HBIG after a follow-up period of 15 to 39 months, favoring lamivudine alone for prophylaxis. Another systematic review, in 2011, of 26 studies, highlighted the importance of recipient anti-HBs status. Although the overall rate of HBV infection in naïve recipients without prophylaxis was 58% versus 11% in those with prophylaxis (lamivudine with or without HBIG), there was no difference and the overall rate of HBV was low in recipients who were anti-HBc–positive/anti-HBs–positive (4% and 3%, respectively, with or without prophylaxis).[26] In contrast, HBV infection occurred in 18% of anti-HBc–negative/anti-HBs–positive recipients without prophylaxis versus 2% with prophylaxis, 14% of anti-HBc–positive/anti-HBs–negative without prophylaxis versus 3% with prophylaxis and 4% of anti-HBc–positive/anti-HBs–positive without prophylaxis and 3% with prophylaxis. Their conclusion was that there is a significant benefit of prophylaxis in HBV-naïve patients and in those anti-HBc–negative/anti-HBs–positive, but that anti-HBc–positive/anti-HBs–positive recipients could be managed with close monitoring, or a short course of antiviral therapy after LT.[26]

With newer antiviral agents, there seem to be a small incremental improvement in decreasing the risk of donor-transmitted hepatitis,[27,28] likely by preventing virologic breakthrough owing to viral resistance. A study from Korea of 66 pediatric LT from anti-HBc–positive donors from 1994 to 2013 showed that 33% of children without lamivudine prophylaxis developed donor-transmitted hepatitis, comparted with 10.8% who did.[29] Although 4 recipients developed lamivudine resistance, there were no graft failures, because alternative antivirals were given. Guidelines recommend using entecavir or tenofovir (disoproxil fumarate or alafenamide) with the choice of prophylaxis guided by cost, renal function, and/or bone health.[30] A study from Hong Kong including patients transplanted from 2000 to 2015 included 416 transplants from anti-HBc–positive donors, including 108 HBsAg-negative recipients and 308 HBsAg-positive recipients. Of the HBsAg-negative recipients, 2.8% developed HBsAg, all among patients receiving lamivudine as opposed to entecavir.[2]

There are sparse data on the role of donor liver biopsies[31,32] and there is insufficient experience with use of novel biomarkers, such as cccDNA measurement, to inform prophylaxis protocols.[33] The primary role of the biopsy would seem to exclude fibrosis.

Kidney–Pancreas, Heart, and Lung Transplantation

One of the first studies of outcomes of anti-HBc–positive donors in kidney recipients was from the University of California at San Francisco; only 1 of 42 kidney recipients (2%) developed HBsAg and none of the recipients developed anti-HBc[1] with no prophylaxis given. A United Network for Organ Sharing (UNOS) database analysis from 1994 to 1999 in 903 kidney transplant recipients who received a kidney from donors who were anti-HBc–positive/HBsAg–negative compared with anti-HBc–negative reported a difference in the development of anti-HBc in the recipient 2.2% versus 1.1%, but not HBsAg 0.65% versus 0.26% and no difference in patient or graft survival.[34] There were no data on prior vaccination/anti-HBs status or oral antiviral use. A quantitative review of 9 studies with 1385 kidney recipients from anti-HBc–positive donors revealed a rate of HBsAg development of 0.28% and anti-HBc and/or anti-HBs development in 3%, with no case of symptomatic hepatitis, adverse effects, or graft or patient survival. The development of anti-HBc did not adversely affect outcomes.[35] Finally, a UNOS database study of 199 pediatric kidney transplant recipients from anti-HBc–positive/HBsAg–negative donors into mostly (80%) HBV naive recipients, with a median follow-up of 7.9 years, showed comparable outcomes compared with those received transplants from HBV-naïve donors.[36]

Similar excellent outcomes have been reported with heart and lung recipients of anti-HBc–positive/HBsAg–negative donors, although the numbers are smaller. In a study of 29 anti-HBc–negative lung recipients given anti-HBc–positive/HBsAg–negative donors, none developed HBsAg or anti-HBc; however, the immune status of the recipients was not reported.[37,38] A study of 17 lung anti-HBc–negative lung recipients who were transplanted with organs from anti-HBc–positive/HBsAg–negative donors, found none developed HBsAg, but 4 of 17 lung transplant recipients (24%) developed anti-HBc, with a recipient anti-HBs titer of greater than 100 IU/L possibly decreasing this risk.[38] A single-center retrospective study from Duke University of 18 heart transplant recipients from anti-HBc–positive donors (75% also anti-HBs–positive) into recipients who were anti-HBc–negative/HBsAg–negative and treated with a median of 6 doses of HBIG and most received lamivudine for up to 12 months, all remained HBsAg negative with undetectable HBV DNA.[39] Another study of 21 anti-HBc–positive donors to HBsAg-negative heart and lung recipients, including 11 heart and 1 heart/lung, and 3 lung transplants, found that no recipients became HBsAg-positive.[22] A UNOS database study of 333 recipients of lungs and hearts from anti-HBc–positive donors revealed no difference in 1- or 5-year post-transplant survival rates.[40]

Regarding prophylaxis, most studies have not used prophylaxis. However, 1 study used a single perioperative dose of 2000 IU of HBIG in 18 of 54 patients receiving kidney transplants from anti-HBc–positive donors. Among 42 recipients who were anti-

HBc–negative before kidney transplantation, none developed HBsAg; 5 recipients (11.9%) who did not receive HBIG developed anti-HBc, compared with none who received prophylaxis. The authors conclusions were that a single dose of HBIG protects against the development of anti-HBc.[41]

RECOMMENDATIONS FOR USE OF ANTI-HEPATITIS B CORE ANTIGEN–POSITIVE, HEPATITIS B SURFACE ANTIGEN–NEGATIVE ORGANS
General

All potential solid organ transplant recipients who do not have therapeutic titers of anti-HBs either through natural immunity or vaccination should be vaccinated. Although an ant-HBs titer of greater than 10 mIU/mL is protective in nontransplant settings, there are some data to suggest that an anti-HBsAb titer of 100 mIU/mL or greater may be better in the context of protection from donor-transmitted HBV.[38,42]

Liver Transplant Recipients

Available data support the long-term safety of adult and pediatric deceased and living donor LT from these donors into recipients who are HBsAg-positive, HBsAg-negative/anti-HBc–positive and –negative for all markers, provided that appropriate prophylaxis is provided (**Fig. 1**). Biopsy of the donor liver does not seem to be standard practice, but should be considered if there are concerns regarding fibrosis, because spontaneous HBsAg loss can occur after decades of chronic HBV infection and absence of HBsAg does not preclude significant fibrosis.

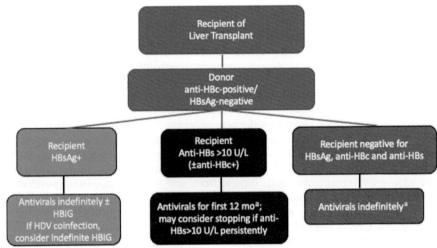

Fig. 1. Prophylaxis for HBsAg-negative nonliver solid organ transplant recipients receiving livers from anti-HBc–positive donors. Prophylaxis recommendations vary by serologic status of the recipient. For recipients who are HBsAg positive, antivirals are indicated for the management of preexisting chronic HBV. For those who are HBV naïve, antivirals should be started at the time of solid organ transplant and continued for at least the first 6 to 12 months and then if anti-HBs titers of greater than 10 U/L are maintained, consideration can be made to stop antivirals. Vaccination with the goal of achieving protective anti-HBs titers should be undertaken after solid organ transplant. For recipients with evidence of protective anti-HBs titers at the time of solid organ transplant, no antiviral therapy is needed. Monitoring of HBsAg and HBV DNA every 3 months for the first year is recommended. [a]Preferred antiviral agents are those with high potency and a high barrier to resistance (entecavir, tenofovir alafenamide, and tenofovir disoproxil).

Liver recipients who are HBsAg positive are treated with institution-specific HBIG protocols and indefinite oral antivirals and nonliver solid organ transplant recipients are treated indefinitely with oral antivirals,[43,44] regardless of the anti-HBc status of the donor, so it is natural to target these donors to recipients with HBV. There are differences between society guidelines for HBV prophylaxis in recipients of livers from anti-HBc–positive/HBsAg–negative donors (**Table 2**). Although some studies show a relatively low risk of HBsAg development in some recipient populations such as anti-HBc–positive/anti-HBs–positive recipients, given the high efficacy and excellent tolerability of highly potent antivirals with a high barrier to resistance (entecavir, tenofovir disoproxil, and tenofovir alafenamide), and the significant risk of morbidity if a patient develops HBsAg, we recommend indefinite antiviral prophylaxis. The administration of HBIG to these recipients does not seem to alter outcomes and is not recommended.

Kidney–Pancreas and Thoracic Organ Recipients

The risk of HBV transmission from anti-HBc–positive donors to HBsAg-negative nonliver recipients is very low, at less than 1%, especially in recipients who have adequate anti-HBs titers (**Fig. 2**). It is prudent to vaccinate potential recipients early to achieve protective anti-HBs titers. As mentioned, there are data that anti-HBs titers of more than 100 U/L at the time of transplant seem to be optimal to decrease recipient risk, providing a "cushion" owing to waning titers during the enhanced immunosuppression

Table 2
Summary of guidelines on anti–HBc-positive organs in solid organ transplantation

Organ Recipient	Donor anti–HBc-Positive/ HBsAg-Negative: If Recipient Status Is:	AST Prophylaxis Guidelines	American Association for the Study of Liver Diseases Prophylaxis Guidelines
Liver	HBsAg positive	Manage using existing guidelines for HBsAg-positive recipient	Manage using existing guidelines for HBsAg-positive recipient
Liver	HBsAg negative **AND** anti-HBc positive/anti-HBs negative OR anti-HBc negative/anti-HBs negative	Indefinite antiviral prophylaxis	Indefinite antiviral prophylaxis
Liver	Anti-HBc positive/anti-HBs positive	Antiviral prophylaxis not recommended	Indefinite antiviral prophylaxis
Nonliver	Anti-HBc positive/anti-HBsAb positive	Antiviral prophylaxis not recommended	Prophylaxis recommended (6–12 mo)
Nonliver	Anti-HBc negative/anti-HBs negative	Consider antiviral prophylaxis up to 1 year	Prophylaxis recommended (6–12 mo)
Nonliver	Anti-HBc positive/anti-HBs negative	Consider antiviral prophylaxis up to 1 year	Prophylaxis recommended (6–12 mo)

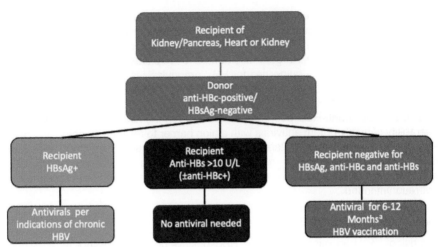

Fig. 2. Prophylaxis for HBsAg-negative LT recipients receiving livers from HBc-positive donors. Prophylaxis recommendations vary by serologic status of the recipient. For recipients who are HBsAg positive, prophylaxis would be antiviral plus HBIG (per institutional approach to HBsAg-positive recipients). For those who are HBV naïve, antivirals should be started at time of LT and continued indefinitely. For those recipients with anti-HBs (naturally or via vaccination), antivirals should be provided for at least the first 6 to 12 months and then if anti-HBs titers of greater than 10 U/L are maintained, consideration can be made to stop antivirals. Monitoring of HBsAg and HBV DNA every 3 months for the first year is recommended. For those with anti-HBs, vaccination with the goal of achieving protective anti-HBs titers should be undertaken after LT. [a]Preferred antiviral agents are those with high potency and a high barrier to resistance (entecavir, tenofovir alafenamide, and tenofovir disoproxil).

early after transplant. Recipient development of anti-HBc has implications if there is a need for enhanced immunosuppression for T-cell–mediated rejection, antibody-mediated rejection or treatment for post-transplant lymphoproliferative disorders, including the use of high-dose corticosteroids, thymoglobulin, and rituximab, and chemotherapy for post-transplant malignancies, all of which may increase the risk of HBsAg development and a flare of hepatitis from HBV.[45]

Although there are differences in society guidelines for HBV prophylaxis in this recipient population (see **Table 2**), the data support that for recipients with anti-HBs titers of greater than 10 IU/mL at the time of transplant, no additional prophylaxis is necessary. One study suggested a benefit in providing a single perioperative dose of HBIG protects against the development of anti-HBc.[41] Alternatively, treating with either entecavir, tenofovir disoproxil, or tenofovir alafenamide for the first 6 to 12 months is recommended, during initial months of immunosuppression. We also recommending monitoring for HBsAg and HBV DNA every 3 months for the first year, testing for the development of anti-HBc and anti-HBs at 1 year and offering vaccination if HBV serologic markers are negative.

NATURAL HISTORY AND OUTCOMES WITH THE USE OF HEPATITIS B SURFACE ANTIGEN–POSITIVE DONORS

The use of HBsAg-positive organs may be particularly relevant in countries with a high prevalence of chronic HBV. These organs are used very infrequently in the United States.[46] With appropriate recipient management, the use of HBsAg-positive donors may be feasible. In general, these donors should be targeted to recipients with chronic hepatitis B or patients in whom the potential risk of acquired HBV are warranted by an urgent need of transplantation. Certainly, appropriate informed consent explaining all the risks with such organs should be obtained from all recipients.

Liver Transplant Recipients

Data are limited. In an early series from Italy, 3 HBsAg-positive recipients transplanted with HBsAg-positive donors all became HBsAg-positive after LT despite receipt of HBV antivirals and high-dose HBIG prophylaxis.[47] Two patients had hepatitis delta virus (HDV) co-infection before LT and both became coinfected with HDV with progressive liver disease, with 1 patient requiring repeat transplantation within 1 year. The recipient without HDV had an uneventful post-transplant course despite HBsAg positivity. In a subsequent similar case report where the recipient was noted to be HBV/HDV co-infected, after LT, treatment with peginterferon failed and ultimately the patient was retransplanted.[48] In addition, other case series mainly from Asia have reported LT with use of HBsAg-positive donors into HBsAg-positive recipients. Although all the recipients remained HBsAg positive, recipient survival was not affected with a follow-up of more than 1 year.[49–51] A large multicentric retrospective study of 282 patients (96% HBsAg-positive) with HBsAg-positive donors and a matched control group of 259 with HBsAg-negative donors showed no difference in postoperative liver dysfunction, early stage or long-term complications, or survival, although HBV recurrence was higher in patients with HBsAg-positive donors.[52] A UNOS analysis from 2016 reported 92 recipients, of whom 24 had HBV-unrelated disease who had HBsAg-positive donors.[53] Allograft and patient survival was comparable between the 2 groups.[53]

Kidney Transplant Recipients

Reports of successful use of HBsAg-positive deceased and living donors into hepatitis B immune kidney transplant recipients has been reported.[14,54–56] Prophylaxis was provided with antivirals, HBIG, and, in some cases, vaccination. Development of HBsAg positivity among the 80 recipients reported in these 3 studies was 1.25%.[54–56] Use of HBsAg-positive organs in HBsAg-positive recipients have also been reported, and, as expected, chronic infection persisted after kidney transplantation and with antiviral therapy yielded excellent graft and patient survival.[57] A more recent retrospective, large, single-center study from China compared HBsAg-negative patients who underwent living donor kidney transplantation from HBsAg-positive donors versus anti-HBc–positive donors.[58] Sixty-three of the HBsAg-positive donor recipients had either natural (prior HBV infection) or vaccine-induced anti-HBs; none became HBsAg positive, but 7 became anti-HBc–positive without any clinical sequelae. In contrast, among 20 recipients of HBsAg-positive donors who were anti-HBs/anti-HBc–negative recipients, 2 (10%) became HBsAg-positive and 1 died of acute liver failure; 5 other patients became anti-HBc positive. The use of HBIG and antiviral therapy was variable in this cohort but even with HBIG and lamivudine prophylaxis, recipients without pretransplant anti-HBs became infected.

Other Solid Organ Recipients

The use of HBsAg-positive organs in heart and lung recipients is very rare. In a single center retrospective review of 412 heart transplant recipients and donors from Taiwan, only 3 patients who were HBsAg negative before transplant received

HBsAg-positive organs.[59] All patients were treated with HBIG prophylaxis perioperatively and 2 had no evidence of HBV infection after transplantation; 1 patient developed HBsAg positivity and was initiated on antiviral therapy with lamivudine.[59] Lung transplant experience with use of HBsAg-positive donors is limited to a single case report.[60] The HBsAg-positive donor had low level of HBV DNA and the recipient had no immunity. The recipient received HBIG immediately before and after transplantation for 7 days and entecavir. HBV serologies 12 months after transplantation demonstrated positive anti-HBc and anti-HBs at a low titer with undetectable HBV DNA.[60] These limited data suggest that effective pretransplant immunization against HBV or combination HBIG plus antivirals can decrease HBV transmission.

RECOMMENDATIONS FOR USE OF HEPATITIS B SURFACE ANTIGEN–POSITIVE ORGANS
General

The American Society of Transplantation states that organs from HBsAg-positive donors may be considered after an individualized risk and benefit assessment (**Fig. 3**).[46] Carefully selected patients may be candidates to receive HBsAg-positive organs. All potential solid organ transplant recipients should be evaluated for the presence of anti-HBs either through immunity or vaccination. If titers are not detected, then the recipient should be vaccinated; titers of more than 100 mIU have been shown to be protective.[42] Appropriate consent should be obtained from all recipients.

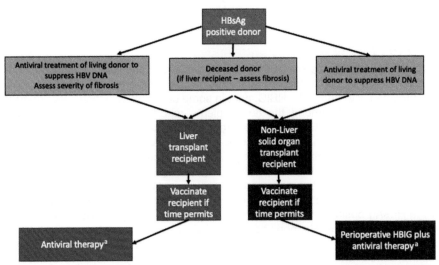

Fig. 3. Prophylaxis for recipients of HBsAg-positive donor. For living donors, antiviral therapy should be used to suppress HBV DNA before donation. For liver recipients, the liver needs to be assessed for level of fibrosis, typically by liver biopsy or elastography. Recipients with hepatitis delta virus (HDV) infection should not receive HBsAg-positive donors. After transplantation, liver recipients require lifelong antiviral therapy; HBIG has no role. For non-liver recipients, perioperative HBIG plus antiviral therapy initially, with assessment of HBV markers at 3 months after transplantation – if the recipient anti-HBs positive with a titer of greater than 10 IU/mL (ideally >100 IU/mL) antiviral therapy can be stopped. If the recipient has seroconverted to HBsAg or anti-HBc positive, long-term antiviral therapy is recommended. [a]Preferred antiviral agent with high potency and a high barrier to resistance (entecavir, tenofovir alafenamide, and tenofovir disoproxil).

Liver Transplant Recipients

The British Transplantation Society guidelines were published in 2018 and are more comprehensive.[61] These indicate that use of HBsAg-positive liver grafts is acceptable in both HBV immune and nonimmune recipients. A histologic evaluation of donor liver should be performed to confirm an absence of significant fibrosis. In addition, the British Transplantation Society recommends that, if the donor HDV status is known and is positive, these organs should be avoided. The presence of HDV in the recipient should also preclude receiving surface antigen–positive organs. The use of high-potency oral antivirals from the time of transplantation will prevent HBV-related graft damage and should be continued indefinitely. The use of HBIG is not recommended in the setting of recipient HBsAg-positivity (ie, recipient with chronic HBV infection) because it does not result in the loss of HBsAg.[61]

Kidney–Pancreas and Thoracic Organ Recipients

The optimal prophylaxis in recipients that are HBsAg negative with a HBsAg positive donor has not been established. Certainly, the use of HBIG perioperatively and high-potency antivirals such as tenofovir would offer the maximum protection. Previous studies have mainly assessed recipients with an anti-HBs levels of greater than 10 IU/L and these patients have shown very low rates of transmission of HBV.[55,56,62–64] Waning anti-HBs titers over time and with immunosuppression may a play role in development of low rates of transmission in these recipients. The risk of de novo HBV infection is low; however, nonimmune recipients should be initiated on antiviral therapy.

Hepatocellular Carcinoma Surveillance in Recipients of Hepatitis B Surface Antigen–Positive Donors

Chronic hepatitis B is a risk factor for hepatocellular carcinoma. Major society guidelines such as American Association for the Study of Liver Diseases[30] and European Association for the Study of the Liver[65] indicate that patients who are HBsAg positive with cirrhosis should undergo screening with an ultrasound examination with and without alfa fetoprotein every 6 months. Whether HCC screening for post-transplant recipients who have become HBsAg positive without advanced fibrosis require screening is unclear. No cases of de novo HCC from donor-acquired HBV infection have been reported. Chronic immunosuppression may theoretically heighten this risk, although the duration of chronic HBV infection and underlying severity of fibrosis are likely the most important risk factors.

CAN ANTIVIRAL PROPHYLAXIS FOR HEPATITIS B VIRUS AFTER LIVER TRANSPLANTATION EVER BE STOPPED?

Livers from donors who are anti-HBc positive, regardless of HBsAg or HBV DNA status, may still harbor residual HBV in the liver as cccDNA and, thus, are at risk for HBV reactivation post-LT. Provision of indefinite antiviral therapy is the surest means of preventing reactivation and HBV-associated hepatitis. However, the pretransplant HBV status of the LT recipient influences the recommendations on HBV prophylaxis. For recipients with preexisting HBV who receive a liver from an HBsAg-negative but anti-HBc–positive donor, HBIG may be considered along with antiviral as a means of preventing reappearance of HBsAg, a factor that is, important, for example, in patients with HDV coinfection (see **Fig. 1**). For recipients of anti-HBc positive donors without preexisting chronic HBV infection and evidence of HBV immunity (anti-HBs positive), the risk of reactivation and hepatitis is decrease, but not completely eradicated.[26] Although a prior consensus guideline indicated that no antiviral prophylaxis be considered in recipients with natural HBV immunity (ie, anti-HBs and anti-HBc) receiving an anti-HBc–positive organ, the strength of this recommendation was weak.[46] The anti-HBs titer that is protective against reactivation in the post-LT setting is not established, but the cut-off used for immunocompetent persons of greater than 10 U/L is insufficient. Additionally, anti-HBs titer can wan over time and under effects of intensive immunosuppression and consequently lead to increased risk of HBV reactivation. For all these reasons, discontinuation of antiviral prophylaxis is not favored. However, if cost or adherence limit the use of antiviral prophylaxis, discontinued in positive LT recipients with anti-HBs titer of greater than 1000 U/L has been suggested with regular monitoring of anti-HBs titers and boosting if needed.[66]

A related but interesting consideration in terms of stopping antiviral prophylaxis is among LT recipients with pretransplant HBV. In this scenario, effective prophylaxis may be able to prevent reinfection of the new liver and these patients potentially be eligible for prophylaxis withdrawal after LT. In a provocative study from Italy of 30 LT recipients with pretransplant chronic HBV (40% who received an anti-HBc–positive donor organ) who were treated for more than 5 years with prophylactic therapy (HBIG plus antivirals) and shown to have undetectable HBV DNA and cccDNA in liver were sequentially withdrawn from HBIG and antivirals. Remarkably, 80% remained without evidence of HBV recurrence and 90% off any HBV therapy with at least 6 years of follow-up and, interestingly, 60% had developed anti-HBs (median titer, 143 U/L).[67] Another study from China reported on the long-term outcomes of 10 patient stopping HBIG and lamivudine owing to nonadherence 13 to 42 months after LT and 9 of the 10 remained without evidence of HBV infection.[68] Donor HBV status was not reported in this latter study. These data challenge our approach to prophylaxis and suggest that a subset of LT patients may be eligible for complete prophylaxis withdrawal. Although interesting, prophylaxis withdrawal in patients with pre-LT HBV infecting treated with HBIG plus antivirals is not currently recommended. Further studies are needed, with novel viral diagnostics potentially of benefit in better characterizing those at risk for recurrence after prophylaxis withdrawal.

VACCINATION IN TRANSPLANT CANDIDATES AND RECIPIENTS

In the prevention of donor-transmitted HBV infection, the recipients anti-HBs status is key to risk mitigation. All transplant candidates should be vaccinated and those who do not respond or who have waning titers after transplantation should undergo repeat vaccination after transplantation. HBV vaccination as early as possible in the disease process requiring a transplant, is a very important measure in mitigating adverse outcomes related to HBV after transplantation.

Although vaccination of healthy infants, adults, and children is successful in more than 90% of cases,[69] patients with chronic diseases requiring transplantation do not fare as well. The results of a systematic review of 11 studies with 961 patients revealed HBV vaccine efficacy in patients with liver cirrhosis to be 16% to 87% (median, 47%) and this did not improve with a higher vaccine dose.[69] A study of 57 patients with advanced liver disease awaiting LT receiving 3 standard doses of the vaccine only showed 16% adequate antibody response[70–72] and several other studies support an efficacy of 20% to 30%.[73] After LT, the response rate to vaccination is also poor. A study of 176 LT recipients revealed success in only 40% with a rapid decline in titers,[74] which may be clinically relevant. Patients on hemodialysis with end-stage renal disease show a 50% to 60% seroprotection rate and anti-HBs titers drop over time. Newer vaccines, such as Hepislav-B, which combines HBsAg with a Toll-like receptor 9 agonist has shown promise in the population with chronic kidney disease, with an increase in anti-HBs titers of more than 100 IU/mL 74% compared with standard vaccine.[75] HBV vaccination in patients with advanced heart failure seems to be approximately 50% effective, and most successful in those who are most stable, because the response correlates with ejection fraction and functional status.[76] Prophylaxis measures would need to be adjusted based on vaccination success rates.

CLINICS CARE POINTS

- Very low risk of HBV transmission using donor with HBV markers if recipient is anti-HBs positive non-liver transplant recipient.

- Risk of transmission with anti-HBc only positive donors is highest in HBV naïve liver recipients and lowest in anti-HBs positive non-liver recipients.

- Selected use of HBsAg+ organs in anti-HBs positive or negative recipients for liver transplantation is being reported, but experience is limited.

- HCC screening is recommended in all HBsAg positive recipients.

- Vaccination against HBV, in appropriate recipients, is an important step in prevention of donor-transmitted HBV infection.

DISCLOSURE

Khemichian: None. Kahn: None; Terrault: Institutional grant support from GSK, Roche-Genentech, Gilead Sciences.

REFERENCES

1. Wachs ME, Amend WJ, Ascher NL, et al. The risk of transmission of hepatitis B from HBsAg(-), HBcAb(+), HBIgM(-) organ donors. Transplant 1995;59(2):230–4.
2. Wong TC, Fung JY, Cui TY, et al. Liver transplantation using hepatitis B core positive grafts with antiviral monotherapy prophylaxis. J Hepatol 2019;70(6):1114–22.
3. Manzarbeitia C, Reich DJ, Ortiz JA, et al. Safe use of livers from donors with positive hepatitis B core antibody. Liver Transpl 2002;8(6):556–61.
4. Prieto M, Gómez MD, Berenguer M, et al. De novo hepatitis B after liver transplantation from hepatitis B core antibody-positive donors in an area with high prevalence of anti-HBc positivity in the donor population. Liver Transpl 2001;7(1):51–8.
5. Valerio L, Barro S, Pérez B, et al. [Seroprevalence of chronic viral hepatitis markers in 791 recent immigrants in Catalonia, Spain. Screening and vaccination against hepatitis B recommendations]. Rev Clin Esp 2008;208(9):426–31.
6. Schweitzer A, Horn J, Mikolajczyk RT, et al. Estimations of worldwide prevalence of chronic hepatitis B virus infection: a systematic review of data published between 1965 and 2013. Lancet 2015;386(10003):1546–55.
7. Siyahian A, Malik SU, Mushtaq A, et al. Prophylaxis for hepatitis B virus reactivation after allogeneic stem cell transplantation in the era of drug resistance and newer antivirals: a systematic review and meta-analysis. Biol Blood Marrow Transpl 2018;24(7):1483–9.
8. Le MH, Yeo YH, Cheung R, et al. Chronic hepatitis B prevalence among foreign-born and U.S.-Born adults in the United States, 1999-2016. Hepatology 2020; 71(2):431–43.

9. Shing JZ, Ly KN, Xing J, et al. Prevalence of hepatitis B virus infection among US adults aged 20-59 Years with a history of injection drug use: national health and nutrition examination survey, 2001-2016. Clin Infect Dis 2020;70(12):2619–27.

10. Wolfe CR, Ison MG, Practice AIDCo. Donor-derived infections: guidelines from the American society of transplantation infectious diseases community of practice. Clin Transpl 2019;33(9):e13547.

11. Jones JM, Gurbaxani BM, Asher A, et al. Quantifying the risk of undetected HIV, hepatitis B virus, or hepatitis C virus infection in Public Health Service increased risk donors. Am J Transpl 2019;19(9):2583–93.

12. Align OPTN policy with U.S. Public health service guideline. Available at: https://optn.transplant.hrsa.gov/media/4225/bp_202012_align_2020_phs_guideline.pdf. Accessed January 26, 2021.

13. Theodoropoulos N, Nowicki MJ, Chinchilla-Reyes C, et al. Deceased organ donor screening for human immunodeficiency virus, hepatitis B virus and hepatitis C virus: discordant serology and nucleic acid testing results. Transpl Infect Dis 2018; 20(1):1–8.

14. Pilmore HL, Gane EJ. Hepatitis B-positive donors in renal transplantation: increasing the deceased donor pool. Transplantation 2012;94(3):205–10.

15. Rehermann B, Ferrari C, Pasquinelli C, et al. The hepatitis B virus persists for decades after patients' recovery from acute viral hepatitis despite active maintenance of a cytotoxic T-lymphocyte response. Nat Med 1996;2(10):1104–8.

16. Pattullo V. Prevention of Hepatitis B reactivation in the setting of immunosuppression. Clin Mol Hepatol 2016;22(2):219–37.

17. Sánchez Ibáñez J, Vilarrodona Serrat A, Seoane Pillado T, et al. Evaluation of occult hepatitis B infection in tissue donors: a multicenter analysis in Spain. Cell Tissue Bank 2019;20(4):513–26.

18. Domen RE, Yen-Lieberman B, Nelson KA, et al. Use of an HBV-DNA hybridization assay in the evaluation of equivocal hepatitis B virus tests in solid organ donors. Prog Transpl 2000;10(1):42–6.

19. Turner DP, Zuckerman M, Alexander GJ, et al. Risk of inappropriate exclusion of organ donors by introduction of hepatitis B core antibody testing. Transplantation 1997;63(5):775–7.

20. Muñoz SJ. Use of hepatitis B core antibody-positive donors for liver transplantation. Liver Transpl 2002;8(10 Suppl 1):S82–7.

21. Dickson RC, Everhart JE, Lake JR, et al. Transmission of hepatitis B by transplantation of livers from donors positive for antibody to hepatitis B core antigen. The national institute of diabetes and digestive and kidney diseases liver transplantation database. Gastroenterology 1997;113(5):1668–74.

22. Proceedings of the 2nd international congress of the society for organ sharing. Vancouver, British Columbia, July 5-7, 1993. Transpl Proc 1993;25(6):2983–3348.

23. Douglas DD, Rakela J, Wright TL, et al. The clinical course of transplantation-associated de novo hepatitis B infection in the liver transplant recipient. Liver Transpl Surg 1997;3(2):105–11.

24. Uemoto S, Sugiyama K, Marusawa H, et al. Transmission of hepatitis B virus from hepatitis B core antibody-positive donors in living related liver transplants. Transplantation 1998;65(4):494–9.

25. Cholongitas E, Papatheodoridis GV, Burroughs AK. Liver grafts from anti-hepatitis B core positive donors: a systematic review. J Hepatol 2010;52(2):272–9.

26. Skagen CL, Jou JH, Said A. Risk of de novo hepatitis in liver recipients from hepatitis-B core antibody-positive grafts - a systematic analysis. Clin Transpl 2011;25(3):E243–9.

27. Chang MS, Olsen SK, Pichardo EM, et al. Prevention of de novo hepatitis B in recipients of core antibody-positive livers with lamivudine and other nucleos(t)ides: a 12-year experience. Transplantatio 2013;95(7):960–5.

28. Wright AJ, Fishman JA, Chung RT. Lamivudine compared with newer antivirals for prophylaxis of hepatitis B core antibody positive livers: a cost-effectiveness analysis. Am J Transpl 2014;14(3):629–34.

29. Lee YJ, Oh SH, Kim KM, et al. De novo hepatitis B virus infection after pediatric liver transplantations with hepatitis B core antibody-positive donors: a single-center 20-yr experience. Pediatr Transpl 2015;19(3):267–72.

30. Terrault NA, Lok ASF, McMahon BJ, et al. Update on prevention, diagnosis, and treatment of chronic hepatitis B: AASLD 2018 hepatitis B guidance. Hepatology 2018;67(4):1560–99.

31. Holt D, Thomas R, Van Thiel D, et al. Use of hepatitis B core antibody-positive donors in orthotopic liver transplantation. Arch Surg 2002;137(5):572–5 [discussion 575-6].

32. Suehiro T, Shimada M, Kishikawa K, et al. Prevention of hepatitis B virus infection from hepatitis B core antibody-positive donor graft using hepatitis B immune globulin and lamivudine in living donor liver transplantation. Liver Int 2005; 25(6):1169–74.

33. Niu Y, Chen X, Feng L, et al. Anti-HBc-positive/HBsAg-negative liver donors pose a higher risk of occult HBV infection but do not cause severe histological damage in liver grafts. Clin Res Hepatol Gastroenterol 2014;38(4):475–80.

34. Fong TL, Bunnapradist S, Jordan SC, et al. Impact of hepatitis B core antibody status on outcomes of cadaveric renal transplantation: analysis of United network of organ sharing database between 1994 and 1999. Transplantation 2002; 73(1):85–9.

35. Mahboobi N, Tabatabaei SV, Blum HE, et al. Renal grafts from anti-hepatitis B core-positive donors: a quantitative review of the literature. Transpl Infect Dis 2012;14(5):445–51.

36. Ruebner RL, Moatz T, Amaral S, et al. Outcomes among children who received a kidney transplant in the United States from a hepatitis B core antibody-positive donor, 1995-2010. J Pediatr Infect Dis Soc 2016;5(4):439–45.

37. Hartwig MG, Patel V, Palmer SM, et al. Hepatitis B core antibody positive donors as a safe and effective therapeutic option to increase available organs for lung transplantation. Transplantation 2005;80(3):320–5.

38. Fytili P, Ciesek S, Manns MP, et al. Anti-HBc seroconversion after transplantation of anti-HBc positive nonliver organs to anti-HBc negative recipients. Transplantation 2006;81(5):808–9.

39. Horan JL, Stout JE, Alexander BD. Hepatitis B core antibody-positive donors in cardiac transplantation: a single-center experience. Transpl Infect Dis 2014; 16(5):859–63.

40. Dhillon GS, Levitt J, Mallidi H, et al. Impact of hepatitis B core antibody positive donors in lung and heart-lung transplantation: an analysis of the United Network for Organ Sharing Database. Transplantation 2009;88(6):842–6.

41. Veroux M, Corona D, Ekser B, et al. Kidney transplantation from hepatitis B virus core antibody-positive donors: prophylaxis with hepatitis B immunoglobulin. Transpl Proc 2011;43(4):967–70.

42. Khiangte B, Kothakota SR, Sasidharan M, et al. Hepatitis B reactivation in liver transplant recipients with hepatitis B virus core antibody positive grafts: a retrospective study. J Clin Exp Hepatol 2020;10(6):548–54.

43. Ahn HJ, Kim MS, Kim YS, et al. Clinical outcome of renal transplantation in patients with positive pre-transplant hepatitis B surface antigen. J Med Virol 2007; 79(11):1655–63.

44. Ko WJ, Chou NK, Hsu RB, et al. Hepatitis B virus infection in heart transplant recipients in a hepatitis B endemic area. J Heart Lung Transpl 2001;20(8):865–75.

45. Smalls DJ, Kiger RE, Norris LB, et al. Hepatitis B virus reactivation: risk factors and current management strategies. Pharmacotherapy 2019;39(12):1190–203.

46. Huprikar S, Danziger-Isakov L, Ahn J, et al. Solid organ transplantation from hepatitis B virus-positive donors: consensus guidelines for recipient management. Am J Transpl 2015;15(5):1162–72.

47. Franchello A, Ghisetti V, Marzano A, et al. Transplantation of hepatitis B surface antigen-positive livers into hepatitis B virus-positive recipients and the role of hepatitis delta coinfection. Liver Transpl 2005;11(8):922–8.

48. Bahde R, Hölzen JP, Wolters HH, et al. Course of a HBsAg positive liver transplantation in a hepatitis B and D virus coinfected recipient. Ann Hepatol 2011; 10(3):355–60.

49. Jiao Z, Zhang Y, Han L, et al. Four-year follow-up of two chronic hepatitis B recipients of hepatitis B surface antigen-positive cadaveric liver grafts from asymptomatic carriers. Hepatol Res 2011;41(9):846–52.

50. Jiang L, Yan L, Li B, et al. Successful use of hepatitis B surface antigen-positive liver grafts in recipients with hepatitis B virus-related liver diseases. Liver Transpl 2011;17(10):1236–8.

51. Choi Y, Choi JY, Yi NJ, et al. Liver transplantation for HBsAg-positive recipients using grafts from HBsAg-positive deceased donors. Transpl Int 2013;26(12): 1173–83.

52. Wei L, Chen D, Zhang B, et al. Long-term outcome and recurrence of hepatitis B virus following liver transplantation from hepatitis B surface antigen-positive donors in a Chinese population. J Viral Hepat 2018;25(12):1576–81.

53. Saidi RF, Jabbour N, Shah SA, et al. Liver transplantation from hepatitis B surface antigen-positive donors. Transpl Proc 2013;45(1):279–80.

54. Singh G, Hsia-Lin A, Skiest D, et al. Successful kidney transplantation from a hepatitis B surface antigen-positive donor to an antigen-negative recipient using a novel vaccination regimen. Am J Kidney Dis 2013;61(4):608–11.

55. Sumethkul V, Ingsathit A, Jirasiritham S. Ten-year follow-up of kidney transplantation from hepatitis B surface antigen-positive donors. Transpl Proc 2009;41(1): 213–5.

56. Jiang H, Wu J, Zhang X, et al. Kidney transplantation from hepatitis B surface antigen positive donors into hepatitis B surface antibody positive recipients: a prospective nonrandomized controlled study from a single center. Am J Transpl 2009;9(8):1853–8.

57. Veroux P, Veroux M, Sparacino V, et al. Kidney transplantation from donors with viral B and C hepatitis. Transpl Proc 2006;38(4):996–8.

58. Wang XD, Liu JP, Song TR, et al. Kidney transplantation from HBsAg+ living donors to HBsAg- recipients: clinical outcomes at a high-volume center in China. Clin Infect Dis 2021;72(6):1016–23.

59. Chen YC, Chuang MK, Chou NK, et al. Twenty-four year single-center experience of hepatitis B virus infection in heart transplantation. Transpl Proc. 2012;44(4): 910–2.

60. Belga S, Kabbani D, Doucette K. Hepatitis B surface antigen-positive donor to negative recipient lung transplantation. Am J Transpl 2020;20(8):2287–8.

61. Andrews P. Hepatitis B and solid organ transplantation. Available at: https://bts.org.uk/wp-content/uploads/2018/03/BTS_HepB_Guidelines_FINAL_09.03.18.pdf. Accessed January 26, 2021.
62. Asuman Yavuz H, Tekin S, Yuksel Y, et al. Donors with hepatitis B surface antigen positivity. Transpl Proc 2015;47(5):1312–4.
63. Tuncer M, Tekin S, Yucetin L, et al. Hepatitis B surface antigen positivity is not a contraindication for living kidney donation. Transpl Proc 2012;44(6):1628–9.
64. Yilmaz VT, Ulger BV, Aliosmanoglu İ, et al. Assessment of long-term outcomes in Hbs Ag-negative renal transplant recipients transplanted from Hbs Ag-positive donors. Ann Transpl 2015;20:390–6.
65. easloffice@easloffice.eu EAftSotLEa, Liver EAftSot. EASL 2017 Clinical Practice Guidelines on the management of hepatitis B virus infection. J Hepatol 2017;67(2):370–98.
66. Lin CC, Yong CC, Chen CL. Active vaccination to prevent de novo hepatitis B virus infection in liver transplantation. World J Gastroenterol 2015;21(39):11112–7.
67. Lenci I, Baiocchi L, Tariciotti L, et al. Complete hepatitis B virus prophylaxis withdrawal in hepatitis B surface antigen-positive liver transplant recipients after long-term minimal immunosuppression. Liver Transpl 2016;22(9):1205–13.
68. Geng L, Lin BY, Shen T, et al. Anti-virus prophylaxis withdrawal may be feasible in liver transplant recipients whose serum HBeAg and HBV DNA are negative. Hepatobiliary Pancreat Dis Int 2016;15(3):316–8.
69. Aggeletopoulou I, Davoulou P, Konstantakis C, et al. Response to hepatitis B vaccination in patients with liver cirrhosis. Rev Med Virol 2017;27(6):1–8.
70. Arslan M, Wiesner RH, Sievers C, et al. Double-dose accelerated hepatitis B vaccine in patients with end-stage liver disease. Liver Transpl 2001;7(4):314–20.
71. Chalasani N, Smallwood G, Halcomb J, et al. Is vaccination against hepatitis B infection indicated in patients waiting for or after orthotopic liver transplantation? Liver Transpl Surg 1998;4(2):128–32.
72. Keeffe EB, Krause DS. Hepatitis B vaccination of patients with chronic liver disease. Liver Transpl Surg 1998;4(5):437–9.
73. Castells L, Esteban R. Hepatitis B vaccination in liver transplant candidates. Eur J Gastroenterol Hepatol 2001;13(4):359–61.
74. Loinaz C, de Juanes JR, Gonzalez EM, et al. Hepatitis B vaccination results in 140 liver transplant recipients. Hepatogastroenterology 1997;44(13):235–8.
75. Fabrizi F, Cerutti R, Dixit V, et al. Hepatitis B virus vaccine and chronic kidney disease. The advances. Nefrologia 2021. https://doi.org/10.1016/j.nefro.2020.08.016.
76. Foster WQ, Murphy A, Vega DJ, et al. Hepatitis B vaccination in heart transplant candidates. J Heart Lung Transpl 2006;25(1):106–9.

Hepatitis B and Health Care Workers

Stephen C. Pappas, MD, JD, FCLM

KEYWORDS

- Health care workers • HBV transmission • Vaccination • Screening
- Booster therapy

KEY POINTS

- The risk of transmission of HBV from a patient to a health care worker is very low as a result of widespread HBV vaccination and adoption of standard precautions.
- Risk of HBV transmission from a health care worker to a patient is extremely low.
- HBV infection in a health care worker neither requires restrictions on professional practice nor requires disclosure of infection status to a patient
- HBV vaccine and vaccination protocols exist that confer lifelong immunity to HBV in health care workers with successful vaccination; a booster dose of HBV vaccine is not required
- Strategies to manage HBV vaccine failure should be discussed with the health care worker on a case-by-case basis

It is hard to believe that less than 50 years have passed between the discovery of the "Australia antigen" and, as evidenced by the articles in this issue, the ability for clinicians to obtain sophisticated hepatitis B virus (HBV) serology and viral load measurement and to provide highly effective antiviral therapy and vaccination protection for HBV infection. By all standards, this is speedy development, particularly relevant for health care workers (HCWs), recognized very early to be at increased risk for HBV infection as an occupational hazard. The risk of HBV transmission in the health care setting is a "two-way street," the most important and common direction being transmission from patients to HCWs, and much less commonly, transmission from HCW to patient. This article reviews the risk of transmission of HBV to HCW from a historical perspective, HBV vaccination focused on the HCW, the need for booster therapy when protective anti-HB surface antibody (anti-HBs) is found to be low or undetectable, options and recommendations when initial vaccination of a HCW fails, mandatory screening for HBV in HCWs, and finally, recommendations for HCWs with chronic HBV infection.

Ben Taub General Hospital, 5th Fl, 5-PO 71 002b, 1504 Ben Taub Loop, Houston, TX 77030, USA
E-mail address: spappas1@comcast.net

Clin Liver Dis 25 (2021) 859–874
https://doi.org/10.1016/j.cld.2021.06.010
1089-3261/21/© 2021 Elsevier Inc. All rights reserved.

liver.theclinics.com

THE RISK OF TRANSMISSION OF HEPATITIS B VIRUS TO HEALTH CARE WORKERS: BACKGROUND AND HISTORICAL PERPSECTIVES

The biology of the HBV creates the "perfect storm" for "silent" transmission; the virus may remain infective on environmental surfaces for up to 7 days,[1] and most relevant to HCW, transmission may occur via "covert" blood exposure with most HCWs unable to recall overt percutaneous exposure.[2] Although blood from persons with HBV infection is regarded as essential to transmission of infection, other body fluids (eg, cerebrospinal fluid, ascites, pleural fluid), if they contain blood, may be associated with HBV transmission.[3] This knowledge was available early on after initial HBV serologic testing was available, and it is important to review several developments that bring us to where we are now in establishing the current risk of HBV transmission in HCW and interventions to decrease this risk.

In the early 1970s the prevalence of HBV infection in HCWs was estimated to be approximately 10 times that of the general population.[4] In 1983 it was estimated that approximately 17,000 HBV infections occurred in HCWs in the United States.[5] At around the same time (1981–1982), highly effective HBV vaccines became available and were recommended in 1982 by the Advisory Committee on Immunization Practices (ACIP) for routine use in HCWs.[6] Several years later, the epidemiology of HBV in the United States and many other countries changed as a result of national efforts to eliminate HBV transmission; this included efforts for universal vaccination of infants and children in 1991 and adolescent "catch up" vaccination in 1995.[7,8] In the period 1990 to 2010 in the United States there was a significant decrease in the number of reported acute HBV infections from 8.9 to 0.9 per 100,000 population; in 2011 the number of new cases of acute hepatitis B was estimated to be approximately 18,800 based on actual reported cases (of which approximately 55% were hospitalized) and accounting for underreporting.[8] In aggregate, these vaccination strategies were associated with a major decline in HBV infection among HCWs.[3,8] These vaccination efforts were in parallel to the adoption of standard precautions (formerly known as *universal precautions*) in hospital and other health care settings as well as the passage of the Needlestick Safety and Prevention Act of 2001, an Occupational Safety and Health Administration (OSHA) mandate initiated to decrease percutaneous injury and blood-borne transmission of infective agents, principally human immunodeficiency virus (HIV), HBV, and other agents potentially posing a risk to HCWs.[3,9] Finally, in 2011 the ACIP emphasized the need for HBV vaccination before exposure for unvaccinated or incompletely vaccinated HCWs with postvaccination serologic testing for protective anti-HBs 1 to 2 months after vaccination.[10]

So where are we now? Based on the historical developments and learnings, we can summarize a few fundamental points regarding the risk for HBV transmission in HCWs currently. Compared with the tremendous amount of new information made available in the period between approximately 1980 and 2012, the period since then has generally seen refinement and confirmation of some of the earlier observations versus major advances in our knowledge base.

With the significant decrease in the prevalence of acute HBV infections in the general population, the risk of HBV in HCWs is currently associated with exposure to patients with chronic HBV, estimated to be approximately 1 million people in the United States.[11] Despite the various interventions and historical developments described earlier in the article, the prevalence of chronic hepatitis B in the United States has remained relatively stable over survey years 1976 to 2010.[3]

Another new wrinkle introduced relates to the fact that whereas initial recommendations related to HCW HBV vaccination were based on HCWs receiving HBV vaccination as adults (usually at the time of hiring as an HCW), many HCWs now received HBV vaccination as an infant or child or during adolescent "catch up" vaccination. Titers of protective anti-HBs are known to decline with time, and any current protocols for testing HCWs for anti-HBs levels before exposure (eg, at the time of hiring to distinguish between vaccine nonresponders vs responders whose anti-HBs titers have declined to less than the protective level) need to consider a population vaccinated up to 25 to 30 years ago.[3] Preexposure testing will need to take into consideration whether past results indicating response are available, whether new results should be obtained at hiring, or whether testing can be undertaken at exposure (eg, if the risk is low) and the exposure is recognized.

VACCINATION OF HEALTH CARE WORKERS

HBV vaccination remains the most important strategy for the protection of HCWs from HBV infection. The currently available vaccines are among the safest and most effective vaccines developed. All HCWs should be vaccinated for HBV; federal OSHA regulations mandate that vaccination should be available for employees within 10 days of their initial assignment placing them in a position reasonably anticipated to present a risk for exposure to blood or body fluids.[3,12] OSHA regulations also mandate a signed declination statement for an HCW declining the offer of HBV vaccination.[12]

Currently available HBV vaccines appropriate for HCWs are included in **Table 1**. The 2013 Centers for Disease Control and Prevention (CDC) guidance for HCW protection by vaccination included only the existing US Food and Drug Administration (FDA)-approved HBV vaccines at that time (ie, Recombivax HB, Engerix-B, Twinrix); more recently Heplisav-B, a single recombinant antigen HBV vaccine with a novel immunostimulatory sequence adjuvant, was approved by the FDA in November 2017.[13] Heplisav-B is administered in a 2-dose, 0 and 1 month regimen.[14] Subsequent review by the ACIP led to the ACIP recommendation that Heplisav-B "may be used as a HepB vaccine in persons aged $\geq$ 18 years recommended for vaccination against HBV."[13] Registration trials for this new HBV vaccine reported increased protection in patients with diabetes, obesity, and older age, populations generally recognized as having a poor response to HBV vaccination.[15,16] Furthermore, a subsequent cost-utility decision analysis Markov modeling study of Heplisav-B suggested that Heplisav-B may result in better outcomes for patients with conditions typically associated with poor vaccination response, as well as for subjects with prior nonresponse to the previously available HBV vaccines.[15] These observations are important because they have implications for dealing with vaccine nonresponse, in addition to consideration of the initial vaccine to be used in the HCW population. Arguably, nonresponse in the HCW is more important than in the general population, and the 2-dose, 4 weeks apart regimen, with slightly increased efficacy is more appealing and likely to be ultimately more cost effective in the HCW.

The safety of HBV vaccines is supported by data from more than 30 years of use for the earlier available vaccines; although safety data for Heplisav-B vaccine are limited to those collected during registration trials and early use since 2017, there is no reason a priori to suspect that the long-term safety profile for that vaccine preparation will be any different compared with the older vaccines.[14] HBV vaccinations are contraindicated in persons with a history of hypersensitivity to yeast or any vaccine component; any person who has experienced anaphylaxis after receiving HBV vaccine should not receive additional doses. In keeping with general principles of good clinical practice, and as recommended by the CDC and other authoritative bodies, health care providers should review vaccine product inserts for precautions, warnings, and contraindications before administering vaccine.

Table 1
Vaccines to prevent hepatitis B

Vaccine	Trade Name (Manufacturer)	Age (y)	Dose	Route	Schedule	Booster
Hepatitis B vaccine, recombinant with novel adjuvant (1018)	Heplisav-B (Dynavax Technologies)	>18	0.5 mL (20 µg HBsAg and 3000 µg 1018)	IM	0, 1 mo	None
Hepatitis B vaccine, recombinant[a]	Engerix-B (GlaxoSmithKline)	0–19 (primary)	0.5 mL (10 µg HBsAg)	IM	0, 1, 6 mo	None
		0–10 (accelerated)	0.5 mL (10 µg HBsAg)	IM	0, 1, 2 mo	12 mo
		11–19 (accelerated)	1.0 mL (20 µg HBsAg)	IM	0, 1, 2 mo	12 mo
		≥20 (primary)	1.0 mL (20 µg HBsAg)	IM	0, 1, 6 mo	None
		≥20 (accelerated)	1.0 mL (20 µg HBsAg)	IM	0, 1, 2 mo	12 mo
Hepatitis B vaccine, recombinant[a]	Recombivax HB (Merck & Co, Inc)	0–19 (primary)	0.5 mL (5 µg HBsAg)	IM	0, 1, 6 mo	None
		11–15 (adolescent accelerated)	1.0 mL (10 µg HBsAg)	IM	0, 4–6 mo	None
		≥20 (primary)	1.0 mL(10 µg HBsAg)	IM	0, 1, 6 mo	None
Combined hepatitis A and B vaccine	Twinrix (GlaxoSmithKline)	≥18 (primary)	1.0 mL (720 ELU HAV + 20 µg HBsAg)	IM	0, 1, 6 mo	None
		≥18 (accelerated)	1.0 mL(720 ELU HAV+20 µg HBsAg)	IM	0, 7, 21–30 d	12 mo

Abbreviations: ELU, ELISA units of inactivated HAV; HAV, hepatitis A virus; HBsAg, hepatitis B surface antigen; IM, intramuscular.
[a] Consult the prescribing information for differences in dosing for hemodialysis and other immunocompromised patients.
From: AM Harris. Hepatitis B. 2019 Available at: https://wwwnc.cdc.gov/travel/yellowbook/2020/travel-related-infectious-diseases/hepatitis-b. Accessed March 3, 2021 (Table4-04 original).

Prevaccination testing for HBV infection is generally not indicated in the HCW solely based on their prior occupational risk.[3] Testing for possible HBV infection (ie, hepatitis B surface antigen [HBsAg], hepatitis B core antibody [HBcAb], HBs antibody [HBsAb]) is reasonable if the HCW is at risk for prior infection based on other risk factors that include, but are not limited to, for example, country of birth where HBsAg prevalence is 2% or more or behaviors associated with increased HBV infection risk (prior intravenous drug use, men who have sex with men). For an individual HCW thought to be at higher risk of HBV infection who declines being tested for HBV infection, the alternative is to proceed with HBV vaccination. If the HCW fails to achieve a response to vaccination (ie, anti-HBs level ≥10 mIU/mL, 1–2 months after the last dose of vaccine), testing for HBV infection could be done at that time.[3]

Incompletely vaccinated HCWs should complete the indicated series for a selected HBV vaccine as outlined in **Table 1**; there is no need to restart the vaccine series. When documentation for some vaccine doses is not available, additional doses should be administered to complete the series. HCWs who lack any documentation of HBV vaccination should be considered unvaccinated. Health care facilities should consider using immunization information systems to obtain documentation of prior HBV vaccination for an HCW to avoid revaccination.[17]

The recommended CDC algorithm for preexposure postvaccination serologic testing is presented in **Fig. 1**. The approach outlined in **Fig. 1** contemplates that "completely vaccinated HCWs with anti-HBs ≥10 mIU/mL are considered hepatitis B immune" and that these HCWs "do not need further periodic testing to assess anti-HBs levels."[3] The decline of protective and anti-HBs levels over time postvaccination has been mentioned earlier. Generally, the consensus has been that once an individual has demonstrated the ability to mount a protective antibody response (ie, ≥10 mIU/mL) on at least one occasion postvaccination, they have long-term protection and do not need further testing of anti-HBs levels.[3] This consensus is based on long-term follow-up, which includes subjects vaccinated in the early days of HBV vaccination as well as subjects more recently vaccinated as a result of universal infant and child and adolescent "catch up" vaccination.[18–21] However, there is no complete agreement as to whether vaccination is associated with life-long immune memory, particularly in the setting where vertical transmission of HBV infection may be high.[22,23] Whether this is relevant to the HCW setting is not entirely clear.

Fig. 1 includes a protective anti-HBs antibody level of ≥10 mIU/mL, generally accepted to be an evidence-based cutoff.[3,24,25] Guidelines for some European countries use a cutoff of 100 mIU/mL, rationalizing this cutoff based on the fact that it is higher than the levels usually seen in the rare situation of an HBV carrier with concurrent positive HBsAg and anti-HBs.[25] The evidence-based data supporting an anti-HBs cutoff of 10 mIU/mL or more seems to be more reasonable, particularly in settings in which HBV prevalence is low.[25,26]

CDC recommendations for postexposure management of HCW based on HBV vaccination status is presented in **Table 2**.[3] At the 2 extremes of HBV vaccination protection, for an HCW who is a documented responder after a complete series for vaccination, no action is needed postexposure. Conversely, in the documented nonresponder HCW, where the source patient is known to be HBV positive, or for whom HBV status is unknown, postexposure prophylaxis includes hepatitis B immune globulin (HBIG) dosing. In between these 2 extremes, various combinations of HBIG, initiation of revaccination or completing vaccination, and postvaccination serologic testing are as outlined in **Table 2**.

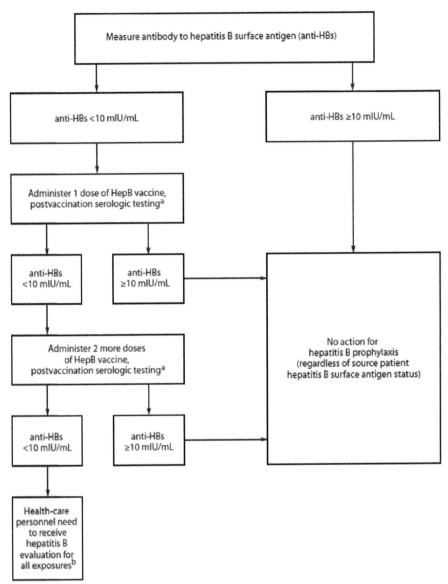

Fig. 1. Preexposure evaluation for health care personnel previously vaccinated with complete, 3-dose HepB vaccine series or more who have not had postvaccination serologic testing. [a]Should be performed 1–2 months after the last dose of vaccine using a quantitative method that allows detection of the protective concentration of anti-HBs ($\geq$10 mIU/mL) (e.g, enzyme-linked immunosorbent assay [ELISA]). [b]A nonresponder is defined as a person with anti-HBs <10 mIU/mL after 26 doses of HepB vaccine. Persons who do not have a protective concentration of anti-HBs after revaccination should be tested for HBsAg. If positive, the person should receive appropriate management or vaccination. (*From* Centers for Disease Control and Prevention. CDC Guidance for evaluating health-care personnel for hepatitis B virus protection and for administering postexposure management. MMWR 2013;62(No. RR-10):1-19.)

Table 2
Postexposure management of health care personnel after occupational percutaneous and mucosal exposure to blood and body fluids, by health care personnel HepB vaccination and response status

Health Care Personnel Status	Postexposure Testing Source Patient (HBsAg)	Postexposure Testing HCP Testing (Anti-HBs)	Postexposure Prophylaxis HBIG[a]	Postexposure Prophylaxis Vaccination	Post-vaccination Serologic Testing[b]
Documented responder[c] after complete series ≥3 doses)	No action needed				
Documented nonresponder[d] after 6 doses	Positive/ unknown	—[e]	HBIG ×2 separated by 1 mo	—	No
	Negative	No action needed			
Response unknown after 3 doses	Positive/ unknown	<10 mIU/mL[e]	HBIG ×1	Initiate revaccination	Yes
	Negative	<10 mIU/mL	None		
	Any result	≥10 mIU/mL	No action needed		
Unvaccinated/ incompletely vaccinated or vaccine refusers	Positive/ unknown	—[e]	HBIG ×1	Complete vaccination	Yes
	Negative	—	None	Complete vaccination	Yes

Abbreviations: anti-HBs, antibody to hepatitis B surface antigen; HBIG, hepatitis B immune globulin; HBsAg, hepatitis B surface antigen; HCP, health care personnel.

[a] HBIG should be administered intramuscularly as soon as possible after exposure when indicated. The effectiveness of HBIG when administered greater than 7 d after percutaneous, mucosal, or nonintact skin exposures is unknown. HBIG dosage is 0.06 mL/kg.

[b] Should be performed 1 to 2 months after the last dose of the HepB vaccine series (and 4–6 months after administration of HBIG to avoid detection of passively administered anti-HBs) using a quantitative method that allows detection of the protective concentration of anti-HBs (≥10 mIU/mL).

[c] A responder is defined as a person with anti-HBs ≥10 mIU/mL after 3 or more doses of HepB vaccine.

[d] A nonresponder is defined as a person with anti-HBs less than 10 mIU/mL after 6 or more doses of HepB vaccine.

[e] HCP who have anti-HBs less than 10mIU/mL, or who are unvaccinated or incompletely vaccinated, and sustain an exposure to a source patient who is HBsAg positive or has unknown HBsAg status, should undergo baseline testing for HBV infection as soon as possible after exposure, and follow-up testing approximately 6 months later. Initial baseline tests consist of total anti-HBc; testing at approximately 6 months consists of HBsAg and total anti-HBc.

From Centers for Disease Control and Prevention. CDC guidance for evaluating health-care personnel for hepatitis B virus protection and for administering postexposure management. MMWR 2013;62(No. RR-10):1-19.

THE NEED FOR BOOSTER THERAPY

A booster dose of HBV vaccine has been defined as "a dose of HBV vaccine given after primary vaccination to provide rapid protective immunity against significant infection (ie, infection leading to test results positive for HBV and/or clinically significant disease)."[27] ("Booster" terminology may also be used to describe a dose of HBV vaccine administered at 12 months as part of an accelerated HBV vaccination regimen [see **Table 1**]; this differs from booster therapy or a challenge dose). Booster therapy should be distinguished from what has been referred to as a "challenge dose" and is generally regarded as "a dose of HBV vaccine to determine the presence of vaccine – induced immunologic memory through generation of an amnestic antibody response."[3] The terms differ essentially only in the intent underlying them. For example, if your intent is to determine whether an HCW has the ability to mount a protective antibody response to a "hypothetical" HBV infection exposure in the future, you would be administering a challenge dose. If your intent is to provide rapid protective immunity, for example, following an actual exposure, you would be administering a booster dose. The nuanced differences are of no clinical relevance because both interventions are for the purpose of generating an amnestic response to HBV infection; this, of course, relates to the previously mentioned decline in the level of protective anti-HBs antibody in the years following HBV vaccination. The decline in levels of protective anti-HBs varies depending on the population and the age at which vaccination was administered.[27] However, as suggested by the previous discussion regarding life-long immunity to HBV infection in vaccine responders with previously demonstrated protective antibody response to HBV vaccination, booster dose or challenge dose administration may be a moot point, particularly because the vast majority of individuals who have received vaccination at age 1 year or more seem to have a high incidence of protective anti-HBs antibody titers; 92.9% health science students previously vaccinated at an average age of 14.5 years had anti-HBs levels 10 mIU/mL or more approximately 9 years later,[28] and several studies have shown that 69% to 96% of persons vaccinated 9 to 22 years earlier, and who had anti-HBs titers less than 10 mIU/mL, demonstrated response to a challenge dose of HBV vaccine.[18,20,21,29] Available data, in aggregate, seem to strongly support that demonstration of the development of a protective level of anti-HBs on at least one occasion following vaccination confers on the HCW continued protection regardless of any subsequent decline in anti-HBs levels. At this time there are no compelling data that booster doses are required in HCWs who are vaccine responders. A small degree of caution is required, however, because the available data are limited to certain timeframes and are largely circumstantial; prospective studies assessing actual infection rates are not available and are unlikely to be performed.

HEPATITIS B VIRUS VACCINATION FAILURE IN HEALTH CARE WORKERS

Nonresponse to HBV vaccination is particularly important for HCWs because they remain at risk for HBV infection following exposure. HBV vaccination nonresponders are defined as subjects who fail to produce and anti-HBs level of 10 mIU/mL or more after revaccination, which includes 2 complete courses of vaccine.[30] Five percent to 10% of immunocompetent subjects receiving 2 complete courses of vaccination meet the definition of nonresponse.[30] A higher incidence of nonresponse has been well described in subjects including, but not limited to, individuals with diabetes, obesity, end-stage renal disease (ESRD) with hemodialysis, HIV or hepatitis C virus (HCV) infection celiac disease, and inflammatory bowel disease.[30,31] HCWs with any of these comorbidities may be expected to have a lower response to initial HBV vaccination. Revaccination for nonresponse in HCW should be undertaken.[3] Approximately 50% of individuals with initial vaccine nonresponse develop protective antibody levels after 1 additional dose of vaccine; 40% of individuals with no response after 1 additional dose develop a response with a further dose.[32] The cumulative response after 3 additional doses (assuming the initial vaccination regimen followed a 3 dose schedule) is approximately 85% increased seroconversion.[30] Similar results have been observed for revaccination with the 2-dose Heplisav-B vaccine, regardless of which vaccine was used for initial vaccination (eg, Recombivax-B, Engerix-B).[16] Heplisav-B may be used for revaccination.[13]

Strategies that should be considered in the HCW with an initial HBV vaccination nonresponse include:

1. Revaccination with the same dose of vaccine as used for initial vaccination; this can be expected to result in an 83% to 87% increased seroconversion.[30] Revaccination with an increased dose has been best studied in the general population with HCV or HIV infection, with a reported 80% increased seroconversion response rate, suggesting there may be little gain from an increased dose regimen.[30]
2. Intradermal dosing of HBV vaccine (as opposed to the usual intramuscular route). The results for intradermal dosing have been mixed, and the strategy does not seem to be more effective in the HIV population. Some data suggest that this may be effective in the setting of ESRD and hemodialysis, comorbidities not likely to be common in HCWs.[30]
3. Revaccination with HBV vaccines with newer adjuvants, for example, Heplisav-B.
4. Coadministration of HBV vaccine with immunostimulatory or immunomodulating agents (eg, levamisole, praziquantel, cimetidine, imiquimod).[30,33]

Unfortunately, beyond revaccination, none of the alternate HBV nonresponder strategies have been shown to be sufficiently effective to justify regular use. These alternate strategies should be discussed on a case-by-case basis if an HCW is particularly motivated to achieve protective levels of anti-HBs, their perceived risk for HBV exposure and infection is high in the occupational setting, and/or they have attendant medical comorbidities justifying a more intense effort to achieve HBV immunity.

SHOULD HEPATITIS B VIRUS SCREENING AND VACCINATION BE MANDATORY FOR HEALTH CARE WORKERS?

The legal and ethical principles for mandating any particular type of screening or vaccination require that any interventions that restrict autonomy must be reasonable and necessary.[34] In addition, mandated screening or vaccination must be based on a platform where screening or vaccination has been recommended by an authoritative body such as the ACIP and, for the vaccination component, the risks, efficacy, and risk/benefit profiles must be well-known and described. As evidenced by recent experience with the coronavirus disease 2019 (COVID-19) pandemic and discussions regarding mandated vaccination, these discussions often "spark intense clashes of feeling."[34] For a severe acute respiratory syndrome coronavirus 2 vaccine mandatory vaccination can be promoted on the basis that COVID-19 disease is not adequately contained with other strategies, whereas the same cannot be said for HBV vaccination in the HCW. Although HBV screening and vaccination in the HCW has been recommended by the ACIP and the safety of HBV vaccination is well described, an ethical question around mandatory screening and vaccination is "who are you protecting by the mandates?" The risk of HBV infection for the HCW is higher than that of the general population, but the risk is still very low, arguably so low that it does not rise to the level justifying restricting autonomy. Furthermore, the risk to the HCW is currently much lower than it was earlier (ie, the problem is not growing or poorly controlled). Finally, the chances of transmission of HBV infection from an HCW to a patient is extremely low.[35] Based on this ethical (and legal) paradigm, mandatory HBV screening and vaccination may not be reasonable or necessary. At present, it may be difficult to justify continuing mandatory HBV vaccination for HCWs in the jurisdictions where it exists (see later discussion).

Procedurally, the legal framework for health care facility HBV vaccination laws rests with the state and is governed by state laws. Each state adopts its own legislation to govern HBV screening and vaccination. Individual institutions may develop additional policies or regulations, often relying on local advisory expert panels, to manage HBV vaccination as long as they do not conflict with state law or abridge rights conferred by the Constitution. Federal law governs HBV vaccination within Veterans Affairs facilities, federal prisons, active-duty military facilities, and immigration detention medical centers.

The CDC Office for State, Tribal, Local and Territorial Support published a Menu of State Healthcare Facility Hepatitis B Vaccination Laws, updated in 2017, which provides an overview of state laws including those applicable to HBV vaccination and screening.[36] In general, as of October 2017, 17 states required that hospitals, long-term care facilities, and ambulatory care facilities have defined HCW programs and policies for the assessment of an HCW's vaccination status and administrative requirements for offering HBV vaccination. Three states require that HCWs in hospitals be vaccinated against HBV (eg, Rhode Island law stating that "evidence of immunity is required for all health care workers…against…Hepatitis B…"),[37] essentially mandating HBV vaccination with exemptions permitted for medical, religious, or philosophic reasons. Four states require similar mandatory HBV vaccination or proof of immunity for HCWs employed in long-term care facilities, with 6 states requiring HBV vaccination or proof of immunity for HCWs working in ambulatory care facilities.[36]

Notwithstanding that mandatory HBV screening and vaccination rules are based on what may be interpreted as "shaky legal and ethical grounds," within an individual institution, it is important that HCWs, administrators, legal and medical staff, and others involved in policy making be aware that internal institution policies, regulations, and State or Federal law as applicable, vary from state to state and institution to institution.

HEALTH CARE WORKERS WITH CHRONIC HEPATITIS B VIRUS

Recommendations for the management of HBV-infected HCWs have been developed in the United States and other countries.[35,38] In 2012, the CDC updated existing 1991 recommendations to incorporate learnings from the adoption of standard precautions in 1996, the increasing use of double-gloving during the performance of so-called exposure-prone procedures (EPPs), and increasing compliance with and developments for modified practices and instrumentation, including avoiding resheathing of needles, puncture-resistant needles, and use of needleless infusion setups.[38] The validity of the updated recommendations is supported by the observation that transmission of HBV infection from HCWs to patients is extremely low.[35]

Overall, in contrast to previous recommendations, current recommendations promulgate the position that as a general principle, chronic HBV infection should not restrict an HCW within their professional practice.[35,38,39] In addition, mandatory disclosure of HBV status to a patient is no longer warranted.[35,38] An HCW's HBV status should remain confidential. However, current CDC recommendations continue to endorse that HCWs should know their HBV infection's status, noting that "providers have an ethical and professional obligation to know their HBV status and to act on such knowledge accordingly."[38] Other aspects of the current recommendations that differ from, or expand on, prior recommendations include what is a "safe" level of HBV infection in an HCW (ie, a level of virus associated with highly unlikely transmission of HBV infection) and what are EPPs? At present, there seems to be general agreement between recommendations in the United States and other countries that HBV DNA levels (as opposed to the presence of hepatitis B e antigen [HBeAg]) should be used to determine "safe" levels of HBV infection in an HCW and that HBV DNA thresholds of 200, 1000, or 2000 IU/mL are appropriate thresholds (European Association for the Study of the Liver Clinical Practice Guidelines recommendations: <200 IU/mL, CDC recommendations: <1000 IU/mL, recommendations in many countries: <2000 IU/mL).[35,38,40,41] EPPs have been defined as those procedures "known or likely to pose an increased risk of percutaneous injury to a healthcare provider that have resulted in provider to patient transmission of HBV"[38] (**Box 1**).

An issue, with both medicolegal and ethical implications, may arise with the recommendations regarding a "safe" level of HBV infection in an HCW performing EPP. Antiviral treatment in an HCW with an accepted medical indication for antiviral treatment is clearly appropriate.[24] However, particularly in the face of an extremely low transmission rate of HBV infection from HCW to patient, is it reasonable to essentially mandate (by excluding HCWs from performing EPPs if their HBV-DNA level is greater than a certain threshold) that an HCW, who would otherwise not need treatment, take HBV antiviral treatment for the sole purpose of reducing HBV-DNA levels less than a certain threshold? Examples of such an HCW would be an HBeAg-negative HCW with persistently normal alanine aminotransferase level and HBV-DNA levels greater than 2000 and less than 200,000 IU/mL, or an immunotolerant patient as defined by existing criteria.[24,40,41] On the one hand, highly effective, well-tolerated, and safe antiviral therapy exists that will reduce HBV-DNA levels to less than threshold levels, allowing the HCW to perform EPP. Furthermore, if the HCW is not taking antiviral treatment (eg, it is not strictly mandated or the HCW opts for more frequent monitoring), transmission of HBV infection to a patient occurring as a result of performing an EPP raises potential medicolegal liability and questions of a breach of ethical obligations. On the other hand, there are no data that the current extremely low transmission rate of HBV infection from HCWs to patients has decreased (or will decrease) as a result of mandatory antiviral treatment of certain HCWs.[40,41] The European guidelines express recommendations on this matter in terms of "...*may* be treated with [antivirals] to reduce transmission risk..."[41]

On balance, in view of the prevailing ethical (and probably legal) obligations for an HCW performing EPP, the current recommendations suggesting antiviral treatment of those HCWs who would otherwise not need treatment seem reasonable and not unduly burdensome. Institutions should document details of the specific antiviral treatment policies to be adopted for the management of HCWs with chronic HBV infection. In practice, it is likely that most HCWs who perform EPP will readily accept the minimal burden of antiviral treatment, otherwise not indicated, for the sole purpose of lowering viremia so that they can perform EPP and mitigate the likelihood of potential legal or ethical challenges.

A summary of recommendations for the known or potential HBV-positive HCW is as follows:

1. HCW who does not achieve protective levels of anti-HBs antibody after revaccination should be tested for HbsAg and antibody to hepatitis B core Ag (anti-HBc) to determine infection status.
2. Prevaccination testing is not indicated except for HCWs at an increased risk of HBV infection.
3. HCWs performing EPPs should receive prevaccination testing for chronic HBV infection.
4. HCWs who perform EPPs should be "guided by review of a duly constituted expert review panel with a balanced perspective... regarding the procedures that they can perform and prospective oversight of their practice."[38,39] As noted earlier,

---

Box 1
Centers for Disease Control and Prevention classification of exposure-prone patient care procedures

Category I. Procedures known or likely to pose an increased risk of percutaneous injury to a health care provider that have resulted in provider-to-patient transmission of HBV

These procedures are limited to major abdominal, cardiothoracic, and orthopedic surgery, repair of major traumatic injuries, abdominal and vaginal hysterectomy, cesarean delivery, vaginal deliveries, and major oral or maxillofacial surgery (eg, fracture reductions). Techniques that have been demonstrated to increase the risk for health-care provider percutaneous injury and provider-to-patient blood exposure include

- Digital palpation of a needle tip in a body cavity

- The simultaneous presence of a health care provider's fingers and a needle or other sharp instrument or object (eg, bone spicule) in a poorly visualized or highly confined anatomic site

Category I procedures, especially those that have been implicated in HBV transmission, are not ordinarily performed by students fulfilling the essential functions of a medical or dental school education

Category II. All other invasive and noninvasive procedures

These and similar procedures are not included in Category I because they pose low or no risk for percutaneous injury to a health care provider or, if a percutaneous injury occurs, it usually happens outside a patient's body and generally does not pose a risk for provider-to-patient blood exposure. These include

- Surgical and obstetric/gynecologic procedures that do not involve the techniques listed for Category I

- The use of needles or other sharp devices when the health care provider's hands are outside a body cavity (eg, phlebotomy, placing and maintaining peripheral and central intravascular lines, administering medication by injection, performing needle biopsies, or lumbar puncture)

- Dental procedures other than major oral or maxillofacial surgery

- Insertion of tubes (eg, nasogastric, endotracheal, rectal, or urinary catheters)

- Endoscopic or bronchoscopic procedures

- Internal examination with a gloved hand that does not involve the use of sharp devices (eg, vaginal, oral, and rectal examination)

- Procedures that involve external physical touch (eg, general physical or eye examinations or blood pressure checks)

From Centers for Disease Control and Prevention. Updated CDC Recommendations for the Management of Hepatitis B Virus–Infected Health-Care Providers and Students. MMWR 2012;61(No. RR-3):1-12.

---

confidentiality of an HCW's HBV serologic status should be maintained at all times during this process.

5. EPPs can continue if a low-threshold HBV DNA level (eg, 1000 IU/mL), adopted by the expert panel, is documented at least every 6 months, with the provision that higher levels may require more frequent monitoring.

6. During periods when HBV DNA levels are more than the threshold, the HCW should not perform EPP.
7. HCWs who perform EPP may consider taking antiviral therapy, which might otherwise not be medically indicated, to lower their HBV-DNA level less than a certain threshold.

It is important for institutions to have documented written policies and procedures for the management of HCW with chronic HBV infection. HCWs with chronic HBV infection should review these policies and procedures to ensure compliance.

SUMMARY

The risk of transmission of HBV infection from the patient to an HCW is now very low, largely as a result of a decreased incidence of HBV in many countries as a result of the adoption of standard (universal) precautions and initiatives for universal HBV vaccination. Highly effective HBV vaccine and vaccination protocols exist that confirm essentially lifelong immunity to HBV with successful vaccination. A booster dose of HBV vaccine does not seem to be required based on currently available data. The problems of vaccination failure or a decision not to receive a vaccine are clearly important but may be less of an issue now than earlier, based on the documented decreased risk of HBV transmission from patient to HCW and the extremely low incidence of HBV transmission from an HCW to a patient, in areas where the prevalence of HBV in the general population is low. With the current epidemiology of HBV infection, the use of standard precautions, highly effective vaccines, and effective viral suppression with antivirals, it is difficult to support mandated HBV screening and vaccination in HCWs who decline or refuse intervention. For HCWs with chronic HBV infection, HBV infection status by itself does not require any restrictions on professional practice; the presence of chronic HBV infection does not require disclosure of infection status to a patient. Further study is required to develop optimal and effective strategies for the management of HBV vaccine nonresponders.

CLINICS CARE POINTS

- Any person who has experienced anaphylaxis after receiving HBV vaccine should not receive additional doses.
- A single dose of HBV vaccine can be used to determine whether a previously vaccinated health care worker with low or undetectable anti-HBs is able to mount a protective antibody response.
- In a health care worker with nonresponse after initial HBV vaccination, revaccination with 2 doses of Heplisav-B vaccine can be expected to produce over 80% increased seroconversion with levels of anti-HBs greater than or equal to 10 mIU/mL.

DISCLOSURE

The author has nothing to disclose.

REFERENCES

1. Bond WW, Favero MS, Petersen NJ, et al. Survival of hepatitis B virus after drying and storage for one week. Lancet 1981;1:550–1.

2. Garibaldi RA, Hatch FE, Bisno AL, et al. Nonparenteral serum hepatitis: report of an outbreak. JAMA 1972;220:963–6.
3. Centers for Disease Control and Prevention. CDC guidance for evaluating health-care personnel for hepatitis B virus protection and for administering postexposure management. MMWR 2013;62(No. RR-10):1–19.
4. US Public Health Service. Updated U.S. Public Health Service guidelines for the management of occupational exposures to HBV, HCV, and HIV and recommendations for postexposure prophylaxis. MMWR 2001;50(No. RR-11):1–50.
5. Beltrami EM, Williams IT, Shapiro CN, et al. Risk and management of blood-borne infections in health care workers. Clin Microbiol Rev 2000;13:385–407.
6. CDC. Recommendation of the immunization practices advisory committee (ACIP). Inactivated hepatitis B virus vaccine. MMWR 1982;31(317–22):27–8.
7. CDC. Hepatitis B virus: a comprehensive strategy for eliminating transmission in the United States through universal childhood vaccination: recommendations of the Advisory Committee on Immunization Practices (ACIP). MMWR 1991;40(No. RR-13):1–25.
8. CDC. Viral hepatitis statistics and surveillance. Available at: http://www.cdc.gov/hepatitis/statistics/index.htm. Accessed February 10, 2021.
9. US Department of Labor. Occupational health and safety administration. Available at. http://www.osha.gov. Accessed February 10, 2021.
10. CDC. Immunization of health-care personnel: recommendations of the advisory committee on immunization practices (ACIP). MMWR Recomm Rep 2011;60(No. RR-7):1–45.
11. CDC. Recommendations for identification and public health management of persons with chronic hepatitis B virus infection. MMWR Recomm Rep 2008;57(No. RR-8):1–20.
12. US Department of Labor. Occupational health and safety administration. Available at: http://www.osha.gov. Accessed March 4, 2021.
13. Centers for Disease Control and Prevention. Recommendations of the advisory committee on immunization practices for use of a hepatitis B vaccine with a novel adjuvant. MMWR Recomm Rep 2018;67(No. RR-15):455–8.
14. Food and Drug Administration. Product approval information: package insert. In: Heplisav-B. Silver Spring, MD: US Department of Health and Human Services, Food and Drug Administration; 2018. Available at: https://www.fda.gov/BiologicsBloodVaccines/Vaccines/ApprovedProducts/ucm584752.htm. Accessed on March 1, 2021.
15. Rosenthal EM, Hall EW, Rosenberg ES, et al. Assessing the cost-utility of preferentially administering Heplisav-B vaccine to certain populations. Vaccine 2020;38(51):8206–15.
16. Halperin SA, Ward B, Cooper C, et al. Comparison of safety and immunogenicity of two doses of investigational hepatitis B virus surface antigen co-administered with an immunostimulatory phosphorothioate oligodeoxyribonucleotide and three doses of a licensed hepatitis B vaccine in healthy adults 18–55 years of age. Vaccine 2012;30(15):2556–63.
17. CDC. Immunization information systems. Available at: https://www.cdc.gov/vaccines/programs/iis/index.html. Accessed on July 21, 2021.
18. Bruce MG, Bruden D, Hurlburt D, et al. Antibody levels and protection after hepatitis B vaccine: results of a 30-year follow-up study and response to a booster dose. J Infect Dis 2016;214(1):16–22.
19. Van Damme P. Long-term protection after hepatitis B vaccine. J Infect Dis 2016;214(1):1–3.

20. Floreani A, Baldo V, Cristofoletti M, et al. Long-term persistence of anti-HBs after vaccination against HBV: an 18 year experience in health care workers. Vaccine 2004;22(5–6):607–10.

21. Coppeta L, Pompei A, Balbi O, et al. Persistence of immunity for hepatitis B virus among Healthcare workers and Italian medical students 20 Years after vaccination. Int J Environ Res Public Health 2019;16(9):1515.

22. Trevisan A. Long-term persistence of immunity after hepatitis B vaccination: a fact, not a fancy. Hum Vaccin Immunother 2017;13(4):916–7.

23. Lao TT. Long-term persistence of immunity after hepatitis B vaccination: is this substantiated by the literature? Hum Vaccin Immunother 2017;13(4):918–20.

24. Terrault NA, Lok ASF, McMahon BJ, et al. Update on prevention, diagnosis, and treatment of chronic hepatitis B: AASLD 2018 hepatitis B guidance. Hepatology 2018;67(4):1560–99.

25. De Schryver A, Lambaerts T, Lammertyn N, et al. European survey of hepatitis B vaccination policies for healthcare workers: an updated overview. Vaccine 2020; 38(11):2466–72.

26. Werner JM, Abdalla A, Gara N, et al. The hepatitis B vaccine protects re-exposed health care workers, but does not provide sterilizing immunity. Gastroenterology 2013;145:1026–34.

27. Leuridan E, Van Damme P. Hepatitis B and the need for a booster dose. Clin Infect Dis 2011;53:68–75.

28. Spradling PR, Williams RE, Xing J, et al. Towers J. Serologic testing for protection against hepatitis B virus infection among students at a health sciences university in the United States. Infect Control Hosp Epidemiol 2012;33:732–6.

29. McMahon BJ, Dentinger CM, Bruden D, et al. Antibody levels and protection after hepatitis B vaccine: results of a 22-year follow-up study and response to a booster dose. J Infect Dis 2009;200:1390–6.

30. Saco TV, Strauss AT, Ledford DK. Hepatitis B vaccine nonresponders: possible mechanisms and solutions. Ann Allergy Asthma Immunol 2018;121(3):320–7.

31. Walayat S, Ahmed Z, Martin D, et al. Recent advances in vaccination of non-responders to standard dose hepatitis B virus vaccine. World J Hepatol 2015; 7(24):2503–9.

32. Averhoff F, Mahoney F, Coleman P, et al. Immunogenicity of hepatitis B vaccines. Implications for persons at occupational risk of hepatitis B virus infection. Am J Prev Med 1998;15:1–8.

33. Hung IF, Yap DY, Yip TP, et al. A double-blind randomized phase 2 controlled trial of intradermal hepatitis B vaccination with a topical Toll-like receptor 7 agonist imiquimod, in patients on dialysis. Clin Infect Dis 2020. https://doi.org/10.1093/cid/ciaa804.

34. Mello MM, Silverman RD, Omer SB. Ensuring uptake of vaccines against SARS-CoV-2. N Engl J Med 2020;383:1296–9.

35. Lewis JD, Enfield KB, Sifri CD. Hepatitis B in healthcare workers: transmission events and guidance for management. World J Hepatol 2015;7(3):488–97.

36. CDC menu state vaccination laws. Available at: https://www.cdc.gov/phlp/docs/menu-hepb.pdf. Accessed March 2, 2021.

37. Section 216-RICR-20-15-7.6 - Minimum Standards for Immunization and Communicable Disease Testing for Health Care Workers. Available at: https://casetext.com/regulation/rhode-island-administrative-code/title-216-department-of-health/chapter-20-community-health/subchapter-15-information-for-health-care-professionals/part-7-immunization-testing-and-health-screening-for-health-care-workers/section-216-

ricr-20-15-76-effective-until-1142021minimum-standards-for-immunization-and-communicable-disease-testing-for-health-care-workers. Accessed on July 21, 2021.

38. Centers for Disease Control and Prevention. Updated CDC recommendations for the management of hepatitis B virus–infected health-care providers and students. MMWR Recomm Rep 2012;61(No. RR-3):1–12.

39. Henderson DK, Dembry L, Fishman NO, et al. SHEA guideline for management of healthcare workers who are infected with hepatitis B virus, hepatitis C virus, and/or human immunodeficiency virus. Infect Control Hosp Epidemiol 2010;31: 203–32.

40. Gerlich WH. Reduction of infectivity in chronic hepatitis B virus carriers among healthcare providers and pregnant women by antiviral therapy. Intervirology 2014;57(3–4):202–11.

41. EASL clinical practice guidelines: management of hepatitis B virus infection. J Hepatol 2017;67:370–98.

Novel Therapies That May Cure Chronic Hepatitis B Virus

Alessandro Loglio, MD[a], Mauro Viganò, MD, PhD[b],
Pietro Lampertico, MD, PhD[a,c],*

KEYWORDS

- Hepatitis B virus • Viral replication cycle • cccDNA • New anti-HBV therapy
- Inhibitors of viral replication • Viral replication Inhibitors • Viral antigen inbibitors
- Immunomodulators

KEY POINTS

- The virus replication cycle consists of several phases that starts with the adhesion of mature virions to the NTCP. After the entry of the Dane particle into the cell, the rcDNA-containing nucleocapsid is released into the cytoplasm and travels to the nucleus where is converted to a covalently close circular DNA (cccDNA).
- cccDNA serves as a template for the transcription of different types of genomic and pgRNA and is the stabilized form for viral replication that is relatively resistant to the action of antivirals and the immune system.
- Long-term NA treatment achieve and maintain viral replication suppression thus preventing CHB progression, however with low rates of HBsA seroclearance.
- None of the NAs that inhibits the DNA-polymerase can directly target and efficiently clear the cccDNA, which persists in the nuclei of the infected hepatocytes allowing treatment to be stopped with no risk of virological relapse.
- New anti-HBV strategies that target directly or indirectly HBsAg, to achieve functional cure (HBsAg loss, and eventually anti-HBs seroconversion) are based on the short-term administration of combination therapies characterized by complementary and synergistics mechanisms of action.
- The new antiviral treatments targeting one or multiple critical steps of viral life could be classified in 3 groups: inhibitors of viral replication (to control viral replication and cccDNA reamplification); viral antigen inhibitors (to inhibit HBV life-cycle process through different mechanism) and immune modulators (to activate and restore immune response to HBV).

[a] Division of Gastroenterology and Hepatology, Foundation IRCCS Ca' Granda Ospedale Maggiore Policlinico, Via F. Sforza 35, 20122 Milan, Italy; [b] Hepatology Division, San Giuseppe Hospital Multimedica Spa, Via San Vittore 12, 20123 Milan, Italy; [c] Department of Pathophysiology and Transplantation, CRC "A. M. and A. Migliavacca" Center for Liver Disease, University of Milan, Via F. Sforza 35, Milan 20122, Italy
* Corresponding author. Division of Gastroenterology and Hepatology, Foundation IRCCS Ca' Granda Ospedale Maggiore Policlinico, CRC "A. M. and A. Migliavacca" Center for Liver Disease, University of Milan, Via F. Sforza 35, Milan 20122, Italy.
E-mail address: pietro.lampertico@unimi.it

Clin Liver Dis 25 (2021) 875–899
https://doi.org/10.1016/j.cld.2021.07.001
1089-3261/21/© 2021 Elsevier Inc. All rights reserved.
liver.theclinics.com

THE HEPATITIS B VIRUS
The Viral Structure

The hepatitis B virus (HBV) is a member of the Hepadnaviridae family, which includes small DNA enveloped viruses that infect primates, rodents, and birds and is the causative factor of chronic hepatitis B (CHB). A common feature of all these viruses is their great specificity by species and cell type, as well as a peculiar genomic and replication organization similar to that of retroviruses.[1]

The HBV virion consists of an external lipid envelope and an internal icosahedral protein capsid containing the viral genome and a DNA polymerase, which also functions as a reverse transcriptase.

The HBV structure is characterized by various antigenic properties: the surface antigen (HBsAg), the envelope antigen (HBeAg), the core antigen (HBcAg), and intracytoplasmic proteins: protein X (HBx) and polymerase (**Fig. 1**).[1]

The Hepatitis B Virus Genome

The relatively small genome of HBV is composed of partially double-stranded relaxed circular DNA (rcDNA) with a length of about 3200 bases, which is composed of a complete coding minus strand and an incomplete noncoding plus strand with a fixed 5′ end and a variable-size 3′ end.[2,3] The relaxed circular configuration of HBV genome (**Fig. 2**) is maintained by the cohesive end regions containing 2 direct repeats: DR1 (nt 1824–1834) and DR2 (nt 1590–1600).[4] Both DR1 and DR2 play the important roles in viral replication and the integration of HBV DNA sequences into host cell genome. DR1 and DR2 at the 5′ end of the plus strand are required for the strand-specific synthesis of DNA.[5]

The coding minus strand contains 4 overlapping open-reading frames (ORFs) (preC/C, P, preS/S, and X), 4 promoters (core promoter [CP, nt 1613–1849] consists of the upper regulatory region [URR, nt 1613–1742] and the basal core promoter [BCP, nt 1742–1849], PreS1 promoter [SP I, nt2718–2808], PreS2 promoter [SP II, nt 2983–3210], and X promoter [XP, nt 1171–1361]), and 2 enhancers (Enhancer I [EN I, nt 957–1361] and Enhancer II [EN II, nt 1685–1773]), as well as polyadenylation [poly(A)] signal (nt 1916–1921).[6–9] Under the regulation of 4 promoters and 2 enhancers, the 3.5, 2.4, 2.1, and 0.7 kb polyadenylated HBV RNAs are generated, respectively.[10,11]

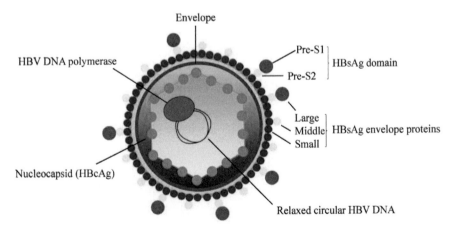

Fig. 1. The virion structure of HBV.

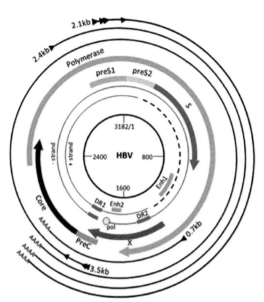

Fig. 2. The relaxed circular configuration of HBV. (*From* Minor MM, Slagle BL. Hepatitis B Virus HBx Protein Interactions with the Ubiquitin Proteasome System. Viruses. 2014; 6(11):4683-4702. https://doi.org/10.3390/v6114683.)

The preC/C ORF and P ORF overlap each other partially. The gene coding for protein C has the pre-Core and Core regions within it. Region C encodes both for the viral nucleocapsid, HBcAg, and for the HBeAg depending on whether the reading is initiated, respectively, from the Core or pre-Core region. The Core protein has the intrinsic property of self-assembling into a capsid structure and contains a highly basic amino acid cluster at the C-terminal end with binding function for RNA and binds with covalently closed circular DNA (cccDNA) to participate in its epigenetic modifications.

The P ORF is responsible for the synthesis of HBV DNA polymerase (P protein) that is functionally divided into 3 domains: the terminal region, which is involved in encapsidation and initiation of strand synthesis negative; reverse transcriptase, which catalyzes DNA synthesis; and the H ribonuclease, which degrades pregenomic RNA (pgRNA) and facilitates replication. Core protein and P protein are translated from pregenomic RNA, whereas HBeAg is translated from precore mRNA. Both pgRNA and precore mRNA are transcriptionally regulated by CP in which the URR regulates the promoter activity and the BCP regulates the transcriptions of both pgRNA and precore mRNA.[6,12–17]

The precursor of HBeAg undergoes proteolytic processing in the endoplasmic reticulum (ER) and generates the mature HBeAg.[18] Although HBeAg is not essential for the viral replication and infection, such a secretory protein has immune regulatory functions in inducing immunologic tolerance and thus favoring the chronicization of the infection.[19,20]

The preS/S ORF is located within P ORF and uses 3 different in-frame AUG start codons to encode 3 envelope glycoproteins including large (L), middle (M), and small (S) HBsAg. L-HBsAg is translated from the 2.4 kb HBV RNA transcriptionally regulated by SP I, and the latter 2 envelope glycoproteins are translated from 2.1 kb HBV RNA transcriptionally regulated by SP II.[21]

The X ORF is the smallest ORF and overlaps with P ORF and encodes a 16.5 kD protein (HBx), which has various functions including signal transduction, transcriptional activation, DNA repair, and inhibition of protein degradation. The mechanism of these activities and the biological functions of HBx within the life cycle of the virus are currently unknown. Despite this, it has been shown that its presence is necessary not only for the infection to be productive in living beings but also in the oncogenetic potential of HBV. HBx is translated from the 0.7 kb HBV RNA, which is transcriptionally regulated by XP.

In addition to the promoter elements, the expressions of these viral genes are also modulated by 2 enhancer elements: EN I and EN II giving the virus tissue selectivity for hepatocytes. EN I is located between ORF S and X and consists of a 5′ modulatory element, a central core domain with actual enhancer activity and a 3′ domain that overlaps with X ORF.[22,23] EN II is located at the upstream of CP and partially overlaps with BCP and URR, which comprises region IIA and IIB potent enhancer elements.[11,12] Both EN I and EN II have the ability to upregulate the activities of the HBV promoters in an orientation-independent manner, in which EN I preferentially upregulates the activities of CP/BCP and XP but has a modest effect on the activities of SP I and SP II, whereas EN II preferentially upregulates the activities of the SP I, SP II, and XP.[12,13,24–26]

Hepatitis B Virus Replication Cycle

The virus replication cycle consists of several phases (**Fig. 3**). The initial phase includes the adhesion of mature virions to the cell membrane. Recently, the HBV virion entry receptor has been identified as the sodium/taurocholate cotransporting polypeptide (NTCP).[27] This polypeptide interacts with the pre-S1 regions of the L-HBsAg protein and mediates the entry of the Dane particle into the cell. On fusion with the host membrane, the rcDNA-containing nucleocapsid is released into the cytoplasm and travels to the nucleus. Once inside, rcDNA is converted to a highly stable episomal DNA known as covalently close circular DNA (cccDNA) via the host DNA repair

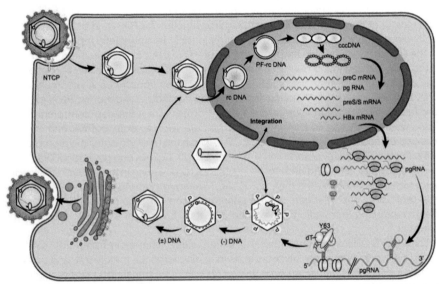

Fig. 3. HBV replication cycle. (*From* Tong, S. and Revill, P., 2016. Overview of hepatitis B viral replication and genetic variability. Journal of Hepatology, [online] 64(1), pp.S4-S16. Available at: https://www.sciencedirect.com/science/article/pii/S0168827816000635?via%3Dihub#f0005 [Accessed 28 July 2021].)

machinery molecule.[28,29] cccDNA serves as a template for the transcription of different types of genomic and pgRNA and is the stabilized form for viral replication that is relatively resistant to the action of antivirals and the immune system.[30] HBV DNA is also found integrated into the host chromosome although integration of viral DNA does not seem to play a direct role in virus replication. Instead, it is thought that HBV DNA integration may render the cellular environment more permissive to virus replication through modulating gene expression. It also likely plays an important role in hepatocellular carcinogenesis.[31]

The 3.5 Kbase transcripts are represented by 2 species with different 5' end groups: pgRNA and pre-Core RNA. The first serves as a template for reverse transcription and messenger RNA for the Core and pol gene; the pre-Core RNA instead controls the translation of the products of the related gene. Polymerase synthesis started at the start codon of the pol gene in the pgRNA, probably due to a ribosomal scanning mechanism. The L-HBsAg, the largest form of the surface antigen, is translated by a 2.4 Kbase subgenomic RNA; the intermediate (M-HBsAg) and small (S-HBsAg) forms by the various 2.1 Kbase RNAs; and the HBxAg protein by the 0.7 Kbase form. S-HBsAg is the major product of the S gene, and the L and M forms represent minor species.

The replication of HBV begins with the encapsidation of the genome. The terminal area of the pol protein interacts with the assembly signal and, together with the Core protein, forms the nucleocapsid. After encapsidation, the pol protein mediates the reverse transcription of pgRNA in the negative strand and consequently the synthesis of the positive strand. The circular shape of the DNA is completed via many strand transfer steps. Once all viral proteins are synthesized and the rcDNA-containing nucleocapsid is formed, it can travel through the cellular secretion pathway and be released as an enveloped and infectious virion. Alternatively, the nucleocapsid can cycle back to the nucleus intracellularly, whereby the recently synthesized rcDNA serves to replenish the cccDNA pool. In this way, cccDNA can be maintained even in the absence of observable viremia.[1,2]

cccDNA AND WHY IT IS SO HARD TO ERADICATE

At the time of hepatocyte infection, the nucleocapsid of the Core is released into the cytoplasm and the viral DNA is transferred to the cell nucleus, where the partially double-stranded rcDNA is converted into a molecule of cccDNA.[32,33] At the biochemical level this transformation requires the removal of the DNA polymerase attached covalently to the 5' end of the minus strand, the removal of the RNA oligomer present in the positive strand of the 5' end - which is then used as a primer for synthesis-, the removal of the terminal of the negative filament, the completion of the positive filament - which has a variable length in the rc form, exploiting the replicative mechanisms of the host cell - and finally the coupling of the 2 filaments.[34]

In the liver of infected individuals, most cccDNA arises from the accumulation of protein-free rcDNA, which is composed of rcDNA from which the polymerase has been removed, but unlike rcDNA it contains almost exclusively mature positive filaments.[32] Masked as a stable nonintegrated minichromosome, cccDNA is not replicated via the viral mechanisms of semiconservative DNA synthesis but uses the cellular RNA-producing transcription systems necessary for protein synthesis and viral replication, which occurs in the cytoplasm after transcription inverse of pgRNA.[35] The cccDNA pool does not derive from the infection by many virions but from the release of many newly formed nucleocapsids from a few cells containing a stable cccDNA pool. In any case, the viral and host factors that control the formation of this are unclear. A negative feedback system may be involved in the production of L-HBsAg such that after the production of an adequate number of 10 to 50 proteins the amplification of the cccDNA is disrupted and redirected to the mature nucleocapsids for envelope production and secretion.

The cccDNA is very stable in quiescent hepatocytes, and the pool of this, once created, can be reduced through various mechanisms that include cell elimination, dilution due to cell proliferation, and "cure" mechanisms involving cytokines. Control of cccDNA by reducing its transcriptional activity has recently been proposed.

In general, cccDNA can persist for the entire lifespan of the hepatocyte without affecting its functionality. On the contrary, cell proliferation can favor the dilution/loss of cccDNA during mitosis, as a selection of the cells that do not contain it can take place through the intervention of T cells.[36] During viral clearance, cytokines are hypothesized to block viral replication and the formation of further cccDNA. The release of infected hepatocytes from both replicative intermediates and cccDNA can occur in 3 ways. In the first, cccDNA is eliminated primarily by cytokines and cell death; however, this pathway is minor in overall viral clearance. In the second, cytokines suppress viral replication in the cytoplasm and prevent the formation of further cccDNA, but these do not act on the preexisting one, which must instead be eliminated by cell death or mitosis (which requires a turnover of about 70% of the mass total liver disease): this pattern is also known as "compensatory death and proliferation." In the third, cccDNA survives mitosis, is distributed binomially to the hepatocyte progeny, and is eliminated only by killing infected cells; in this way it is necessary that the hepatic cell pool is completely replaced 2.5 times before clearance is achieved: this pattern is also known as "cell death".[32]

A computer model based on observations in the marmot liver treated with Entecavir showed that in addition to cell death, a combination of cytokine suppression and mitotic loss is also needed for cccDNA to be lost. Traces of cccDNA were found in the liver of chronically infected marmots even in cells that had lost the pool, as the viral DNA is able to integrate into the host's genome[37] and as the destruction of the cccDNA, but not of the cell that contained it, is not entirely effective in eliminating the viral genome. Because the death and regeneration of hepatocytes normally occurs in the marmot liver, an alternative hypothesis proposed is that in the surviving hepatocytes both the integration and the cccDNA are present; the latter is lost but not the integrated heritage. On the other hand, some studies have shown how levels, although very low, of cccDNA can persist indefinitely,[38,39] providing a possible explanation of the immune response to HBV that persists even after the infection is resolved.

Because polymerase inhibitors do not directly affect cccDNA, a decrease in its levels is assumed to result from the lack of sufficient viral nucleocapsids in the nucleus, given the potent inhibition of DNA synthesis in the cytoplasm and a reduced number of virions in the blood. In this scenario, cccDNA depletion requires many years of treatment with analogues and is believed to lead to the selection of resistances.[40]

The nuclear molecules of hepadnaviridae cccDNA are organized in a chromatinlike structure as a viral minichromosome that presents the typical characteristics of chromosomes when observed under an electron microscope. In fact, 2 populations of minichromosomes can be found, corresponding to a whole or a half nucleosome, based on transcriptional regulation. It has been shown that the HBV minichromosome contains both histone and nonhistone proteins.[35]

The development of highly selective real-time polymerase chain reaction allowed to further investigate the replicative activity and efficacy of antiviral therapy in treated patients by determining both serum and intrahepatic HBV DNA levels, including quantification of cccDNA in biopsy samples. Several studies have shown that the share of the latter varies considerably according to the stage of infection; in fact the patients who had seroconverted to anti-HBe showed lower levels of cccDNA.[32] The lower viremia of these patients also seems to be determined not only by lower levels of cccDNA but also by a lower replicative efficiency, also demonstrated by the relative share of rcDNA. Quantitative measurement of viral RNA also indicated that stability at a lower level of pgRNA found in HBeAg-negative patients was responsible for the lower virion production observed at the DNA level.[41]

In experimental models with transgenic mice and chimpanzees it has been shown that proinflammatory cytokines such as interferon-1 (IFN-1) and tumor necrosis factor-α can effectively suppress viral replication through noncytolytic patterns, which also contributes to the reduction of the cccDNA pool. In the chronic phase of the disease, however, these mechanisms may prove ineffective; in the absence of cell division, the long half-life of the hepatocytes guarantees the survival of cccDNA in infected cells. It is likely that the complex interchange between the virus and the host, which occurs in the various stages of chronic infection, promotes the selection of some variants of HBV. An in vivo virological study has demonstrated the continued accumulation of viral genetic diversity in patients who seroconvert to anti-HBe as a product of immunologic pressure.[42] Transcription of pgRNA is under the control of the BCP; mutations in this region and in the pre-Core region are common in HBeAg-negative subjects, and these have been shown to regulate viral replication in vitro. The occurrence of mutations within the regulatory regions of the virus can have effects on replication in vivo, but at the moment most of the studies concerning these events are on in vitro models, in which the structure and organization of the cccDNA cannot be replicated.

The transcriptional regulation of genes is based on nuclear enzymatic activities that constantly modify chromatin to make it permissive or refractory to the activation of genes. Given that the cccDNA has a nucleosomal organization in infected cells and is the template for cellular polymerases to produce viral messenger RNAs, the acetylation and deacetylation of histones could regulate the expression of cccDNA.[34] It has also been shown that nucleos(t)ide analogues (NAs) have no effect on cccDNA acetylation.[32] The long-term stability and persistence of cccDNA in the hepatocyte nucleus is the molecular basis for occult HBV infection, a form characterized by the persistence of HBV DNA in liver tissue and serum in the absence of HBsAg positivity, and the risk of viral reactivation in case of immunosuppression.[43]

Despite the significant progress into the control of HBV infections and prevention of CHB progression[44] with very high rates of persistently undetectable serum HBV DNA but detectable serum HBsAg achieved by NA, none of these drugs that inhibits the DNA-polymerase can directly target and efficiently clear the cccDNA, which persists in the nuclei of the infected hepatocytes, and for this reason the "complete sterilizing cure" or "clinical cure" of CHB (ie, undetectable HBsAg in serum and eradication of HBV DNA including viral intrahepatic cccDNA and integrated HBV DNA allowing treatment to be stopped with no risk of virological relapse) may not be feasible.[45]

ENDPOINTS OF THERAPY AND TARGETED POPULATIONS

While the current antiviral paradigm aims to achieve and maintain long-term suppression of viral replication, HBV DNA less than 10 to 15 IU/mL, new anti-HBV strategies target directly or indirectly HBsAg, to achieve functional cure, that is, HBsAg loss, and eventually anti-HBs seroconversion. The former strategy requires the long-term administration of NA monotherapy, whereas the latter would be based on the short-term administration of combination therapies characterized by complementary and synergistics mechanisms of action. *Partial cure* refers to sustained virological suppression after stopping NA, even if patients are still HBsAg positive.

Safe and well-tolerated, with high barrier to resistance, third-generation NA inhibits conversion of pgRNA to dsDNA but, because of the refractory nature of the intracellular cccDNA, fewer than 1% of HBV patients *per* year will achieve HBsAg loss,[46] therefore needing a long-term, maybe for life, treatment.

There are many advantages in reaching the functional cure for NA-suppressed patients: stop NA safely (even in compensated cirrhotics), less monitoring (for noncirrhotic population), reduction of safety issues related to NA, save money (for NA withdrawal, etc.), reduction of infected cells and/or cccDNA, and maybe a lower HCC risk. In an NA-naïve population, a short-term finite therapy achieving HBsAg loss could allow to expand the anti-HBV treatment criteria, to "cure" many more patients and to reach the target of WHO in eradicating HBV within 2030.

PROPOSED STRATEGIES FOR NOVEL HEPATITIS B VIRUS THERAPIES

Because cccDNA is the main cause that CHB is difficult to cure, the elimination, or at the very least, transcriptional control of cccDNA is an ideal goal for the cure of CHB. The new antiviral treatments targeting one or multiple critical steps of viral life cycle (**Fig. 4**) may be an alternative approach to long-term NA administration and could be classified in 3 groups (**Fig. 5**):

1. Inhibitors of viral replication (to control viral replication and cccDNA reamplification);
2. Viral antigen inhibitors (to inhibit HBV life-cycle process through different mechanism);
3. Immune modulators (to activate and restore immune response to HBV).

The cccDNA inhibitor compounds should be the fourth group, the most important to achieve HBV sterilizing cure by directly targeting cccDNA, however still in preclinical development, and these newer liver-targeted delivery systems should overcome the potential off-target toxicities associated with antisense oligos.[47]

While **Table 1** summarizes drugs under evaluation, next sections focus on new anti-HBV compounds in clinical phases of development.

Inhibitor of Viral Replication

Although inhibition of viral replication is already the aim of current anti-HBV therapies based on long-term administration of NA, there is evidence that low-level ongoing intrahepatic viral replication continues despite, for example, ETV or TDF administration, drugs both potent and almost resistant-free. This residual intrahepatic viremia may lead to continuous de-novo infection of the hepatocytes, contributing to HBsAg positivity as well as to HCC development.

One new strategy could be to target the HBV core protein, a unique viral protein that is essential for the HBV nucleocapsid assembly. Its inhibition would suppress the production of HBV virions (primary mechanism of action) but also reduce cccDNA replenishment (secondary mechanism of action) (see **Fig. 4**). HBV core protein allosteric modulators (CpAMs) have different chemical structures and induce allosteric conformational changes in the core protein subunits, therefore making capsids unable to encapsidate viral RNA.[48] Three classes of CpAMs have been described according to allosteric modulation: (1) "misdirectors", such as heteroaryl-dihydropyrimidine derivatives, that misdirect core protein dimers to assemble non-capsid polymers (Class I); (2) "accelerators of capside assembly", such as

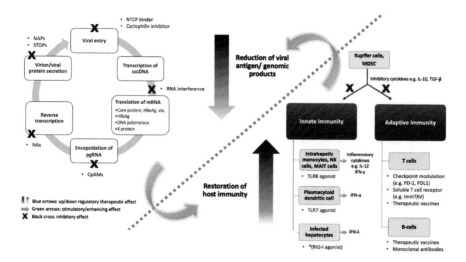

Fig. 4. HBV life cycle and antiviral drugs under evaluation. Therapeutic approaches currently in clinical development in chronic hepatitis B infection. [a]RIG-I agonists once entered a phase 2 clinical trial but this was terminated due to a safety issue. cccDNA, covalently closed circular DNA; CpAMs, core protein allosteric modulators; CTLA-4, cytotoxic T lymphocyte–associated protein 4; HBeAg, hepatitis B e antigen; HBsAg, hepatitis B surface antigen; IFN, interferon; IL, interleukin; ImmTAV, immune-mobilizing monoclonal T-cell receptor against viruses; MAIT, muscosal-associated invariant T cells; MDSC, myeloid-derived suppressor cell; mRNA, messenger RNA; NAs, nucleos(t)ide angalogues; NAPs, nucleic acid polymers; NK, natural killer; NTCP, sodium taurocholate co-transporting polypeptide; PD-1, programmed death-1; PD-L1, programmed death-ligand 1; pgRNA, pregenomic RNA; RIG-1, retinoic acid–induced gene-I; TLR, toll-like receptor. (*From* Mak L-Y, Seto W-K, Yuen M-F. Novel Antivirals in Clinical Development for Chronic Hepatitis B Infection. Viruses 2021;13:1169. https://doi.org/10.3390/v13061169.)

phenylpropanamides; and (3) "noneffector for empty capside", such as sulfamoyl-benzamides. The last 2 compounds that induce the assembly of empty capsids or capside unable of encapsidate RNA represents Class II CpAMs. At least 7 different compounds belong to this class, as well as some new-discover allosteric modulators. A CpAM-based strategy would have the advantage of being administered orally but the disadvantage of requiring a combination therapy with nucleoside analogue to minimize the risk of resistance.[49,50]

In an ongoing phase II study, 125 NA-naïve and 125 ETV-suppressed patients with CHB will be randomly allocated 4:1 to receive 120 mg of Class 1 CpAM GLS4 + 100 mg ritonavir (TID) + ETV or ETV monotherapy for 96 weeks. In an interim analysis, out of 77 patients who received treatment greater than 12 weeks, 12.5% patients in the GLS4/ritonavir group achieved a 1.5 Log HBsAg decline at week 24 compared with none of ETV group. In the naive patients, GLS4/ritonavir was more effective at week 24 than ETV in suppressing pgRNA (2.63 vs 0.27 Log IU/mL) and HBsAg levels (0.43 vs 0.21 Log IU/mL). In NA-suppressed cohorts, the mean declines of pgHBV RNA were 1.59 versus 0.15 Log IU/mL, whereas HBsAg 0.11 versus 0 Log IU/mL, respectively. A grade 3 increase of alanine aminotransferase (ALT) levels was observed in 7.1% patients under GLS4/ritonavir + ETV (vs 2.6% in ETV).[51]

The efficacy and safety of combination of NA with CpAM Class II JNJ-6379 at 2 different daily dose (75 mg vs 250 mg vs pbo) is under evaluation in a phase II study.

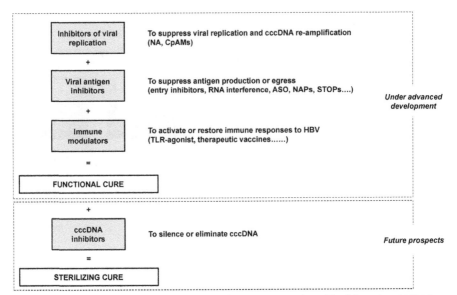

Fig. 5. The possible future curative regimens for hepatitis B. (*Modified from* Seto WK, Yuen MF. New pharmacological approaches to a functional cure of hepatitis B. Clin Liver Dis (Hoboken). 2016 Oct 27;8(4):83-88. doi: 10.1002/cld.577. eCollection 2016 Oct)

Of 172 patients in the combination arms (88 naive; 84 NA-treated), 48% were Asian and 34% HBeAg-positive. Even the degree of HBsAg reduction was relatively modest (0.4 Log) in HBeAg-positive treatment-naïve patients at week 24; JNJ-6379 75 mg and 250 mg + NA showed a higher HBV RNA median decline from baseline (2.82 and 3.13 Log cp/mL) over NA + placebo (1.43 Log cp/mL). In NA-naïve cohort, HBV RNA became undetectable at week 24 in 16/27 (59%), 19/25 (76%), and 9/20 (45%) of patients treated with 75 mg versus 250 mg versus pbo + NA. Moreover, combination was effective in suppression of HBV DNA and safe, therefore under evaluation also with a third new compound (small interfering RNA [siRNA]).[52]

ABI-H0731 (vebicorvir), a first-generation HBV Class 2 core protein inhibitor that has demonstrated effective antiviral activity in patients with CHB in a phase 1b clinical trial,[53] entered in phase II studies (study 201 and 202). Study 202 evaluated 25 HBeAg-positive treatment-naïve CHB patients that were randomized 1:1 to ETV versus ETV + ABI-H0731 for 24 weeks.[54] The 12 patients treated with combination regimen showed a significantly faster and deeper reduction in HBV DNA levels, as early as week 2 ($P = .03$) compared with ETV cohort; this difference in HBV DNA level between Combination versus NA arm increased over time (median −1 Log at week 12, and −2 Log at week 24). All patients on combination arm achieved a rapid decline in HBV RNA levels, and, among subjects with abnormal ALT at entry, a more rapid ALT normalization was seen in combination than in ETV arm: 5/7 versus 0/5 by week 4 ($P<.05$) and 7/7 versus 2/5 by week 12 ($P<.05$). Study 201 enrolled 73 NUC-suppressed CHB patients, both HBeAg negative and positive, who were randomized to NA + ABI-H0731 versus NA. Among patients with detectable baseline HBV RNA (N = 37), this biomarker became less than LOQ (200 copies/mL) at week 16 in 60% of NA + ABI-H0731 subjects compared with 0% on NA monotherapy. However, no HBsAg decline greater than 0.5 Log was observed at week 24. In terms of safety, ABI-H0731 was well tolerated, without significant ALT flares and only 3 grade 1 to 2

Table 1
Novel anti-hepatitis B virus drugs under clinical development

Antiviral Group	Main Mechanism	Subtype	Drug	Phase	Delivery	Clinical Trial Number
Inhibitors of viral replication	Inhibition of Capsid formation (CpAM)	Class 1	GLS-4 (Morphothiadin) ritonavir	2	Oral	NCT04147208
		Class 2	JNJ-6379	2		NCT03361956
		Class 2	ABI-HB07311 (vebicorvir)	2		NCT03780543
		Class 2	ABI-H2158	2		NCT04398134
		Class 2	EDP-514	1		NCT04470388
		NA	QL-007	1		NCT03244085
		Class 2	ZM-H1505R	1		NCT04220801
		Class 2	ABI-H3733	1		NCT04271592
		Class 2	ALG-000184	1		NCT04536337
		Class 1	R07049359 (RG7907)	1		NCT02952924
Viral antigen inhibitors	Entry-inhibitor	NTCP binding	Bulevirtide	3	SC	NCT03852719
	RNA interference	Cyclophilin Inhibitor	CRV-431	1	Oral	NCT03596697
		siRNA	JNJ3959	2	SC	NCT04129554
			AB-729	2		NCT04820686
			VIR-2215	2		NCT03672188
			RG6346	1/2		NCT03772249
		ASO	G5K-S36-nonGalNAc	2	SC	NCT04449029
			GS K-404-GalNAc	2		NCT03020745
			RO7062931-GalNAc	1		NCT03038113
	Inhibition of HBsAg release	Nucleic acid polymer (NAP)	REP2139	2	IV	NCT02565719
		STOPS	ALG-010133	1	SC	NCT04485663
	Interaction with host nuclear receptors	FXR agonist	EYP001	2	Oral	NCT04465916
Immune modulation	Enhancement of innate immunity	TLR-7 agonist	Vesatolimod (GS-9620)	2	Oral	NCT02166047
			R07020531 (RG-7854)	1		NCT02956850
		TLR-8 agonist		2	Oral	NCT03491553

(continued on next page)

Table 1
(continued)

Antiviral Group	Main Mechanism	Subtype	Drug	Phase	Delivery	Clinical Trial Number
	Enhancement of adaptative immunity	Checkpoint inhibitor	Selgantolimod (GS-9655)			
			ASC22 (anti-PDL 1)	2	SC	NCT04465890
			APG-1387 (apoptosis inducer)	2	IV	NCT04568265
			Cemiplimab (anti-PDI)	1,2		NCT04046107
			IMC-1109 V (soluble T-cell receptor. ImmTAV molecule)	1/2		NCT03973333
			Nivolumab (anti-PDI)	1		ACTRN1261150011 33527 (Australian-NZ registry)
		Therapeutic vaccine	HeberNasvac (ABX-203)	3	Intranasal	NCT02249988
			GS-4774	2	SC	NCT01943799
			HepTcell	2	IM	NCT04684914
			TG-1050	1	SC	NCT02428400
			AIC649	1	IV	NA
		Monoclonal antibody	GC1102	2	IV	NCT03801798
			VIR-3434	1	SC/IV	NCT04423393

Abbreviations: ASO, antisense oligonucleotide; CpAM, core protein allosteric modulator (class 1: forming aberrant unstable capsids; class 2: forming empty capsids); FXR, farnesoid X receptor; IM, intramuscular; IV, intravenous; NTCP, sodium taurocholate cotransporting polypeptide; SC, subcutaneous; siRNA, small interfering RNA; STOPS, S-antigen transport-inhibiting oligonucleotide polymers; TLR, toll-like receptor.

self-limited rashes.[54] In the 211 study, 26 HBeAg-positive and 43 HBeAg-negative virally suppressed CHB patients with mild liver fibrosis who received ABI-H0731 + NA for 76 weeks were analyzed. Among these patients, 23 and 18 subjects, respectively, met the stopping criteria (HBsAg positivity but HBV DNA + pgRNA <20 IU/mL and HBeAg negative or HBeAg 5 IU/mL for 6 months at week 52): mean age of 46 years, 71% men, 78% Asian, 80% on TDF, and 20% on ETV. Because all patients experienced a virological relapse and none achieved HBsAg seroclearance[55] following drug discontinuation to achieve a finite HBV treatment, the clinical development of this compound was halted by the company in February 2021.

Class 2 ABI-H2158 in under evaluation in phase 2 trial but no clinical results are available.

Viral Antigen Inhibitors

Many compounds targeting different HBV life-cycle steps are under evaluation (see **Fig. 4** and **Table 1**).

Interference of hepatitis B virus RNA

RNA interference is a natural process by which an siRNA duplex directs sequence-specific posttranscriptional silencing by binding to complementary mRNA, triggering its elimination. siRNAs are administered subcutaneously, because they are rapidly digested in the gut and their intravenous administration is often associated with infusion reactions, and their conjugation with N-acetylgalactosamine (GalNAc) enhances hepatic uptake. Because the HBV genome is compact with multiple overlapping reading frames, a single siRNA can silence multiple transcripts, potentially blocking the production of the core, X-, polymerase, and surface proteins, and directly inhibit HBV replication and indirectly restore HBV-specific immunity.[56,57] Although first-developed siRNA targets cccDNA-derived pgRNA (the predominant source of HBsAg in younger HBeAg-positive patients) and not integrated HBs (the predominant source of HBsAg in older HBeAg-negative patients), thus being less effective in HBeAg-negative patients, a second-generation (ie, ARC521) that targets both integrated and cccDNA have been developed.[58] Most siRNAs are given at monthly doses and achieve potent and robust on-treatment HBsAg responses.

JNJ-3989 has shown promising reduction in virologic parameters (HBV DNA, RNA, HBcrAg, HBeAg) in 114 patients in phase I/II study, when it was named ARO-HBV. The phase II AROHBV1001 study that enrolled 56 patients with CHB, both HBeAg positive than negative, and both NUC treated than untreated, assessed the safety and efficacy of 3 doses of JNJ-3989 administered weekly to monthly, at different doses (100, 200, 300 or 400 mg/each), in some patients with a loading dose (bi-weekly treatments). All patients received NA from baseline, and after JNJ-3989 dosing ends. No serious AEs have been reported, and injection site AEs (all mild) occurred in ~12% out of 171 injections. Mean HBsAg decline was about 2 Logs in all different treatment arms, and a more frequent administration did not increase HBsAg loss rate. The nadir in HBsAg levels was reached around 4 months after JNJ-3989 introduction (88% patients reached an HBsAg <100 IU/mL), and HBsAg rebound was very slow (>4 months).[59]

To assess the sustained response in HBsAg, HBV RNA, HBeAg, and HBcrAg levels, all patients enrolled in the AROHBV1001 study were followed for 1 year after the last dose of JNJ-3989. Thirty-nine percent (15/38) of patients maintained a sustained response (defined as $\geq$1 Log IU/mL reduction in HBsAg level from day 0 to day 392). Reductions in HBV RNA, HBcrAg, and HBeAg levels were generally more pronounced in HBsAg sustained responders than in nonresponders. Doses up to 400 mg were well tolerated and seemed to have a good long-term safety profile, with one patient who experienced abdominal pain and another muscle pain as adverse events (none of grade 3 nor 4) in the 8 patients in 400 mg arm.[60]

In a phase II study, 24 noncirrhotic (18 HBeAg− and 6 HBeAg+), virologically suppressed CHB patients received 2 subcutaneous doses of VIR-2218 or placebo on day 1 and day 29 (doses from 20 to 200 mg) and followed-up for 12 weeks after the second dose and additional 32 weeks for participants achieving prespecified HBsAg declines. Maximum mean HBsAg Log IU/mL declines ranged from 1.03 to 1.65 for doses between 20 and 200 mg in HBeAg-negative patients and from 1.16 to 1.57 for HBeAg-positive ones, respectively. Most participants achieved maximum HBsAg decline by week 16, suggesting that VIR-2218 may silence transcripts from both cccDNA and integrated DNA. No significant changes in HBV DNA nor HBV RNA were detected, whereas a decline in qHBeAg and HBcrAg levels were observed in HBeAg-positive subjects receiving 200 mg VIR-2218. Treatment was well tolerated.[61]

IONIS-HBVRx, also known as GSK3228836, is an investigational antisense oligonucleotide (ASO) drug designed to specifically recognize all HBV RNAs and reduce the production of viral proteins, by inducing cleavage of HBV RNAs in the nucleus and cytoplasm via RNase H1. A phase II, double-blinded, randomized (3:1), placebo-controlled, dose-escalation (150 and 300 mg) study aimed to examine the safety and tolerability of IONIS-HBVRx subcutaneous administration to 31 treatment-naive CHB patients and the effects of subsequent NA treatment. At EASL 2020 meeting have been presented results of 12 naive versus 5 NA-treated Asian patients who introduced GSK836 300 mg by subcutaneous injections on days 1, 4, 8, 11, 15, and 22; from day 29 all naive patients introduced TDF or ETV for 6 months. HBeAg was negative in 50% of naive and 100% of NA-treated cohort at baseline. Five out of seventeen patients had injection site reactions, some lasting greater than 4 days. Reductions of HBsAg greater than 3 Log IU/mL were observed in 3 of 4 patients on stable NA regimens and in 3 of 12 naive patients, and prolonged HBsAg loss was observed in 1 NA-treated and 1 NA-naive patient. However, post-ASO ALT flare/elevation (higher in NA-naive group, up to 15xUNL) occurred in both naive than NA-treated group, which likely indicates infected hepatocyte clearance.[62] Longer administration of GSK3228836 is under evaluation in another phase II clinical trial, in both naive than NA-treated patients.

Inhibitors of viral entry

Bulevirtide (BLV, previously named Myrcludex-B), the first entry inhibitor of HBV/HDV in liver cells, blocks the interaction between sodium/NTCP) and large-HBsAg. Approved at the subcutaneous dose of 2 mg daily for the treatment of Hepatitis Delta by EMA in 2020, BLV treatment is still in a preclinical phase for patients with HBV monoinfection. A randomized, open-label multicentre phase 1b/2a clinical trial evaluated daily BLV administration versus ETV in 48 patients (97% Caucasian, 67% men) with naïve HBeAg-negative CHB, assigned at 6 treatment groups of 8 patients each, under subcutaneous injections of Myrcludex-B at 0.5 mg, 1 mg, 2 mg, and 5 mg daily doses for 12 weeks, 10 mg/d for 24 weeks, and ETV 0.5 mg monotherapy for 24 weeks (NCT02881008 Clinical Trial). No one showed HBsAg greater than 0.5 Log decline during 24 weeks of BLV 10 mg versus ETV. At week 12, HBV DNA was negative in 25%, 0%, 25%, 12.5%, and 75% under increasing dose of BLV, while 100% under ETV, whereas ALT normalized in 42.9%, 57.1%, 50%, 50%, 66.7%, and 57.1%, respectively. No cccDNA reduction was observed 12 weeks after 24 weeks of treatment with BLV 10 mg in 5 patients.

In HDV trials, the combination of PegIFN alpha2a and BLV for 48 weeks induced a greater decline of HBsAg (>1 Log IU/mL and/or HBsAg negativity) compared with either PegIFN alpha-2a or BLV monotherapy. The safe profile is excellent, as only a dose-related, however fully asymptomatic, increase in bile acids has been observed.[63,64] Therefore, many investigational preclinical trials are evaluating BLV as a useful HBV entry inhibitor strategy.

Inhibitors of HBsAg release

Nucleic acid polymers (NAPs) are a broad spectrum of antiviral agents that block the release of HBsAg from liver cells, thus allowing host-mediated HBV clearance by restoring functional control of HBV infection. The host protein interaction with NAPs that drives their antiviral effects is under evaluation, and the interaction targeted by NAP REP 2139 within infected cells has not yet been elucidated, and clinical trials are ongoing also on HDV coinfected patients.[65–67] In monotherapy, REP 2139 has been evaluated in phase I study (REP 102 study), enrolling 12 Bangladeshi naïve patients with HBeAg-positive CHB, 83% men, 50% genotype C, median age 21 years, and HBV-DNA 8 Logs cp/mL. REP 2139-Ca exposure was scheduled for 40 weeks of 500 mg weekly intravenous infusions (with hair loss, dysphagia, and dysgeusia, which were considered related to heavy metal exposure endemic at the trial site): 3 patients started ETV or TDF for nonresponse in monotherapy, whereas 9 of 12 patients who showed an initial virologic response and were transitioned to combined treatment with Peg-INF2a or thymosin alpha 1 for 13 to 26 weeks experienced HBsAg loss and seroconversion. Eight of nine patients achieved HBV DNA less than 116 copies/mL after all treatment withdrawal, whereas viral rebound occurred after 12 to 123 weeks in 7 patients.[68] Therefore, this drug should be promising in combination strategy: REP-2139 + PegIFN achieve significant declines in HBV DNA and HBsAg, and increased rates of anti-HBs seroconversion in 5 patients enrolled in another phase II trial (both HBeAg positive than negative, naïve or under ETV, adding-on Peg-IFN).

Immune Modulation

Because a vigorous and multispecific host immune response, mainly CD8+ T-cell mediated, against HBV is the major determinant of spontaneous clearance following an acute infection,[69] several approaches were evaluated that were thought to activate antiviral immunity against HBV, through the stimulation of antiviral effector cells (T cells, B cells, and dendritic cells), the generation of "new" T cells (therapeutic vaccines), or the recovery of exhausted T cells (typical of chronic HBV infection). This hypothesis is indeed supported by the widespread use of PegIFNalfa in the treatment of HBV, a potent immunomodulator.

Toll-like receptor agonist

The activation of toll-like receptor 7 (TLR-7) in plasma dendritic cells engages innate and adaptive effector cells, as well as antiviral cytokine responses. Clinical studies on the orally bioavailable TLR-7 agonist, GS-9620, and TLR-8 showed some enhancement of innate and HBV-specific immune responses, however, with no peculiar changes in HBV DNA nor HBsAg levels.[70,71]

Vesatolimod is a TLR-7 agonist, safe and well tolerated in patients with CHB, both naive than virally suppressed by NA. Although consistent dose-dependent pharmacodynamic induction of interferon-stimulated genes was demonstrated, it did not result in clinically significant HBsAg decline. In a phase II, double-blind, randomized, placebo-controlled study, 162 patients stratified by HBsAg levels and HBeAg status were randomized 1:3:3:3 to once-weekly oral placebo or vesatolimod (GS-9620; 1-, 2-, or 4-mg doses) for 4, 8, or 12 weeks per cohort. Most of the patients were men (76%) and HBeAg negative (79%) at baseline. Most (41%–80%) experienced more than or equal to 1 adverse event during the study, with the majority mild or moderate in severity. No significant declines in HBsAg were observed at the primary (week 24) or secondary endpoints (weeks 4, 8, 12, and 48). Interferon-stimulated gene (ISG)-15 induction was dose dependent and consistent after repeat dosing, returning closer to baseline by 1 week after treatment at all dose levels; no patient demonstrated significant serum IFNα expression at any timepoint evaluated. Multivariate analyses showed that greater than or equal to 2-fold ISG15 induction is associated with 2- or 4-mg vesatolimod dose and female sex.[72] One hundred ninety-two CHB-naive patients, stratified by HBeAg status and ALT level, were randomized 2:2:2:1 to receive oral vesatolimod (1-, 2-, or 4-mg) or placebo once weekly for 12 weeks in a phase II study; TDF was administered for 48 weeks. Primary endpoint was HBsAg decline at week 24 from baseline. Most patients were men (64.1%) and HBeAg negative (60.9%) at baseline. Many patients (60.4%–69.1%) experienced more than or equal to 1 treatment adverse event in vesatolimod arms, however mild or moderate in severity. No significant differences in HBsAg changes were observed and no patients experienced HBsAg loss, whereas 3 patients experienced HBeAg-seroconversion at week 48. HBV DNA suppression rates were similar across all treatment arms at week 24. ISG15 induction was dose dependent and did not correlate with HBsAg changes. A small proportion of patients exhibited dose-dependent IFNα induction that correlated with grade of influenza-like adverse events.[73]

The TLR-8 recognizes pathogen-derived single-stranded RNA fragments to trigger innate and adaptive immune responses; TLR-8 agonist has greater than 100-fold TLR-7 selectivity.[74] Selgantolimod (formerly GS-9688) induces cytokines in human peripheral blood mononuclear cells that are able to activate antiviral effector function by multiple immune mediators (HBV-specific CD8+ T cells, CD4+ follicular helper T cells, natural killer cells, and mucosal-associated invariant T cells). Although reducing the frequency of some immunoregulatory subsets, it enhances the immunosuppressive potential of others, highlighting potential biomarkers and immunotherapeutic targets to optimize the antiviral efficacy of GS-9688.[75] In a multicenter, double-blind, phase 2 study 67 patients with CHB were randomized in 2 cohorts (39 HBeAg-positive) to oral GS-9688 3 mg, 1.5 mg, and placebo (2:2:1) once a week for 24 weeks + TAF. Baseline characteristics were similar between groups: 98.5% Asian, 58% men, with a median age of 47 (35–54) years, HBsAg 4.1 (3.5–4.7) Log IU/mL, and HBV DNA level of 7.5 (5.4–8.3) Log IU/mL. No patients achieved the greater than or equal to 1 Log decline in HBsAg levels at week 24, and only 3 (6%) GS-9688-treated patients showed a decline greater than or equal to 0.5 Log at week 48. Most patients showed a decline of immune cell subsets in the circulation 4 hours after GS-9688 administration, concurrent with increases of circulating IL-12p40 and IL-1RA. However, these parameters reverted to baseline values at 24 hours postdosing, and nausea (26%), vomiting (17%), and fatigue (15%) were associated to new treatment. Therefore, further evaluation of GS-9688 in combination with immunomodulatory and antiviral agents is planned.[76]

Therapeutic vaccines

Many immunogenic and recombinant vaccines have been developed (against pre-S1, pre-S2, and T-cell peptide), generating HBV-specific B-cell and T-cell responses and protection in HBV-naïve individuals, however with no clinical or virological efficacy in patients with CHB (both naive than under NA treatment).[77] Here are summarized studies with available clinical results.

The therapeutic vaccine GS-4774, engineered using the Tarmogen (targeted molecular immunogen) platform and expressing surface, core, and X proteins, showed an

HBV-specific T-cell–mediated responses (core and X proteins) in untreated HBV patients but did not provide a significant reduction in HBsAg levels in virally suppressed patients.[78,79]

In a phase II study CHB-naïve patients were randomly assigned (1:2:2:2) to groups given oral TDF 300 mg daily alone (n = 27; controls) or with 2, 10, or 40 yeast units GS-4774 (n = 168), administered subcutaneously every 4 weeks until week 20 for a total of 6 doses. The primary endpoint was HBsAg change at week 24. GS-4774 was safe and well tolerated but did not reduce levels of HBsAg. However, it showed a strong immune stimulatory effect on CD8+ T cells: production of interferon gamma, tumor necrosis factor, and interleukin-2 increased significantly at weeks 24 and 48, compared with baseline, in HBV-specific CD8+ T cells from patients given GS-4774 but not from controls. GS-4774 had greater effects on CD8+ than CD4+ T cells, which were not affected at all or very weakly by TDF with or without GS-4774.[80] Its strong immune stimulatory effect on CD8+ T cells might be used in combination with other antiviral agents to boost the antivirus immune response.

ABX-203 is a new vaccine formulation (developed ad NASVAC by CGB, Cuba) combining HBV surface and core antigens. Simultaneous administration of intranasal and subcutaneous drug increases the immune response. In a phase I trial, 6 patients with CHB who had prior PEG-IFN treatment received ABX-203 intranasally every 2 hours, for a total of 10 doses and followed-up for 5 years. HBsAg seroclearance occurred in 2 out of 6 patients during follow-up, and 2 patients had ALT flare.[81] In phase III trial, 276 subjects with CHB (94% Asian, 72% men, HBsAg >1000 IU/mL at baseline, mean age 50 years) under NA from 4.8 ± 2.4 years were randomized in 2 cohorts: for 6 months, Group 1 (N = 184) added 5 intranasal ABX203 100 ug administrations every 2 weeks, followed by 5 administrations of intranasal + subcutaneous vaccine every 2 weeks, whereas Group 2 (N = 92) maintained NA alone. After 24 weeks of treatment, NA was stopped in all patients, evaluating the percentage of patients who maintained HBV DNA undetectable during 24 weeks of follow-up. No differences occurred in Group 1 versus 2 (6.9% vs 11.7%, $P = .20$), and ALT values (74% vs 80%) and HBsAg declined, even if viral rebound (HBV DNA >2000 IU/mL) occurred much earlier in patients treated with TDF (>70% at week 12) versus entecavir (<10% at week 12) irrespective of ABX203 treatment. Future studies need to investigate if alternative vaccine regimens (ie, after stopping NA) may induce off-therapy viral control.[82]

Combination of Three Approaches

Even though preliminary results of each phase II study are promising, the combination of 3 complementary strategies, that is, inhibition of viral replication plus inhibition of antigen production/release plus immunostimulation, could increase the goal for the functional cure (see **Fig. 5** and **Table 2**).

A phase II study evaluated the combination of NAP (REP 2139 or REP 2165) + TDF + Peg-IFN (ie, experimental therapy) for 48 weeks. After 24 months of TDF, 40 patients were assigned to groups to receive 48 weeks of experimental therapy or 24 weeks of control therapy (TDF + pegIFN) followed by 48 weeks of experimental therapy. Similar levels of HBsAg, anti-HBs, and HBV DNA were observed in patients treated with REP 2139 or REP 2165. An increase in ALT levels was significantly more frequent and greater in the NAP groups, however with no symptoms, correlated with the initial decrease in HBsAg, and normalized during therapy and follow-up. After 48 weeks, the combination strategy cleared HBsAg in 60% of patients, with 35% of the patients achieving also HBsAg seroclearance. During treatment-free follow-up, virologic control persisted in 13 of 40 participants after 48 weeks, whereas functional

Table 2
Results of new anti-hepatitis B virus strategies tested in phase II studies

Drug in Phase-II Development	CHB Population	Strategy	Control Group	Interesting Results
GLS-4	NA-naive	CpAM + ritonavir + ETV	ETV	HBsAg decline: 0.43 vs 0.21 Log IU/mL at wk 24 pgRNA suppression: 2.63 Log vs 0.27 Log IU/mL at wk 24
	NA-treated	CpAM + ritonavir + ETV	ETV	HBsAg decline: 0.11 vs 0 Log IU/mL at wk 24 pgRNA suppression: 1.59 Log vs 0.15 Log IU/mL at wk 24
JNJ-6379	Both	CpAM 75 mg + NA	NA	HBV RNA decline: 2.82 vs 1.43 Log cp/mL at wk 24 in HBeAg + NA-naive
		CpAM 250 mg + NA	NA	HBV RNA decline: 3.13 vs 1.43 Log cp/mL at wk 24 in HBeAg + NA-naive
		CpAM + NA	NA	HBsAg decline: 0.40 vs 0 Log IU/mL at wk 24 in HBeAg + NA-naïve
JNJ-3989	Both	siRNA + NA	NA	2 Log mean HBsAg decline, 4 mo after 3 monthly administrations of JNJ
VIR-2218	NA-treated	siRNA + NA	/	HBsAg decline: 1.65 Log IU/mL after 2 200 mg dose in HBeAg- HBsAg decline: 1.57 Log IU/mL after 2 200 mg dose in HBeAg+
GSK3228836	NA-naive	ASO followed by NA	/	HBsAg decline: >3 Log IU/mL in 3 out of 12 patients[a]
	NA-treated	ASO + NA		HBsAg decline: >3 Log IU/mL in 3 out of 4 patients
REP 2139	NA-treated	NAP + TDF + PegIFN	/	HBsAg <0.05 IU/mL in 60% of patients after 48 wk
REEF-1 study	NA-treated	CpAM JNJ-6379 + siRNA JNJ-3989 + NA	/	Study ongoing. HBsAg decline: 1.7 Log IU/mL at day 113[b], and profound suppression of HBV RNA, HBV DNA, HBsAg
/	NA-treated	Stop NA-to-Flare	NA	Functional cure in 10%–20% after 2–3 y of NA withdrawal, vs <1% per year[c]

Others: TLR-7 and TLR-8 agonists are under evaluation in combination with immunomodulators/antivirals due to increase in Interferon-Stimulated-Gene only; therapeutic vaccine GS-4774 is under evaluation in combination with immunomodulators/antivirals due to great effect on CD8+ T cells.

[a] ALT flare up to 15xULN.
[b] Preliminary results in 12 patients under JNJ-3989 high-dose 200 mg for 3 monthly administrations.
[c] Under evaluation after new compounds use.

cure persisted in 14/40 participants (with anti-HBsAg positive).[83] These results, although very promising, require to be validated by independent investigators.

The combination strategy of NA + siRNA + CpAM has been evaluated in the ongoing phase IIb study 73763989HPB2001 (REEF-1; NCT03982186), which enrolled 471 NA-treated patients with CHB without advance fibrosis to evaluate the dose-response relationship for antiviral activity of 3 dose levels of siRNA JNJ-3989 + NA and to compare the efficacy of combination regimens of JNJ-3989 + NA ± CpAM JNJ-6379 after 48 weeks of treatment. The primary endpoint will be the proportion of participants meeting the NA treatment completion criteria at week 48 (ALT <3x upper limit of normal and HBV DNA < LLOQ and HBeAg-negative and HBsAg <10 IU/mL) in order to stop all treatment including NA and to evaluate the proportion of participants with sustained reduction, suppression, and/or HBsAg seroclearance during the 48 weeks of follow-up. Preliminary results of this triple combination in 12 patients under high-dose JNJ-3989 (200 mg for 3 monthly doses) + CpAM + NA led to mean HBsAg 1.7 Log reduction on day 113, with a profound suppression of HBV DNA, HBV RNA, and HBcrAg.[84]

DRUGS IN DEVELOPMENT (PHASE I STUDIES)

There are several immunomodulators, therapeutic vaccines, and checkpoint inhibitors under evaluation in phase I.

A liver-targeted ASO that inhibits synthesis of hepatitis B surface antigen and all other HBV proteins is GSK3389404. In a phase I study, subcutaneous administration of 4 single-dose cohorts (10 mg, 30 mg, 60 mg, and 120 mg) and 3 multiple ascending-dose cohorts (30 mg, 60 mg, and 120 mg once weekly for 4 weeks) each composed 6 subjects under GSK3389404 and 2 subjects to placebo. The most frequent treatment-related AEs were injection site reactions (19.0%). GSK3389404 dosing has been tested up to 120 mg for 4 weeks with an acceptable safety and pharmacokinetic profile, supporting further clinical investigation in patients with CHB.[85]

AB-729 is a (GalNAc)-conjugated siRNA drug that blocks all HBV RNA transcripts, including HBx. In a phase I study, 5 noncirrhotic (4 Caucasian), HBeAg-negative naïve CHB subjects with HBV DNA greater than 1000 IU/mL, mean age 43 years, ALT 32 (SD 13 U/L), HBsAg 2336 (317–6451), and HBV DNA 86,840 (1220–360,560 IU/mL) received a single 90 mg subcutaneous dose of AB-729, showing a reduction in all measured viral markers, including HBsAg, HBV DNA, HBV RNA, and HBcrAg, with suppression lower than baseline levels up to 44 weeks postdose in 4/5 subjects. Grade 1 ALT alteration occurred in 2 patients and dizziness and grade 1 injection site bruising in one patient.[86] AB-729 is now in phase IIa development.

CRV431 is a cyclophilin inhibitor that inhibits HBV entry without interfering with the NTCP transporter. The anti-HBV mechanisms remain unknown but is thought that drug could neutralize the effect on the peptidyl–prolyl isomerase activity resulting in interference with protein unfolding, leading to a reduction in liver HBV DNA levels and serum HBsAg level without toxicities.[87]

Because in patients with CHB T-cell receptors are overexpressed, therefore limiting the T-cell effector function, PD-1 and PD-1 ligand (PD-L1) inhibitors (mainly expressed on HBV T cells in the liver and on hepatocytes, respectively) could be used as potential therapies to restore T-cell exhaustion, although with a risk of possible immune-mediated hepatic flares.[88] In a phase Ib study, patients received either a single dose of nivolumab (a checkpoint inhibitor, anti-PD1) at 0.1 mg/kg (n = 2) or 0.3 mg/kg (n = 12) or 40 yeast units of GS-4774 at baseline and week 4 and 0.3 mg/kg of nivolumab at week 4 (n = 10). All patients retained T cell PD-1 receptor occupancy 6 to 12 weeks postinfusion, with a mean total across 0.1 and 0.3 mg/kg cohorts of 76%.

Patients receiving 0.3 mg/kg nivolumab without and with GS-4774 had mean HBsAg declines of −0.30 (95% confidence interval [CI] −0.46 to −0.14) and −0.16 (95% CI −0.33 to 0.01) Log IU/ml, respectively. One patient seroconverted HBsAg at week 20 after an ALT flare (grade 3) at week 4 that was accompanied by a significant increase in peripheral HBsAg-specific T cells at week 24.[89] Currently, there are 4 phase 1 studies evaluating the risk of nivolumab, HBV reactivation, and ALT flare in the HCC/oncologic setting.

SUMMARY

In conclusion, novel anti-HBV strategies that aimed to stop viral replication, antigen production, or release and stimulate the immune system are under clinical assessment. Phase II studies are promising but not yet conclusive, as no antiviral strategy has been able so far to clear HBsAg, leading to functional cure, in most patients. It is likely that a combination of different compounds tackling different steps of the HBV replication couple with potent and possibly selective immunomodulators, even pegIFN in selected clinical settings, may serve the purpose of achieving functional cure. The therapeutic paradigms in HBV are therefore changing, from targeting HBV DNA to targeting HBsAg and HBV DNA, but keeping in mind that these new strategies must display an excellent safety profile.[90]

CLINICS CARE POINTS

- Long-term NA treatment maintain HBV-DNA suppression, thus preventing liver disease progression, but with low rates of HBsA seroclearance.
- cccDNA is difficult to eradicate with NA therapy alone, thus representing a risk factor for persistence of HBV and ALT flare after NA withdrawal.
- To achieve functional cure, ie. HBsAg loss, promising anti-HBV strategies are based on the short-term administration of combination therapies characterized by complementary and synergistics mechanisms of action:
  1) Viral replication inhibitors (to control viral replication and cccDNA reamplification);
  2) Viral antigen inhibitors (to inhibit directly or undirectly viral antigen production or egress through different mechanisms);
  3) Immune modulators (to activate and restore immune response to HBV)

ACKNOWLEDGMENTS

This work was supported by a grant from "Ricerca Corrente RC2021/105-01", Italian Ministry of Health.

CONFLICT OF INTEREST

A. Loglio: speaker bureau for MYR Pharma. M. Viganò, speaker bureau for Gilead and Abbvie. P. Lampertico: advisor and speaker bureau for BMS, Roche, Gilead Sciences, GSK, MSD, Abbvie, Janssen, Arrowhead, Alnylam, Eiger, MYR Pharma, Antios, Aligos.

REFERENCES

1. Liang TJ. Hepatitis B: the virus and disease. Hepatology 2009;49(5 Suppl): S13–21.

2. Lamontagne RJ, Bagga S, Bouchard MJ. Hepatitis B virus molecular biology and pathogenesis. Hepatoma Res 2016;2:163–86.

3. Glebe D, Bremer CM. The molecular virology of hepatitis B virus. Semin Liver Dis 2013;33:103–12.

4. Nassal M. Hepatitis B virus replication: novel roles for virus-host interactions. Intervirology 1999;42:100–16.

5. Wei Y, Neuveut C, Tiollais P, et al. Molecular biology of the hepatitis B virus and role of the X gene. Pathol Biol 2010;58:267–72.

6. Ganem D, Schneider RJ. Hepadnaviridae: the viruses and their replication. Fields Virology 2001;2:2923–69.

7. Hollinger FB, Liang TJ. Hepatitis B virus. In: Knipe DM, Howley PM, Griffin DE, et al, editors. Fields virology. 4th edition. Philadelphia: Lippincott-Raven Publishers; 2001. p. 2971–3036.

8. Karayiannis P. Hepatitis B virus: virology, molecular biology, life cycle and intrahepatic spread. Hepatol Int 2017;11:500–8.

9. Hao R, Xiang K, Peng Y, et al. Naturally occurring deletion/insertion mutations within HBV whole genome sequences in HBeAg-positive chronic hepatitis B patients are correlated with baseline serum HBsAg and HBeAg levels and might predict a shorter interval to HBeAg loss and seroconversion during antiviral treatment. Infect Genet Evol 2015;33:261–8.

10. Tong S, Revill P. Overview of hepatitis B viral replication and genetic variability. J Hepatol 2016;64:S4–16.

11. Kim DH, Kang HS, Kim KH. Roles of hepatocyte nuclear factors in hepatitis B virus infection. World J Gastroenterol 2016;22:7017–29.

12. Moolla N, Kew M, Arbuthnot P. Regulatory elements of hepatitis B virus transcription. J Viral Hepat 2002;9:323–31.

13. Quarleri J. Core promoter: a critical region where the hepatitis B virus makes decisions. World J Gastroenterol 2014;20:425–35.

14. Zlotnick A, Venkatakrishnan B, Tan Z, et al. Core protein: a pleiotropic keystone in the HBV lifecycle. Antiviral Res 2015;121:82–93.

15. Clark DN, Hu J. Unveiling the roles of HBV polymerase for new antiviral strategies. Future Virol 2015;10:283–95.

16. Jones SA, Hu J. Hepatitis B virus reverse transcriptase: diverse functions as classical and emerging targets for antiviral intervention. Emerg Microbes Infect 2013; 2:e56.

17. Nassal M. Hepatitis B viruses: reverse transcription a different way. Virus Res 2008;134:235–49.

18. Venkatakrishnan B, Zlotnick A. The structural biology of hepatitis B virus: form and function. Annu Rev Virol 2016;3:429–51.

19. Chen MT, Billaud JN, Sällberg M, et al. A function of the hepatitis B virus precore protein is to regulate the immune response to the core antigen. Proc Natl Acad Sci U S A 2004;101:14913–8.

20. Ou JH, Laub O, Rutter WJ. Hepatitis B virus gene function: the precore region targets the core antigen to cellular membranes and causes the secretion of the e antigen. Proc Natl Acad Sci U S A 1986;83:1578–82.

21. Sheu SY, Lo SJ. Preferential ribosomal scanning is involved in the differential synthesis of the hepatitis B viral surface antigens from subgenomic transcripts. Virology 1992;188:353–7.

22. Quasdorff M, Protzer U. Control of hepatitis B virus at the level of transcription. J Viral Hepat 2010;17:527–36.

23. Huan B, Siddiqui A. Regulation of hepatitis B virus gene expression. J Hepatol 1993;17(Suppl 3):S20–3.

24. Li Y, Ito M, Sun S, et al. LUC7L3/CROP inhibits replication of hepatitis B virus via suppressing enhancer II/basal core promoter activity. Sci Rep 2016;6:36741.

25. Zhang Q, Cao G. Genotypes, mutations, and viral load of hepatitis B virus and the risk of hepatocellular carcinoma: HBV properties and hepatocarcinogenesis. Hepat Mon 2011;11:86–91.

26. Seeger C, Ganem D, Varmus HE. Genetic and biochemical evidence for the hepatitis B virus replication strategy. Science 1986;232:477–85.

27. Yan H, Zhong G, Xu G, et al. Sodium taurocholate cotransporting polypeptide is a functional receptor for human hepatitis B and D virus. Elife 2012;1:e00049.

28. Schreiner S, Nassal M. A role for the host DNA damage response in hepatitis B virus cccDNA formation—and beyond? Viruses 2017;9:125.

29. Zeisel MB, Lucifora J, Mason WS, et al. Towards an HBV cure: state-of-the-art and unresolved questions-report of the ANRS workshop on HBV cure. Gut 2015;64:1314–26.

30. Nassal M. HBV cccDNA: viral persistence reservoir and key obstacle for a cure of chronic hepatitis B. Gut 2015;64:1972–84.

31. Tu T, Budzinska MA, Shackel NA, et al. HBV DNA integration: molecular mechanisms and clinical implications. Viruses 2017;9:75.

32. Levrero M, Pollicino T, Petersen J, et al. Control of cccDNA function in hepatitis B virus infection. J Hepatol 2009;51:581–92.

33. Tuttleman JS, Pourcel C, Summers J. Formation of the pool of covalently closed circular viral DNA in hepadnavirus-infected cells. Cell 1986;47:451–60.

34. Pollicino T, Belloni L, Raffa G, et al. Hepatitis B virus replication is regulated by the acetylation status of hepatitis B virus cccDNA-bound H3 and H4 histones. Gastroenterology 2006;130:823–37.

35. Newbold JE, Xin H, Tencza M, et al. The covalently closed duplex form of the hepadnavirus genome exists in situ as a heterogeneous population of viral minichromosomes. J Virol 1995;69:3350–7.

36. Mason WS, Litwin S, Xu C, et al. Hepatocyte turnover in transient and chronic hepadnavirus infections. J Viral Hepat 2007;14:22–8.

37. Mason WS, Xu C, Low HC, et al. The amount of hepatocyte turnover that occurred during resolution of transient hepadnavirus infections was lower when virus replication was inhibited with entecavir. J Virol 2009;83:1778–89.

38. Penna A, Artini M, Cavalli A, et al. Longlasting memory T cell responses following self-limited acute hepatitis B. J Clin Invest 1996;98:1185–94.

39. Rehermann B, Ferrari C, Pasquinelli C, et al. The hepatitis B virus persists for decades after patients' recovery from acute viral hepatitis despite active maintenance of a cytotoxic T-lymphocyte response. Nat Med 1996;2:1104–8.

40. Zoulim F. Assessment of treatment efficacy in HBV infection and disease. J Hepatol 2006;44:S95–9.

41. Volz T, Lutgehetmann M, Wachtler P, et al. Impaired intrahepatic hepatitis B virus productivity contributes to low viremia in most HBeAg-negative patients. Gastroenterology 2007;133:843–52.

42. Lim SG, Cheng Y, Guindon S, et al. Viral quasi-species evolution during hepatitis Be antigen seroconversion. Gastroenterology 2007;133:951–8.

43. Raimondo G, Allain JP, Brunetto MR, et al. Statements from the Taormina expert meeting on occult hepatitis B virus infection. J Hepatol 2008;49:652–7.

44. European Association for the Study of the Liver. EASL 2017 clinical practice guidelines on the management of hepatitis B virus infection. J Hepatol 2017; 67:370–98.

45. Lok AS, Zoulim F, Dusheiko G, et al. Hepatitis B cure: from discovery to regulatory approval. J Hepatol 2017;67:847–61.

46. Trepo C, Chan HL, Lok A. Hepatitis B virus infection. Lancet 2014;384:2053–63.

47. Ramanan V, Shlomai A, Cox DB, et al. CRISPR/Cas9 cleavage of viral DNA efficiently suppresses hepatitis B virus. Sci Rep 2015;5:10833.

48. Zhang X, Cheng J, Ma J, et al. Discovery of novel hepatitis B virus nucleocapsid assembly inhibitors. ACS Infect Dis 2019;5:759–68.

49. Klumppa K, Lama A, Lukacs C, et al. High-resolution crystal structure of a hepatitis B virus replication inhibitor bound to the viral core pro- tein. Proc Natl Acad Sci U S A 2015;112:15196–201.

50. Yuen MF, Kim DJ, Weilert F, et al. NVR 3–778, a first-in-class HBV core inhibitor, alone and in combination with peg-interferon (PegIFN), in treatment-naive HBeAg-positive patients: early reductions in HBV DNA and HBeAg (abstract). J Hepatol 2016;64:S210–21.

51. Zhang M, Zhang J, Tan Y, et al. Efficacy and safety of GLS4/ritonavir combined with entecavir in HBeAg-positive patients with chronic hepatitis B: interim results from phase 2b, multi-center study. J Hepatol 2020;73:S878–9.

52. Janssen H, Hou J, Asselah T, et al. Efficacy and safety results of the phase 2 JNJ-56136379 JADE study in patients with chronic hepatitis B: interim week 24 data. J Hepatol 2020;73:S129–30.

53. Huang Q, Cai D, Yan R, et al. Preclinical profile and characterization of the Hepatitis B virus core protein inhibitor ABI-H0731. Antimicrob Agents Chemother 2020;64:e01463-20.

54. Xiaoli MA, Lalezari J, Nguyen T, et al. Interim safety and efficacy results of the ABI-H0731 phase 2a program exploring the combination of ABI H0731 with Nuc therapy in treatment naive and treatment suppressed chronic hepatitis B patients. J Hepatol 2019;70:e130.

55. Gane E, Sulkowski M, Ma X, et al. Viral response and safety following discontinuation of treatment with the core inhibitor vebicorvir and a nucleos(t)ide reverse transcriptase inhibitor in patients with HBeAg positive or negative chronic hepatitis B virus infection. J Hepatol 2021;75:S736.

56. Chen Y, Cheng G, Mahato RI. RNAi for treating hepatitis B viral infection. Pharm Res 2008;25:72–86.

57. Flisiak R, Jaroszewicz J, Lucejko M. siRNA drug development against hepatitis B virus infection. Expert Opin Biol Ther 2018;18:609–17.

58. Yuen M, Chan H, Liu K, et al. Differential reductions in viral antigens expressed from cccDNA vs integrated DNA in treatment naïve HBeAg positive and negative patients with chronic HBV after RNA interfer- ence therapy with ARC-520. J Hepatol 2016;64:S390.

59. Yuen MF, Locarnini S, Lim TH, et al. Short term RNA interference therapy in chronic hepatitis B using JNJ-3989 brings majority of patients to HBsAG <100 IU/ml threshold. J Hepatol 2019;70:e51.

60. Gane E, Locarnini S, Lim TH, et al. Short-term treatment with RNA interference therapy, JNJ-3989, results in sustained hepatitis B surface antigen suppression in patients with chronic hepatitis B receiving nucleos(t)ide analogue treatment. J Hepatol 2020;73:S20.

61. Gane E, Lim Y, Cloutier D, et al. Safety and antiviral activity of VIR-2218, an X-targeting RNAi therapeutic, in participants with chronic hepatitis B infection: week 48 follow-up results. J Hepatol 2021;75:S287–8.

62. Yuen MF, Heo J, Jang JW, et al. Hepatitis B virus (HBV) surface antigen (HBsAg) inhibition with ISIS 505358 in chronic hepatitis B (CHB) patients on stable nucleos (t)ide analogue (NA) regimen and inNA -naive CHB patients: phase 2a, randomized, double-blind, placebo-controlled study. J Hepatol 2020;73:S49.

63. Kang C, Syed YY. Bulevirtide: first approval. Drugs 2020;80:1601–5.

64. Urban S, Bartenschlager R, Kubitz R, et al. Strategies to inhibit entry of HBV and HDV into hepatocytes. Gastroenterology 2014;147:48–64.

65. Jansen L, Vaillant A, Stelma F, et al. Serum HBV-RNA levels decline significantly in chronic hepatitis B patients dosed with the nucleic-acid polymer REP 2139-CA. J Hepatol 2015;62:S250.

66. Quinet J, Jamard C, Vaillant A, et al. Achievement of surface antigen clearance in the liver by combination therapy with REP2139-CA and nucleoside analogues against chronic hepatitis B. J Hepatol 2016;64:S285.

67. Vaillant A. REP 2139: antiviral mechanisms and applications in achieving functional control of HBV and HDV Infection. ACS Infect Dis 2019;5:675–87.

68. Al-mahtab M, Bazinet M, Vaillant A. Safety and efficacy of Nucleic Acid Polymers in monotherapy and combined with immunotherapy in treatment-naive bangladeshi patients with HBeAg+ chronic hepatitis B infection. PLoS One 2016;11(6): e0156667.

69. Rehermann B, Nascimbeni M. Immunology of hepatitis B virus and hepatitis C virus infection. Nat Rev 2005;5:215–29.

70. Lanford RE, Guerra B, Chavez D, et al. GS-9620, an oral agonist of toll-like receptor-7, induces prolonged suppression of hepati- tis B virus in chronically infected chimpanzees. Gastroenterology 2013;144:1508–17.

71. Gane E, Lim Y, Gordon S, et al. The oral toll-like receptor-7 agonist GS-9620 in patients with chronic hepatitis B virus infection. J Hepatol 2015;63:320–8.

72. Janssen HL, Brunetto MR, Kim YJ, et al. Safety, efficacy and pharmacodynamics of vesatolimod (GS-9620) in virally suppressed patients with chronic hepatitis B. J Hepatol 2018;68:431–40.

73. Agarwal K, Ahn SH, Elkhashab M, et al. Safety and efficacy of vesatolimod (GS-9620) in patients with chronic hepatitis B who are not currently on antiviral treatment. J Viral Hepat 2018;25:1331–40.

74. Mackman RL, Mish M, Chin G, et al. Discovery of GS-9688 (Selgantolimod) as a potent and selective oral Toll-Like Receptor 8 agonist for the treatment of chronic hepatitis B. J Med Chem 2020;63:10188–203.

75. Gane E, Dunbar PR, Brooks A, et al. Efficacy and safety of 24 weeks treatment with oral TLR8 agonist, selgantolimod, in virally-suppressed adult patients with chronic hepatitis B: a phase 2 study. J Hepatol 2020;73:S52.

76. Janssen1 HLA, Lim YS, Kim HJ, et al. Safety and efficacy of oral TLR8 agonist, selgantolimod, in viremic adult patients with chronic hepatitis B. J Hepatol 2021;75:S757–8.

77. Vandepapeliere P, Lau GKK, Leroux-Roels G, et al. Therapeutic vaccination of chronic hepatitis B patients with virus suppression by anti- viral therapy: a randomized, controlled study of co-administration of HBsAg/AS02 candidate vaccine and lamivudine. Vaccine 2007;25:8585–97.

78. Gaggar A, Coeshott C, Apelian D, et al. Safety, tolerability and immunogenicity of GS-4774, a hepatitis B virus-specific thera- peutic vaccine, in healthy subjects: a randomized study. Vaccine 2014;32:4925–31.

79. Lok A, Pan C, Han S-H, et al. Randomized phase II study of GS-4774 as a therapeutic vaccine in virally suppressed patients with chronic hepatitis B. J Hepatol 2016;65:509–16.

80. Boni C, Janssen HL, Rossi M, et al. Combined GS-4774 and Tenofovir therapy can improve HBV-specific T-cell responses in patients with chronic hepatitis. Gastroenterology 2019;157:227–41.

81. Aguilar JC, León Y, Lobaina Y, et al. Five-year follow-up of chronic Hepatitis B patients immunized by nasal route with the therapeutic vaccine HeberNasvac. Euroasian J Hepatogastroenterol 2018;8:133–9.

82. Wedemeyer H, Hui AJ, Sukeepaisarnjaroen W, et al. Therapeutic vaccination of chronic hepatitis B patients with ABX203 (NASVAC) to prevent relapse after stopping NUCs: contrasting timing rebound between tenofovir and entecavir. J Hepatol 2017;66:S101.

83. Bazinet M, Pantea V, Placinta G, et al. Safety and efficacy of 48 Weeks REP 2139 or REP 2165, Tenofovir Disoproxil, and Pegylated Interferon Alfa-2a in patients with chronic HBV infection naive to nucleos(t)ide therapy. Gastroenterology 2020;158:2180–94.

84. Yuen MF, Locarnini S, Given B, et al. First clinical experience with RNA interference [RNAI]-based triple combination therapy in chronic hepatitis B (CHB): JNJ-73763989 (JNJ-3989), JNJ-56136379 (JNJ-6379) and a nucleos(t)ide analogue (NA). Hepatology 2020;72:1489A.

85. Han K, Cremer J, Elston R, et al. A randomized, double-Blind, placebo-controlled, first-time-in-human study to assess the safety, tolerability, and pharmacokinetics of single and multiple ascending doses of GSK3389404 in healthy subjects. Clin Pharmacol Drug Dev 2019;8:790–801.

86. Gane E, Sevinsky H, Yuen M-F, et al. A single dose of the GalNAc-siRNA, AB-729, results in prolonged reductions in HBsAg, HBcrAg, HBV DNA and HBV RNA in the absence of nucleos (t)ide analogue therapy in HBeAg negative subjects with chronic hepatitis B infection. J Hepatol 2021;75:S762–3.

87. Gallay P, Ure D, Bobardt M, et al. The cyclophilin inhibitor CRV431 inhibits liver HBV DNA and HBsAg in transgenic mice. PLoS One 2019;14:e0217433.

88. Liu J, Zhang E, Ma Z, et al. Enhancing virus-specific immunity in vivo by combining therapeutic vaccination and PD-L1 blockade in chronic hepadnaviral infection. PLoS Pathog 2014;10:e1003856.

89. Gane E, Verdon DJ, Brooks AE, et al. Anti-PD-1 blockade with nivolumab with and without therapeutic vaccination for virally suppressed chronic hepatitis B: a pilot study. J Hepatol 2019;71:900–7.

90. Revill PA, Chisari FV, Block JM, et al. A global scientific strategy to cure hepatitis B. Lancet Gastroenterol Hepatol 2019;4:545–58.

UNITED STATES POSTAL SERVICE®
Statement of Ownership, Management, and Circulation
(All Periodicals Publications Except Requester Publications)

1. Publication Title	2. Publication Number	3. Filing Date
CLINICS IN LIVER DISEASE	016 – 754	9/18/2021

4. Issue Frequency	5. Number of Issues Published Annually	6. Annual Subscription Price
FEB, MAY, AUG, NOV	4	$319.00

7. Complete Mailing Address of Known Office of Publication (Not printer) (Street, city, county, state, and ZIP+4®)

ELSEVIER INC.
230 Park Avenue, Suite 800
New York, NY 10169

Contact Person
Malathi Samayan

Telephone (Include area code)
91-44-4299-4507

8. Complete Mailing Address of Headquarters or General Business Office of Publisher (Not printer)

ELSEVIER INC.
230 Park Avenue, Suite 800
New York, NY 10169

9. Full Names and Complete Mailing Addresses of Publisher, Editor, and Managing Editor (Do not leave blank)

Publisher (Name and complete mailing address)

Dolores Meloni, ELSEVIER INC.
1600 JOHN F KENNEDY BLVD. SUITE 1800
PHILADELPHIA, PA 19103-2899

Editor (Name and complete mailing address)

KERRY HOLLAND, ELSEVIER INC.
1600 JOHN F KENNEDY BLVD. SUITE 1800
PHILADELPHIA, PA 19103-2899

Managing Editor (Name and complete mailing address)

PATRICK MANLEY, ELSEVIER INC.
1600 JOHN F KENNEDY BLVD. SUITE 1800
PHILADELPHIA, PA 19103-2899

10. Owner (Do not leave blank. If the publication is owned by a corporation, give the name and address of the corporation immediately followed by the names and addresses of all stockholders owning or holding 1 percent or more of the total amount of stock. If not owned by a corporation, give the names and addresses of the individual owners. If owned by a partnership or other unincorporated firm, give its name and address as well as those of each individual owner. If the publication is published by a nonprofit organization, give its name and address.)

Full Name	Complete Mailing Address
WHOLLY OWNED SUBSIDIARY OF REED/ELSEVIER, US HOLDINGS	1600 JOHN F KENNEDY BLVD. SUITE 1800 PHILADELPHIA, PA 19103-2899

11. Known Bondholders, Mortgagees, and Other Security Holders Owning or Holding 1 Percent or More of Total Amount of Bonds, Mortgages, or Other Securities. If none, check box ▶ ☐ None

Full Name	Complete Mailing Address
N/A	

12. Tax Status (For completion by nonprofit organizations authorized to mail at nonprofit rates) (Check one)
The purpose, function, and nonprofit status of this organization and the exempt status for federal income tax purposes:

☒ Has Not Changed During Preceding 12 Months
☐ Has Changed During Preceding 12 Months (Publisher must submit explanation of change with this statement)

PS Form **3526**, July 2014 [Page 1 of 4 (See instructions page 4)] PSN: 7530-01-000-9931   PRIVACY NOTICE: See our privacy policy on www.usps.com.

---

13. Publication Title		14. Issue Date for Circulation Data Below
CLINICS IN LIVER DISEASE		MAY 2021

15. Extent and Nature of Circulation			Average No. Copies Each Issue During Preceding 12 Months	No. Copies of Single Issue Published Nearest to Filing Date
a. Total Number of Copies (Net press run)			108	101
b. Paid Circulation (By Mail and Outside the Mail)	(1)	Mailed Outside-County Paid Subscriptions Stated on PS Form 3541 (Include paid distribution above nominal rate, advertiser's proof copies, and exchange copies)	41	37
	(2)	Mailed In-County Paid Subscriptions Stated on PS Form 3541 (Include paid distribution above nominal rate, advertiser's proof copies, and exchange copies)	0	0
	(3)	Paid Distribution Outside the Mails Including Sales Through Dealers and Carriers, Street Vendors, Counter Sales, and Other Paid Distribution Outside USPS®	37	35
	(4)	Paid Distribution by Other Classes of Mail Through the USPS (e.g., First-Class Mail®)	0	0
c. Total Paid Distribution (Sum of 15b (1), (2), (3), and (4))		▶	78	72
d. Free or Nominal Rate Distribution (By Mail and Outside the Mail)	(1)	Free or Nominal Rate Outside-County Copies included on PS Form 3541	15	14
	(2)	Free or Nominal Rate In-County Copies Included on PS Form 3541	0	0
	(3)	Free or Nominal Rate Copies Mailed at Other Classes Through the USPS (e.g., First-Class Mail)	0	0
	(4)	Free or Nominal Rate Distribution Outside the Mail (Carriers or other means)	0	0
e. Total Free or Nominal Rate Distribution (Sum of 15d (1), (2), (3) and (4))		▶	15	14
f. Total Distribution (Sum of 15c and 15e)		▶	93	86
g. Copies not Distributed (See Instructions to Publishers #4 (page #3))		▶	15	15
h. Total (Sum of 15f and g)		▶	108	101
i. Percent Paid (15c divided by 15f times 100)			83.87%	83.72%

* If you are claiming electronic copies, go to line 16 on page 3. If you are not claiming electronic copies, skip to line 17 on page 3.

16. Electronic Copy Circulation		Average No. Copies Each Issue During Preceding 12 Months	No. Copies of Single Issue Published Nearest to Filing Date
a. Paid Electronic Copies	▶		
b. Total Paid Print Copies (Line 15c) + Paid Electronic Copies (Line 16a)	▶		
c. Total Print Distribution (Line 15f) + Paid Electronic Copies (Line 16a)	▶		
d. Percent Paid (Both Print & Electronic Copies) (16b divided by 16c × 100)	▶		

☒ I certify that 50% of all my distributed copies (electronic and print) are paid above a nominal price.

17. Publication of Statement of Ownership

☒ If the publication is a general publication, publication of this statement is required. Will be printed
in the **NOVEMBER 2021** issue of this publication.
☐ Publication not required.

18. Signature and Title of Editor, Publisher, Business Manager, or Owner

Malathi Samayan - Distribution Controller

Malathi Samayan

Date 9/18/2021

I certify that all information furnished on this form is true and complete. I understand that anyone who furnishes false or misleading information on this form or who omits material or information requested on the form may be subject to criminal sanctions (including fines and imprisonment) and/or civil sanctions (including civil penalties).

PS Form **3526**, July 2014 (Page 3 of 4)   PRIVACY NOTICE: See our privacy policy on www.usps.com

Moving?

Make sure your subscription moves with you!

To notify us of your new address, find your **Clinics Account Number** (located on your mailing label above your name), and contact customer service at:

Email: journalscustomerservice-usa@elsevier.com

800-654-2452 (subscribers in the U.S. & Canada)
314-447-8871 (subscribers outside of the U.S. & Canada)

Fax number: 314-447-8029

Elsevier Health Sciences Division
Subscription Customer Service
3251 Riverport Lane
Maryland Heights, MO 63043

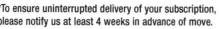

Printed and bound by CPI Group (UK) Ltd, Croydon, CR0 4YY

03/10/2024

01040403-0001